AF884956

BEHAVIORAL HEALTH

FOR CASE MANAGEMENT

BEHAVIORAL HEALTH

FOR CASE MANAGEMENT

Blue Bayou Press

DR. ELLEN FINK-SAMNICK
DBH, MSW, LCSW, ACSW, CCM, CCTP, CRP, FCM

Behavioral Health for Case Management is an independent publication and has not been authorized, or otherwise approved by the owners of the trademarks or organizations referred to in this product.

The author is not affiliated with or endorsed by any organization. All names and acronyms are trademarks of their owners.

Although the author and publisher have made every effort to ensure that the information in this book was correct at press time, the author and publisher do not assume and hereby disclaim any liability to any party for any loss, damage, or disruption caused by errors or omissions, whether such errors or omissions result from negligence, accident, or any other cause.

Because of the dynamic nature of the Internet, any web addresses or links contained in this book may have changed since publication and may no longer be valid. The author of this book does not dispense medical advice or prescribe the use of any technique as a form of treatment for physical, emotional, or medical problems without the advice of a physician, either directly or indirectly. The intent of the author is only to offer information.

Copyright © 2026 Dr. Ellen Fink-Samnick DBH, MSW, LCSW, ACSW, CCM, CCTP, CRP, FCM

All rights reserved. No part of this book may be used or reproduced by any means, graphic, electronic, or mechanical, including photocopying, recording, taping, or by any information storage retrieval system without the prior written permission of the publisher except in the case of brief quotations embodied in critical articles and reviews.

To request permission, contact the publisher at Info@BlueBayouPress.com

ISBN Paperback: 978-1-943889-21-1
Library of Congress Control Number: 2025927175
Edited by Andrea Morris, aripemango.com

Published in the United States by HCP2HCP an imprint of Blue Bayou Press, LLC,
Crestview, FL 32536
BlueBayouPress.com

DEDICATION

To every case manager—

Physical and behavioral health are forever joined. Their collective impact on the human condition is among our grandest challenges.

Embrace all available research and knowledge to advance your practice mastery. Only then can our patients and their families reap the true reward of our professional expertise.

ACKNOWLEDGMENTS

To Steven Samnick: You are forever my rock, my heart, and my home. My gratitude for your never-ending patience, love, unconditional support, and that keen ability to proactively provide me safety from every storm.

To Kevin Samnick: You endowed me with the honor of parenthood, providing me the greatest gift which I never thought possible. In doing so, you have inspired me in more ways than I could ever imagine.

To my enduring village—your constant support and wisdom provide me strength to move past any obstacle: Lorraine Brown Dwyer, Cara English, Michael Garrett, Donna Hatfield, Lisa Haley, Irene and Andy Ilachinski, Lisa and Robert Justus, Abby Kass, Lynn and Steven Muller, Mindy and Bill Owen, Suzanne and James Powell, Dana and Joseph Simon, Hussein Tahan, Teri and Dave Treiger, Alan Weintraub, and Julie Wolf.

To my massive professional hood—you are colleagues, friends, and mentors who have partnered with me on this wild journey. You challenge my thinking and, in doing so, empower my energies. Special nods to: Stefany Almaden, Eric Bergman, Alan Boardman, Jeannie Boling, Elaine Bruner, U. Grant Baldwin, Jr., Michelle Brusio, Raine Arndt-Couch, Janet Coulter, Stefani Daniels, Cha-Loe Davis, Mary Detweiler, Allison Earl, Mark Evans, Lisa Simmons-Fields, Vivian Greenway, Ronald Hirsch, Gerri Lamb, Cheri Lattimer, Anne Llewelyn, Kathleen Moreo, Colleen Morley, Catherine Mullahy, Mary Beth Newman, Patricia Noonan, Lisa Parker-Williams, Melanie Prince, Heaven Provo, Jenny Quigley-Stickney, Nancy Skinner, June Stark, Connie Sunderhaus, Lew Vierling, Samantha Walker, and Rosie Zawia.

To Deanna Cooper and Abi Carmen: We bonded over a shared vision to advance the knowledge of case management professionals. Our journey continues to ensure their access to the most vital intel. I am forever grateful for our friendship.

To my brother, Mark Fink, and sister-in-law, Beth Fink: You are my consummate safety net, always there to catch me when I falter.

To my nieces, Samantha Pilecki and Melisa Caruso and their families: You are my heart and my legacy. Never underestimate your individual power, prowess, and potential.

To my mother, Barbara Fink: My love and gratitude for modeling the importance of doing something right or not at all. This reach goal is one I strive to attain daily.

To my father, Dr. Herbert Fink: My actions remain guided by memories of your unwavering commitment to family and friends, but equal attention to the professional domains of ethics, education, and expertise. Your ability to prioritize this delicate balance remains my north star.

CONTENTS

SECTION 2 BEHAVIORAL HEALTH CONDITIONS AND MANAGEMENT

SECTION 3 THE TREATMENT PROCESS

LIST OF TABLES

LIST OF FIGURES

LIST OF BOXES

FOREWORD

By Dr. Ronald Hirsch

Medical care in the 21st century is amazing. We now have effective treatments for diseases that not long ago were considered uniformly fatal. In 2017 we saw the first FDA approval of a CAR-T therapy for leukemia that reengineers a patient's own cancer cells to become cancer fighting cells, making a resolutely fatal disease treatable. Then 2023 brought the introduction of CRISPR therapy to cure sickle cell disease. In 2024, we saw reports of stem cell therapy curing HIV infections.

Despite these amazing advances, the burden of chronic disease continues unabated. The incidence of hypertension, diabetes, obesity, emphysema, and many other diseases still lead to chronic illness, hospitalizations, morbidity, and mortality. And it should come as no surprise to anyone that the cost per capita for health care in the United States is higher than any other country in the world, with health-related outcomes that are far from the best.

Access to medical care is also a huge issue in the U.S. The reasons are myriad, spanning the piecemeal way health insurance is provided, to the high costs of care even with insurance. Difficulty navigating the healthcare system and its language and cultural barriers are also pressing realities.

While these issues are daunting, the challenges are amplified when it comes to behavioral healthcare. Unlike many physical health issues, where objective measures, such as cholesterol level or imaging, determine severity and need for treatment, behavioral health is purely subjective. Patients cannot be "sent to the lab" to measure the degree their past life experiences and trauma are affecting them now. A diagnostic test like x-ray or CT scan won't help the provider determine the best treatment for the patient.

The effects of behavioral health on the individual can vary tremendously. Veterans may respond differently to certain stressors than civilians, due to their past experiences. Persons with cognitive, developmental, or physical disabilities, who have faced a lifetime of challenges, may manifest their response to a new behavioral health issue differently than persons who've been consistently able-bodied. Some LGBTQIA+ individuals have faced discrimination and stigma throughout their lives, which affects their trust of others. As a result, members of this community may be unforthcoming about their need for care, may delay seeking care, or may not adhere to treatment.

In addition, there are additive effects when behavioral and physical health collide. The patient with diabetes whose depression affects his ability to maintain a healthy diet and exercise routine has an increased risk of adverse effects from their diabetes. These issues, along with not consistently taking medications as directed, lead to complications that may worsen the underlying depression. These interactions cannot always be measured but require careful consideration when providing comprehensive patient care.

Behavioral health issues for adults are a challenge, but they pale in comparison to the effects on children. A child whose educational pathway deviates due to a behavioral health issue may suffer lifelong effects. Behavioral health issues in the child's parents, siblings, and relatives can result in behavioral health issues for the child, which consequently obstruct that child's development. Illness morbidity rises, as do mortality rates.

Yet little is taught about the nuances of behavioral health in our nursing schools, medical schools, colleges, or continuing education offerings, despite the importance in the lives of every patient and every person who works in health care.

Case managers, as defined by the Case Management Society of America, are "healthcare professionals who serve as patient advocates, supporting, guiding, and coordinating care for patients, families and caregivers as they navigate their health and wellness journeys. They serve as the center of communication, connecting individuals/caregivers with members of the healthcare team and community to impact acute and chronic disease management and improve population health" (2022).

As such, to provide comprehensive care coordination to every patient, it is crucial that case managers have a strong foundation in behavioral health. They must understand the many presentations and nuances of behavioral health, and the more invasive mental illness. They must be familiar with industry-vetted screening tools to best assess severity of symptom presentation and diagnosis. Sound screening and assessment also drives the care available to various populations, which is often dependent on payment source. While ensuring proper care is provided to all patients, it is also crucial for case managers to be aware of the varying quality and outcome measures used by external agencies.

In addition, every hospital faces staffing shortages, often limiting access to social work professionals to assess issues of behavioral health and formulate a treatment plan. While social workers have a unique skill set, the role of the case manager in starting the assessment process cannot be understated, helping pave the way for the social worker, once available, to provide their expertise. This team approach provides patients access to the needed care, along with avoiding delays that can increase the length of stay and cost of care, two metrics by which every case management program is measured. No one can argue with the goal of providing better care to each patient in a more efficient manner.

To that end, it is fantastic to see Dr. Ellen Fink-Samnick has, in this book, chosen to address and educate on these many aspects of behavioral health for case managers. As with her other publications, Ellen is able to educate in a way that is both practical and applicable to the daily work of every case manager, and in a comprehensive manner. I am proud to recommend *Behavioral Health for Case Management* by Dr. Ellen Fink-Samnick as required reading for every case manager entering the workforce today and for all experienced case managers, as learning in heathcare never ends.

REFERENCES

- Case Management Society of America. (2022). *Standards of Practice for Case Management.*

PREFACE

Over the years case management colleagues have posed one request to me consistently: *Teach me everything you know about behavioral health*. Although many students take an introductory course on behavioral health during their professional education, once working they quickly learn that the content had provided only an overview. The competencies of condition-specific clinical screening, assessment, intervention, and treatment planning are taught at a foundational level and don't teach the practical applications required for success as a case manager.

REVELATIONS AND REALIZATIONS

Early in my case management career I learned of a critical gap in professional education: that my nursing colleagues were required to take few or no courses on behavioral health. I had been attending a national conference, chatting with a group of acute care case managers about recent challenges. All their problems involved a presentation of a client's or family member's mental health. The comments surprised me:

- "I never learned about mental health in nursing school."
- "The closest thing I had in college on this stuff was an intro course in psychology."
- "I never realized that MSW students take a course dedicated to diagnosing with the DSM."
- "It would be great to know a few therapy techniques, especially to manage challenging family situations!"
- "Motivational interviewing helps, but what do you use when it doesn't work?"
- "I'd give anything to better understand why I need to do a PASARR! What am I actually screening for?"

I was baffled…*How could this possibly be?* As a social worker in healthcare who regularly engaged with nurses and other professionals, I had assumed their academic training included the basics of mental health. Of course, we all know what happens when we assume! I could not have been more wrong.

Soon after, I attended a presentation on case management by Mary Gambosh, one of our profession's true matriarchs. She discussed the rapidly emerging roles for case managers and the expanding scope of practice encompassing physical and mental health assessment. I was captivated by Mary's presentation persona: authentic, informative, and direct. Following the presentation, I approached Mary and nervously waited my turn to speak with this icon of case management practice. Yet Mary's welcoming presence was the antidote for my nerves. "Your session got me thinking, particularly as a 'non-nurse,'" I said. A smile crossed Mary's face when I shared that my discipline of origin was social work.

Mary acknowledged that her wish for nurses entering case manager roles was to have access to a social worker's brain. She discussed her respect for social work's training and walked through assorted theoretical foundations. Among them was Engel's (1977) biopsychosocial model, which informs practitioners how physical and mental illness stem from the interaction of biological, psychological, and sociological factors. Mary attributed this model to fueling her success in workers' compensation.

Mary detailed her tough adjustment to interviewing and assessing clients with traumatic life-changing injuries. She admitted to having little training on the factors influencing client motivation for change, or identification of the common behavioral health coping responses, such as agitation, anxiety, and depression. Mary had basic comprehension of these concepts from her years in direct care. But she felt that more dedicated training to mental health was sorely needed for nurses to work successfully in case management. Mary hoped that her discipline of origin could borrow from social work's curriculum to better navigate client and family dynamics during an illness course, and to address the high prevalence of mental illness and substance use associated with health conditions. She was increasingly aware that pain management, self-medicating, and addiction were major factors to address with her injured workers.

FAST FORWARD

Mary and I crossed paths again 10 years later. She had retired but continued to present and to inspire audiences of new and seasoned case managers. I was surprised when Mary greeted me warmly by name and made time to speak with me privately for several minutes. "You're among the few social workers in case management leadership roles, so you're not easy to forget," she said.

I had much to share with Mary since our first dialogue. I had recently signed my first contract in higher education for George Mason University's Department of Social Work and was scheduled to teach Human Behavior in the Social Environment. I shared with Mary that this synthesis course was required for all students in what was then the School of Health and Human services, which included nursing and social work. Mary's eye's opened wide, and her smile was even wider. I knew the opportunity before me: to provide students entering healthcare a solid foundation of behavioral health knowledge, just as Mary and I had discussed a decade prior. Mary validated my feelings about the importance of behavioral health knowledgé in the course and the implications for case managers. She was elated.

Mary was a visionary who saw our profession's true promise: to achieve successful outcomes through keen initial assessment that would contribute to enhanced care coordination. Her enthusiasm empowered me and furthered my commitment to educate students and the workforce about how human behavior and behavioral health manifest across developmental life stages.

Fast forward 20 years. My conversations with Mary have echoed countless times, now with other case managers and their leadership. Some were nurses, but there were individuals from other non-behavioral health professions, too: physicians; physical, occupational, and vocational therapists; pharmacists; respiratory therapists; and others. Every conversation discussed the benefit of case management's whole-person perspective, while also acknowledging that knowledge of behavioral health was vital to accomplishing whole-person care.

CHANGING TIMES AND WORKFORCE MANDATES

Higher education accrediting organizations have the tough job of defining the knowledge requirements for each healthcare profession. They must keep pace with shifting physical, behavioral, and psychosocial health realities. They must also deep-dive into how the latest issues translate to professional competencies and practice behaviors. From this, students are taught evidence-based theories and knowledge according to the competencies of their chosen discipline's scope of practice (e.g., assessment, diagnosis, ethics, evaluation, intervention, treatment planning, public policy).

Among the latest mandates are psychosocial realities imposed by social determinants of health and mental health. By now, most individuals are aware of their outsized impact: associated with over 80 percent of a persons' health status and many poor clinical outcomes, and especially associated with the prevalence of chronic illness manifestation, morbidity, and mortality in marginalized and minoritized populations. Outcomes are exacerbated by the political determinants of health: the upstream impact of macro-level legislation, policies, and regulatory requirements that created, magnify, and sustain barriers to care (Dawes, 2020). These factors combine to intensify health disparities and contribute to sky-high National Health Expenditures, which are expected exceed $5.3 trillion by 2026 (McGough et al., 2024).

Case managers are entering the workforce in droves from across the disciplinary landscape. Population requirements are driving case management program design, with considerable focus on integration of behavioral health programming. Mental health spending has risen 53 percent since 2020 (Cantor et al., 2023). The U.S. behavioral health market is projected to grow from $83.70 billion to $115.21 billion by 2030; the global market is on a similar track, **valued at $162.31** billion **in 2023 and projected to exceed $310.82** billion **by 2033 (Precedence Research, 2024).**

The Bureau of Labor Statistics (2024) projects a continuing rise in mental health-related occupations. The number of professionals in substance use disorders, behavioral disorders, and mental health are projected to increase as much 19 percent over the next decade, a much faster rate than the 3 percent average for all professions. MCOs and commercial health plans have added these positions to bolster attention on consumers' integrated care needs. These numbers are yielding a rise in case management-focused behavioral health programs that target chronic illness, substance use and addiction, and severe mental illness case management positions.

With case management's growth across every sector and practice setting, the mandate for the workforce is clear. There is no good health without good mental health, and case managers must be able to see it all. They require a foundation in practical behavioral health knowledge, ripe for instant application. They must demonstrate keen proficiency for screening behavioral health conditions, along with mastery of therapy interventions and techniques.

Trial by fire can no longer be the norm for new case managers. Proactive training and workforce orientation must replace the reactive approach. The latter leads to case manager frustration, poor employee retention, and greater healthcare utilization for their patients (Adepoju, 2022). Knowledge is a far more reliable, efficient, and effective resource than searching how-to videos on the internet.

YOUR PRACTICAL AND APPLICABLE REMEDY

Behavioral Health for Case Management will provide case managers a critical foundation to approach whole-person care with confidence. The book contains the most relevant knowledge, theories, interventions, and techniques to inform professionals across disciplines, settings, and levels of practice. Here are my guiding thoughts to organize and prioritize your learning.

1. Consider this book your principal behavioral health resource to:

- Onboard and educate your case management staff, whether novice, experienced, or in leadership roles
- Adopt as an academic textbook
- Understand and distinguish terms used across behavioral health, mental health, and mental illness
- Clarify reimbursement and payment models
- Ascertain relevant quality metrics and benchmarking data
- Identify regulatory requirements and practices
- Screen and assess common behavioral health conditions
- Interview clients and implement conversation maps across behavioral health conditions
- Identify short-term behavioral health interventions and techniques
- Understand how trauma factors into behavioral health conditions
- Identify resources specific to your client population and practice setting
- I am confident at least one of these reasons for being speak to you!

2. The term *patient* is used throughout the book as a generic name for users of case management services. Exceptions occur for direct quotes or references that directly apply other naming (e.g., client, member, consumer, beneficiary).
3. The terms *behavioral health*, *mental health*, and *mental illness* appear throughout the book. The terms are not synonyms and have distinct definitions detailed in Chapter 1.
4. The term *healthcare* refers to the general industry and encompasses health and behavioral health systems and the overall sector where care is rendered. It should also be recognized that behavioral health treatment may occur external to the healthcare sector, as in education (e.g., schools), business (e.g., employee assistance programs), or elsewhere.
5. The book content aligns with the American Psychological Association's Inclusive Language Guidelines (2023), prioritizing culturally respectful language and acknowledging case management's support of the values of diversity, equity, inclusion, and belonging.
6. This book views case management as interdisciplinary in practice—comprising case managers from varied disciplines across health and behavioral health professions.
7. This book also views case management as interprofessional in scope, supporting the individual expertise of case managers and the collective wisdom of their treatment teams. The interprofessional approach enables diverse clients and populations to receive inclusive and quality-driven care, aligned with the Quintuple Aim, which calls for client and patient-centric care rendered at the right time and the right cost by professionals who embrace the work and advance health equity (Itchhaporria, 2021).
8. This book is primarily written for case management professionals, but the content will inform any member of the care process.
9. This book has three sections to set your behavioral health foundation.
    - **Section 1:** Bolster Your Foundation
    - **Section 2:** Behavioral Health Conditions and Management
    - **Section 3:** The Treatment Process

Each chapter has distinct behavioral learning objectives and a list of essential terms; the terms are italicized at their first appearance in the chapter. Content in early sections of the book sets the foundation for the complex information in latter chapters. Case scenarios offer readers opportunities to apply the content and engage in critical thinking. Tables, figures, and callouts foster recall of vital information. Contemplation questions at the end of each chapter promote continuous learning; I suggest working through them in conversation with colleagues, in group sessions, and when readying your unit for the next regulatory survey. *Behavioral Health for Case Management* is your essential guide to this valuable brain trust.

Ready, set, learn.

REFERENCES

- American Psychological Association. (2023). Inclusive Language Guidelines, 2nd edition. Retrieved December 4, 2024, from https://www.apa.org/about/apa/equity-diversity-inclusion/language-guidelines
- Adepoju, O.E., Kim, L.H., & Starks, S.M. (2022). Hospital length of stay in patients with and without serious and persistent mental illness: Evidence of racial and ethnic differences. *Healthcare*, *10*(6), 1128. https://doi.org/10.3390/healthcare10061128
- Bureau of Labor Statistics. (2024). Occupational Outlook Handbook: Substance Abuse, Behavioral Disorders, and Mental Health Counselors. Retrieved September 3, 2024, from https://www.bls.gov/ooh/community-and-social-service/substance-abuse-behavioral-disorder-and-mental-health-counselors.htm
- Cantor, J.H., McBain, R.K., Ho, P.C., Bravata, D.M., & Whaley, C. (2023). Telehealth and in-person mental health service utilization and spending, 2019 to 2022. *JAMA Health Forum*, *4*(8), e232645. https://doi.org/10.1001/jamahealthforum.2023.2645
- Centers for Medicare and Medicaid Services. National Health Expenditure Data, Projected, CMS.gov. Retrieved May 22, 2024, from https://www.cms.gov/data-research/statistics-trends-and-reports/national-health-expenditure-data/projected
- Dawes, D. (2020). *The Political Determinants of Health.* Johns Hopkins University Press: Baltimore, MD.
- Engel, G.L. (1977). The need for a new medical model: A challenge for biomedicine. *Science*, *196*(4286), 129-136. https://doi.org/10.1126/science.847460
- Institute of Medicine. (2001). *Crossing the Quality Chasm: A New Health System for the 21st Century.* The National Academies Press: Washington, D.C. https://doi.org/10.17226/10027.
- Itchhaporia, D. (2021). The evolution of the Quintuple Aim: Health equity, health outcomes, and the economy. *Journal of the American College of Cardiology*, *78*(22), 2262-2264. https://doi.org/10.1016/j.jacc.2021.10.018
- McGough, M., Winger, A., Kurani, N., & Cox, C. (2024). How Much Is Health Spending Expected To Grow? Retrieved May 23, 2025, from https://www.healthsystemtracker.org/chart-collection/how-much-is-health-spending-expected-to-grow/
- Precedence Research. (2024). U.S. Behavioral Health Market Size, Share, and Trends 2024-2034. Retrieved September 4, 2024, from https://www.precedenceresearch.com/us-behavioral-health-market

SECTION 1

BOLSTER YOUR FOUNDATION

CHAPTER 1

FOUNDATIONAL CONCEPTS

CHAPTER 2

REGULATIONS AND REQUIREMENTS

CHAPTER 3

CORE QUALITY MEASURES, VALUE-BASED CARE MODELS, AND REIMBURSEMENT

INTRODUCTION TO SECTION 1

A solid foundation in behavioral health is essential for case managers. The foundation is built on several key pillars of knowledge, including proficiency in foundational terminology and an understanding of the behavioral health workforce, where new roles emerge in response to increasing patient needs and evolving clinical specializations.

Case managers must also be well-versed in the diagnostic tools utilized across behavioral health, particularly those relevant to utilization management, such as coding for reimbursement. Their responsibilities are further anchored in comprehension of regulations, standards, and quality measures. This framework ensures care delivery complies with legal requirements, accreditation criteria, benchmarks, safeguards for patient rights, documentation integrity, and evidence-based protocols.Futhermore, as value-based care models further prioritize outcomes, efficiency, and accountability, case managers will see improvements to symptom management, care coordination, patient engagement, and overall functioning. Case managers who understand these changes, whether novice or leader, will demonstrate practice excellence.

Collectively, these pillars of knowledge form the core of effective, sustainable, and person-centered behavioral health case management. They reinforce every case manager's professional obligation to uphold industry standards, including the quality North Star known as the Quintuple Aim. Ultimately, patient-centered care is delivered on time and cost-effectively by dedicated professionals, ensuring access by all individuals and populations in need.

CHAPTER 1

FOUNDATIONAL CONCEPTS

INTRODUCTION

The mental health of society is among the healthcare industry's hottest topics. Case managers intervene with patients, their family members, and other individuals who display a variety of mental health conditions and symptoms. They present with *psychopathology*, or the presentation of mental health symptoms and features, amid physical disease and injury, known as *pathophysiology*. These conditions and symptoms can turn ordinary case management tasks into complex, time-consuming pursuits.

BEHAVIORAL LEARNING OBJECTIVES

1. Define key terms related to behavioral health, mental health, and mental illness
2. Distinguish between behavioral health, mental health, and mental illness
3. Identify established resources used to diagnose mental health conditions
4. Understand the types of behavioral health professionals
5. Explain key factors impacting patient access to mental healthcare
6. Distinguish between the four types of mental health stigmas

ESSENTIAL TERMS

- Adherence
- Anticipated stigma
- Any mental illness (AMI)
- Applied Behavioral Analysis
- Behavioral analyst
- Behavioral health
- Behavioral Risk Factor Surveillance System (BRFSS)
- Comorbid conditions
- Compliance
- Co-occurring disorders
- *Diagnostic and Statistical Manual of Mental Disorders* (DSM)
- Dual diagnosis
- Experienced stigma
- Ghost networks
- Internalized stigma

- *International Classification of Diseases* (ICD)
- Mental disorders
- Mental health
- Mental illness
- Modifiable risk factors
- Pathophysiology
- Perceived stigma
- Psychopathology
- Quintuple Aim
- Severe and persistent mental illness (SPMI)
- Severe mental illness (SMI)
- Specifiers

TERMS AND DEFINITIONS

The healthcare industry is notorious for countless terms and abbreviations. Behavioral health has its own distinct terminology, including many words used synonymously. Let's set the foundational behavioral health vocabulary for case managers, beginning with mental health, behavioral health, and mental illness (Table 1.1).

Table 1.1: *Definitions*

Term	Definition
Behavioral health	An umbrella term that includes mental health The connection between behaviors and the health and well-being of body, mind, and spirit Includes how behaviors and habits for eating, drinking, or exercising affect physical or mental health (e.g., in the form of depression, anxiety, or stress)
Mental health (WHO, 2022)	A state of wellbeing in which the individual realizes his or her own abilities, can cope with the normal stresses of life, can work productively and fruitfully, and is able to contribute to his or her community
Mental illness (APA, 2024; NIMH, 2024)	Refers collectively to diagnosable mental disorders involving Significant changes in thinking, emotion, or behavior, and/or Distress or problems functioning in social, work, or family activities Mental disorders vary in degree of severity, ranging from mild to moderate to severe.

American Psychiatric Association, 2024; National Institute of Mental Health, 2024; World Health Organization, 2022

MENTAL HEALTH

Mental health is a general reference to a person's overall wellbeing and their functioning in daily activities. It spans academic, occupational, and social interactions. The concept of mental health also considers the quality of an individual's relationships. For example, how might a person's ability to cope with stress play out with their workplace colleagues? How does adversity, such as unemployment, family violence, or an unexpected healthcare concern, affect a person's familial relationships?

Case managers may find themselves in the path of a negative response to stress. Well-meaning professionals often bear patients' frustration, anxiety, or depression.

BEHAVIORAL HEALTH

Behavioral health has several interpretations. The phrase encompasses mental health and also serves as a less-stigmatizing term for the domain. (We will revisit stigma later in the chapter.) The term behavioral health can also imply a discussion on *modifiable risk factors*, or high-risk health behaviors that exacerbate health conditions. Modifiable risk factors include sedentary lifestyles, poor nutrition, and other daily patterns that exacerbate illness morbidity and mortality, as well as impulsive or addictive activities such as smoking, substance use, gambling, unprotected sex, or sex with multiple partners. Persons subjected to trauma or physical violence, including intimate partner violence, may also be considered in discussions of high-risk health factors. (Trauma is addressed in Chapter 11.)

Prevention is a primary focus of behavioral health in the U.S. Twenty-seven percent of healthcare spending, or $730.4 billion, is attributed to five modifiable risk factors: high body mass index (BMI), high systolic blood pressure, high fasting plasma glucose, dietary risks, and tobacco smoke. Over 45 percent of those resources are dedicated to persons over age 65. Of particular note: The proportion of total health burden attributed to the five modifiable risk factors was substantially higher than the proportion of healthcare spending attributed to them—46.2 percent versus 27.0 percent (Bolnick et al., 2020). Spending breakdown by risk factor is shown in Table 1.2.

The Behavioral Risk Factor Surveillance System (BRFSS), from the Center for Disease Control and Prevention's (CDC) National Center for Chronic Disease Prevention and Promotion, is a clearinghouse for data on risk behaviors and preventive health practices for U.S. adults. Data are tracked across the 50 states, District of Columbia, and three U.S. territories. BRFSS tracks the following behaviors: tobacco use, alcohol consumption, physical activity and diet, sexual practices, and disease screening. The BRFSS is the primary data source for population health tools and systems, including the CDC's Population Level Analysis and Community Estimates (PLACES), the CDC's Chronic Disease Indicators, and the U.S. Department of Health and Human Services' Healthy People initiative. Further information is available on the BRFSS website, found in the resource list at the end of this chapter.

Stop and think about how mental health, modifiable risk factors, and overall wellness interweave. How much does anxiety impact obesity? What about the relationship between depression and congestive heart failure? It's not uncommon for a depressed patient to overeat or not follow his or her prescribed low-sodium diet, causing fluid overload. How does stress exacerbate asthma or diabetes? Internalized or repressed emotions can increase inflammation in the lungs, and the stress hormones adrenaline, cortisol, and norepinephrine raise blood sugar and glucose levels.

Healthcare industry attention to the connections between behavioral health and physical health has prompted a revolution in health prevention and wellness, especially for chronic illnesses.

Table 1.2: *Modifiable risk factors and attributed spending*

Modifiable Risk Factor	Attributed Spending
High body-mass index	$238.5 billion
High systolic blood pressure	$179.9 billion
High fasting plasma glucose	$171.6 billion
Poor diet	$143.6 billion
Tobacco use	$130 billion

Bolnick et al., 2020

MENTAL ILLNESS

Mental illness and *mental disorder* are synonymous terms referring to any clinically significant disturbance in a person's cognition, behavior, or ability to regulate emotions. These disorders are diagnoseable and are described in the latest edition of the *Diagnostic and Statistical Manual of Mental Disorders*, 5th edition, text revision, also known as DSM-5-TR. Further information on the DSM-5-TR appears later in this chapter.

Two general framings of mental illness exist: *any mental illness* and *severe mental illness*. Any mental illness (AMI) refers to any mental, behavioral, or emotional disorder. These diagnoses vary in how much they impact a person's life and functioning, ranging from no impairment to mild, moderate, or severe impairment.

Severe mental illness (SMI) is a subset of AMI referring to mental, behavioral, or emotional disorders resulting in serious functional impairment. SMI disorders can substantially interfere with, or limit, one or more major life activities, such as academic performance, employment, or social interactions (National Institute of Mental Health, 2024). This category is also referred to as *severe and persistent mental illness* (SPMI). SMI may produce psychotic symptoms (e.g., hallucinations, delusions), and they encompass the diagnoses in Figure 1.1.

Some 15.4 million people 18 years and older are diagnosed with an SMI, roughly 6 percent of the U.S. population (National Institute of Mental Health, 2024). The onset of SMI typically occurs between 15 and 30 years old and can be followed by years of costly care; lifetime cost burdens can reach upwards of $1.85 million per person (National Institute of Mental Health, 2024; Seabury et al., 2019). Roughly 66 percent of persons diagnosed with an SMI receive appropriate treatment for their condition (Mental Health America, 2024).

Mental Health America (2024) analyzes the realities faced by AMI populations on an annual basis. The measures the organization captures are in Box 1.1, with the full report accessible from its website.

Figure 1.1: *SMI diagnoses*

- **Bipolar disorder**
- **Borderline personality disorder**
- **Major depressive disorder**
- **Obsessive compulsive disorder (OCD)**
- **Panic disorder**
- **Post traumatic stress disorder (PTSD)**
- **Schizophrenia**

Box 1.1: The State of Mental Health in America report: Tracking annual outcomes by state for the following domains

1. Data and rankings for adults
   - Adults with AMI
   - Adults with substance use disorder in the past year
   - Adults with serious thoughts of suicide
   - Adults with AMI who are uninsured
   - Adults with AMI with private insurance that did not cover mental or emotional disorders
   - Adults reporting 14+ mentally unhealthy days a month and unable to see a doctor due to cost
   - Adults with substance use disorder who needed but did not receive treatment
2. Data and rankings for youth (6-17 years of age)
   - Youth with at least one major depressive episode in the past year
   - Youth with serious thoughts of suicide
   - Youth with Medicaid who did not receive mental health services
   - Youth with private insurance that did not cover mental or emotional problems
   - Students identified with an emotional disturbance for an individualized educational program
   - Youth with a major depressive episode who reported treatment or counseling helped them
   - Youth who are flourishing
3. Access to care, for all rankings
4. Mental health workforce availability

Mental Health America, 2024

CO-OCCURRING CONDITIONS, COMORBIDITY, AND DUAL DIAGNOSES

When patients present with one or more illnesses, diseases, or disorders simultaneously, they have *co-occurring* or *comorbid conditions. Dual diagnosis* is another term used.

Co-occurring disorders refer to co-existing mental illness and substance use disorders, such as major depressive disorder and alcohol use disorder. Though the term primarily refers to a combination of substance use and mental disorder, it can also refer to other groupings of disorders, such as mental illness and intellectual disability.

Patients with co-occurring disorders typically experience chronic physical and behavioral health manifestation, exacerbation, and regression, often due to deficiencies in their healthcare. Individuals in this population often appear on case management's radar due to recurrent emergency department (ED) visits, hospitalizations, and readmissions. These patients also typically experience health-related social needs, such as financial challenges, family discord, housing insufficiency, isolation, transportation challenges, sexual and physical victimization, and incarceration.

ESTABLISHED RESOURCES FOR DIAGNOSIS

The DSM-5-TR and the International Classification of Diseases are the two main evidence-based classification systems used to diagnose mental health conditions, mental illnesses, and associated circumstances. The system a case manager uses is based on his or her role and practice setting. Employers may require that case managers be familiar with both classification systems.

> ***Author's Note***
>
> *People diagnosed with an SMI are also highly vulnerable to chronic and acute physical illnesses. They are more prone to develop one or more chronic illnesses, particularly head, neck, esophageal, and colon cancers; cardiovascular disease; chronic obstructive pulmonary disease; diabetes; and liver disease. When substance use also occurs, the effect on illness morbidity and mortality is profound and results in higher rates of hospitalization and readmission (Launders et al., 2022). This topic is further addressed in Chapter 7.*

DIAGNOSTIC AND STATISTICAL MANUAL FOR MENTAL DISORDERS (DSM)

The DSM, published by the American Psychiatric Association, is a comprehensive system for standardizing diagnoses and classifying mental disorders. The DSM's numeric coding system aligns with the medical diagnostic codes used by providers, institutions, and agencies for data collection and billing. Mental health professionals in the U.S. use the most recent edition to guide mental health diagnosis, treatment planning, and research.

Updates to the DSM typically occur every 10-20 years and incorporate changes in symptom manifestation and presentation, coding updates for diagnoses, and other considerations. Minor updates, called text revisions (TR) are published periodically in response to industry mandates. In the case of DSM-5-TR, a diagnosis of prolonged grief disorder was added in response to high COVID-19 death counts. Box 1.2 summarizes the updates published in DSM-5-TR. Further information is available on the book's website, included in the resource list at the end of the chapter. (Note: Referring to the manual as DSM-V-TR is a common industry error. The Roman numeral naming system was discontinued starting with the 2013 publication of DSM-5.)

In the DSM, each diagnosis is assigned a numeric code and a specifier. Specifiers clarify the course, severity, or special features of a disorder. They designate number of symptoms and current severity, distinguishing mild, moderate, moderate-severe, or severe depressive disorders, for example. They also denote whether a disorder presents with two, three, four, or five symptoms, or four or five symptoms with motor agitation.

Professionals use the most current edition of DSM to assess and apply specifiers per diagnosis. Box 1.3 shows the diagnosis code and a sample specifier for attention deficit disorder/hyperactivity disorder.

Box 1.2: DSM-5-TR updates

- Updates to diagnostic criteria
- Accounting for variations in symptom presentation to help clinicians assess influences of culture on diagnosis
- Addition of new disorders, such as prolonged grief disorder
- Updates to coding systems in preparation for codes alignment with the International Classification of Diseases (ICD-11)
- Comprehensive descriptions of diagnostic features, prevalence, risk factors, and comorbidity information to aid thorough clinical assessments

Box 1.3: Example of specifiers in DSM-5-TR, using attention deficit disorder/hyperactivity disorder

Specify presentation:

- F90.2: Combined presentation
- F90.0: Predominantly inattentive presentation
- F90.1 Predominantly hyperactive/impulsive presentation

Specify course:

- Include general information on the diagnosis development and course to provide a picture of how the disorder affects the patient's life
- For example: 'In partial remission: while full criteria were previously met, fewer than full criteria have been met for the past 6 months. Symptoms still result in impairment in social, academic, or occupational function.'

Specify current severity:

- Mild
- Moderate
- Severe

Adapted from American Psychiatric Association, 2022

INTERNATIONAL CLASSIFICATION OF DISEASES (ICD)

The International Classification of Diseases (ICD) is a coding system developed by the World Health Organization (WHO) and the U.S. National Center for Health Statistics. The current version is the International Classification of Diseases, Tenth Revision, Clinical Modification (ICD-10-CM). The Eleventh Revision (ICD-11) was approved by the World Health Assembly in 2019 and became eligible for adoption by member countries in 2022. But U.S. industry concerns about expanding the already-complex coding system mean implementation won't occur here until late 2025 through 2027.

The ICD-10-CM classifies diseases, injuries, and medical procedures and assures a level of global comparability. Codes are alphanumeric and up to seven characters long. Most ICD diagnoses for mental health conditions are categorized as "Mental, behavioral and neurodevelopmental disorders" and span codes F01-F99, commonly referred to as "F codes." "Z" codes in the ICD-10 also reference mental health, as "Factors influencing health status and contact with health services."

Table 1.3: lists ICD-10 codes for mental health conditions. The significance of each code character is displayed, with an example, in Box 1.4. Web-based tools to search codes are accessible via the National Center for Health Statistics and the Centers for Medicare and Medicaid Services websites.

Table 1.3: *ICD-10-CM mental health conditions*

Numeric Code Classification	Disorders
F01-F99	**Mental, behavioral, and neurodevelopmental disorders**
F01-F09	Mental disorders due to known physiological conditions
F09	Unspecified mental disorder due to known physiological condition
F10-F19	Mental and behavioral disorders due to psychoactive substance use
F20-F29	Schizophrenia, schizotypal, delusional, and other non-mood psychotic disorders
F30-F39	Mood (affective) disorders
F40-F48	Anxiety, dissociative, stress-related, somatoform and other nonpsychotic mental disorders
F50-F59	Behavioral syndromes associated with physiological disturbances and physical factors
F60-F69	Disorders of adult personality and behavior
F70-F79	Intellectual disabilities
F80-F89	Pervasive and specific developmental disorders
F90-F98	Behavioral and emotional disorders with onset usually in childhood or adolescence
F99	Unspecified mental disorder
G30-G32	**Other degenerative diseases of the nervous system**
Z10-Z100	**Additional relevant codes**
Z13.30	Screening examination for mental health and behavioral disorders, unspecified
Z71.1	Person with feared complaint in whom no diagnosis is made
Z71.9	Counseling, unspecified
Z81.8	Family history of other mental and behavioral disorders
Z91.4	Personal history of psychological trauma, not elsewhere classified

World Health Organization, 2004

Box 1.4: ICD-10-CM code characters and an example

Example: *F10.231 Alcohol dependence with severe withdrawal with delirium, initial*

Character 1: Provides the general broad category under which a disorder falls

[In example code F10.231, *F* **refers to mental, behavioral, and neurodevelopmental disorders]**

Characters 2 and 3: Describes the main diagnosis group of disease or injury

[*10* **specifies the substance—in this case, alcohol]**

The decimal (.): Separates the category or main diagnosis group from its subcategory or specific details

Character 4: Presents information about the diagnosis, severity, or anatomical location

[*2* **signifies dependence as severe]**

Character 5: Specifies complications related to the diagnosis, or if a recurrent episode

[*3* **signifies withdrawal as a complication]**

Character 6: Reserved for particular purposes, such as whether a patient has recovered, is receiving ongoing treatment, or has had further complication

[*1* **signifies delirium]**

Character 7: Uses a word rather than a number to reflect whether a diagnosis is provisional or confirmed, or the encounter type

[initial, subsequent, or sequela]

National Center for Health Statistics, 2024

TYPES OF BEHAVIORAL HEALTH PROFESSIONALS

Behavioral health workers come from many health professions, from traditional counselors and psychotherapists to addiction specialists, applied behavioral analysts, and behavioral health consultants. The domain is complex, and roles are often defined by federal, state, and organizational requirements that could fill volumes.

This section summarizes types of behavioral health professionals within case management positions, as well as behavioral health professionals with whom case managers may interact. Table 1.4 offers a snapshot of academic degrees and credentials required. Detailed information on the academic, regulatory, and professional scope of each role is included in the chapter resources list. SAMHSA, the Substance Abuse and Mental Health Services Administration, part of the U.S. Department of Health and Human Services, provides a Behavioral Health Workforce Career Navigator (2024). The interactive, state-by-state map offers the following information on behavioral health roles: regulatory board or credentialing, licensure levels, licensure exam requirements, supervision requirements, multi-state compacts, and licensure renewal requirements. State-specific scope of practice requirements for licensed professionals can be accessed from the relevant state regulatory board.

Table 1.4: *Behavioral health professions and roles*

Profession	Education	Licensure Credential
Addiction Medicine	MD: Doctor of Medicine Fellowship or certification in Addiction Medicine	
Counseling	MA: Master of Arts in Counseling MEd: Master of Education in Counseling MMFT: Master of Marriage and Family Therapy MAPC: Master of Arts in Professional Counseling MS or MSC: Master of Science in Counseling	LCDC: Licensed Chemical Dependency Counselor LMHC: Licensed Mental Health Counselor LMFT: Licensed Marriage and Family Therapist LPC: Licensed Professional Counselor
Nursing	ADN: Associate Degree in Nursing BSN: Bachelor of Science in Nursing MSN: Master of Science in Nursing DNP: Doctor of Nursing Practice PhD: Doctor of Philosophy in Nursing	LPN: Licensed Practical Nurse RN: Registered Nurse APRN: Advanced Practice Registered Nurse
Physician Assistant	MS-PAS or MPAS: Master of Science in Physician Assistant Studies MCHS: Master of Clinical Health Studies	PA: Physician Assistant
Psychiatry	DO: Doctor of Osteopathic Medicine MD: Doctor of Medicine	
Psychology	BA: Bachelor of Arts in Psychology MA: Master of Arts in Psychology DBH: Doctor of Behavioral Health PhD: Doctor of Philosophy in Psychology PsyD: Doctor of Psychology	Licensed Psychologist
Social Work	BSW: Bachelor's in Social Work MSW: Master's in Social Work MSSW: Master of Science in Social Work DBH: Doctor of Behavioral Health DSW: Doctor of Social Work PhD: Doctor of Philosophy in Social Work	LBSW: Licensed Baccalaureate Social Worker LMSW: Licensed Master of Social Work LGSW: Licensed Graduate Social Worker LCSW: Licensed Clinical Social Worker (also: LCSW-C, LICGS, LICSW)

NURSES

Psychiatric-mental health (PMH) registered nurses (RN) and advanced practice registered nurses (APRN) are among the largest group of behavioral health professionals in the U.S., behind social workers. They hold a master's or doctoral degree with specialized training, and they render comprehensive mental healthcare to individuals, families, groups, and communities. Further information on this specialty is available through the American Psychiatric Nurses Association.

Many other nurse case managers were prepared for increasing roles in behavioral health through interprofessional synthesis courses during their schooling. Nurse case managers take on behavioral health and integrated care roles at health plans, acute settings, and community-based agencies. Standards for nursing education are defined by the American Association of Colleges of Nursing.

PHYSICIAN ASSISTANTS

Physician assistants (PA) examine, diagnose, and treat patients under the supervision of a physician. They're found in many care settings, including primary and specialty care offices, outpatient clinics, hospitals and other acute care settings, and community health sites. PAs typically hold a master's degree from an accredited academic program, with licensure required in all states. Further information on a PA career is available from the American Academy of Physicians Associates.

PSYCHIATRISTS

Psychiatrists are medical doctors who diagnose, treat, and prevent mental health conditions. They also recommend patients for intensive treatment, such as inpatient therapy. Psychiatrists can weigh in, through consultations, on a patient's clinical capacity. They cannot decide legal capacity, also known as competence, which is decided instead by judges and courts. (See Chapter 2 for more on legal capacity.)

ADDICTION MEDICINE PHYSICIANS

Addiction medicine physicians are medical doctors with advanced training in prevention, evaluation, diagnosis, and treatment of substance use disorders. Addiction medicine physicians must hold licensure in the state(s) where they practice. Information is available through the American Society of Addiction Medicine.

PSYCHOLOGISTS

Psychologists are trained academically at higher education institutions (as opposed to medical settings). Their scope of practice varies across the states. Master's-level education psychologists engage in psychological testing, research, and behavioral analysis. Many work as school counselors. To practice independently as a psychotherapist, they must attain a doctoral degree and, often, further specialization. Neuropsychologists have a doctorate in psychology with additional training in neuropsychology. Case managers may interact with neuropsychologists when serving patients who have endured traumatic brain injury or another neurological event.

Psychologists are unique as non-medical professionals: With a terminal degree (e.g., DBH, EdD, PhD, PsyD), they are legally allowed to prescribe medications in some states (including Louisiana,

New Mexico, Illinois, Iowa, and Idaho). Other clinically licensed professionals have advocated for prescribing privileges, but only psychologists have been successful. More information on the academic and career pathway of psychologists can be accessed from the American Psychological Association.

SOCIAL WORKERS

SAMHSA has long identified social workers as the largest group of mental health and behavioral health providers in the U.S. (American Board of Clinical Social Work, n.d.). The scope of social workers' practice is defined by multiple factors, including academic degree, specialization, level of licensure, and legal scope of practice for that licensure in their state. The variation in these factors is often confusing for case managers, members of the care team, and patients and their families.

Bachelor's in Social Work

Social workers with a baccalaureate degree (BSW) have basic knowledge of behavioral health assessment and interventions, such as crisis intervention, motivational interviewing, and short-term solution-focused therapy. They are taught to assess child and adult abuse, neglect, and exploitation, and to make referrals to local agencies, such as protective services. BSWs working as case managers are proficient in primary-level case management functions: coordination of discharge resources, linkage with social services, and assessment of the psychosocial needs of patients and families.

Master's in Social Work

The roles of social workers with a master's degree (MSW) are often misunderstood, so I'll first correct several misconceptions. Though very many do, not all MSWs work in the clinical domain conducting clinical mental health assessments, diagnosing patients using the DSM, or intervening in challenging family dynamics. Instead, some master's-level practitioners specialize in community planning, public policy advocacy, or non-profit agency management. MSWs also do *not* lack foundational clinical knowledge. Like other professionals, their responsibilities are bound by their education, training, expertise, and licensure. They cannot accept physician orders or prescribe medications, just as nurses cannot diagnose, assess, or treat mental illness unless educated and trained to do so.

In practice, master's level social work is broadly grounded in Engel's biopsychosocial model (1977). The model explains that physical and mental illness stem from the interaction of biological, psychological, and sociological factors. Many MSW practitioners receive advanced training in psychopathology and symptom presentation for distinct categories of mental illness. Others are well-versed in pathophysiology, psychopharmacology, and other medical literacy domains, which can make these professionals a common addition to case management teams in ambulatory and community-based programs, health systems, health plans, continuing and long-term care, and home healthcare. MSW social workers may seek clinical licensure, which allows for reimbursement of independent assessment, diagnosis, and treatment. That decision can be impacted by several factors, from professional aspirations to licensure scope of practice in the practitioner's state.

Licensed clinical social workers

Social workers licensed at the clinical level are allowed by law to diagnose mental health conditions, provide psychotherapy and counseling, and be reimbursed for independent practice. Professional credentialing varies across the states, but case managers will be most familiar with abbreviations LCSW, LCSW-C, or LICSW. More information on the scope of clinical social work is available from the National Association of Social Workers and Association of Social Work Boards. Facts on social work academic curriculums across baccalaureate and master's programs are accessible through the Council on Social Work Education.

OTHER COUNSELING PROFESSIONALS

Other counseling and behavioral health professionals interact with case managers. Most have master's degrees in counseling, allowing them to engage in psychotherapy and related areas, such as mental status exams. Credentials for this group include licensed associate clinicians (LAC), who must work under direct supervision of a licensed therapist; and licensed professional counselors (LPC), licensed mental health counselors (LMHC), and licensed marital and family therapists (LMFT), all of whom may practice independently. Those who wish to further specialize in the substance use and addiction arena may obtain specialty credentialing and certifications, such as substance use disorder counselor, certified addiction counselor, or licensed addiction counselor (SubstanceAbuseCounselor.org, n.d.). Many of these clinicians complete their terminal degree (e.g., DBH, PhD, PsyD) to advance in academia, research, or other professional pursuits. Further access to the state to state requirements for these credentials appears in the resources list.

Addiction counselors, mental health technicians, peer recovery specialists

Society's escalating mental health needs mandate an expanded workforce. New job titles address the full scope of patient needs, especially in programs for patients with SMI, co-occurring disorders, and other mental health conditions. We now have, for example, behavioral or mental health technicians, case management assistants, and support specialists to assist licensed professionals. These positions are often held by persons with lived experience recovering from addiction or mental illness (called 'peer recovery specialists'), or by early-career practitioners (having earned associate's degrees). Most such support positions require a high school diploma or GED at minimum; others require a bachelor's degree.

Many such support roles are involved in substance use intervention and require specialty certifications, which can vary across the states. Certifications include certified alcohol drug counselor, certified behavioral health technician, certified mental health technician, or certified peer recovery specialist, to name a few. Figure 1.2 displays some of these emerging roles.

Figure 1.2: *Lived experience and other roles in behavioral health*

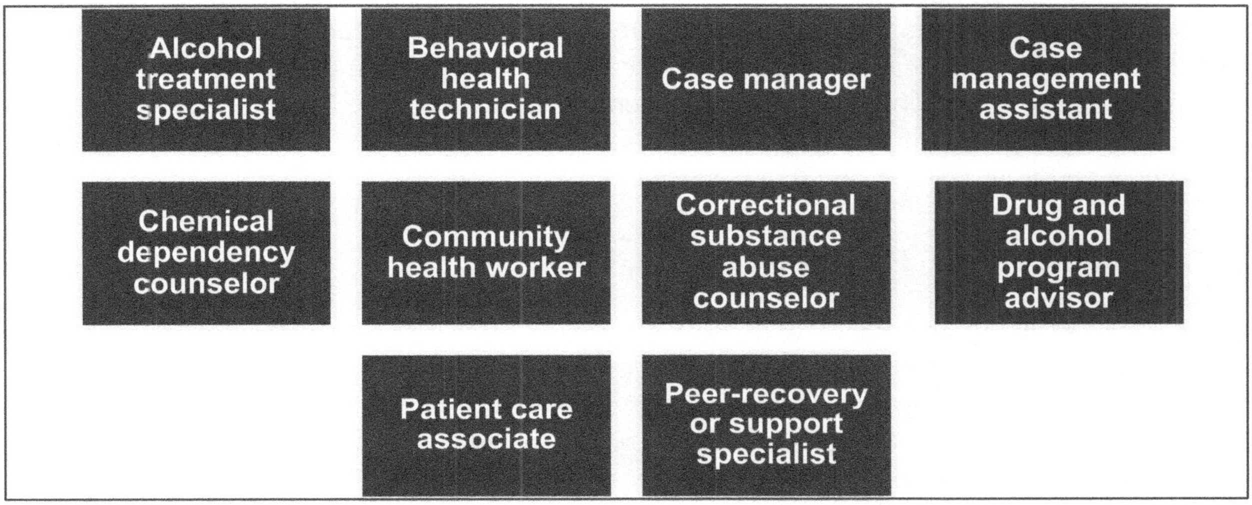

Applied behavioral analysts

Applied behavioral analysis (ABA) is a growing specialty across practice sectors, particularly for patients with neurodevelopmental disorders (e.g., intellectual disability, communication disorders, autism spectrum disorder, or attention deficit disorder with hyperactivity). Applied behavioral analysis encompasses behavior assessment, intervention design and planning, and plan implementation and adjustments. Specialized behavioral techniques include positive reinforcement, shaping, prompt fading, and task analysis, to name a few. The patient's progress is closely monitored, and there's a high level of collaboration between the ABA professional and other providers.

To become a board-certified behavioral analyst (BCBA), a master's degree in a behavioral science field (e.g., behavioral analysis, education, or psychology) is required, followed by passing the certification exam to practice independently. Many BCBAs earn their terminal doctoral degree. Further information on the levels of practice for this specialty are available via the Behavioral Analyst Certification Board.

Qualified mental health professionals

Qualified mental health professional (QMHP) denotes persons trained and experienced in human services—such as social work, psychology, psychiatric rehabilitation, sociology, counseling, vocational rehabilitation, human services counseling, or other degrees deemed equivalent by the state regulatory entity—and who've worked one year full-time or completed an internship. They work in a variety of settings, from community mental health centers to day treatment or residential programs, intensive home-based services, or intensive community-based services. QMHPs provide mental health services to children and adults who may be at imminent risk of placement due to mental health issues, emotional disturbance, or substance abuse. The role is regulated by a professional board in each state, though *which* board varies. In some states, oversight is performed by the Board of Counseling.

CONSIDERATIONS FOR CASE MANAGERS

Those familiar with my work know I align each aspect of a case manager's role with ethics. Mental health intersects directly with case management's ethical principles, particularly when considering patient autonomy and the right to self-determination regarding treatment. Case managers must also uphold their obligation to not harm a patient (known as 'nonmaleficence'), due to biases, stigmas, or other discriminatory actions.

CLINICIAN BIAS AND TREATMENT NON-ADHERENCE VERSUS NON-COMPLIANCE

Bias is present during almost 80 percent of clinical decisions for patients with an SMI (Crapanzo et al., 2023). Bias shows up in labels or nicknames practitioners use, for example. Patients with mental health disorders are commonly referred to as 'non-compliant' when they fail to follow treatment plans, implying intent to disobey. ED readmissions are often derogatorily labeled 'frequent flyers.'

In actuality, barriers to care may be out of a patient's control. They may have few options to access timely follow-up care, prescription drugs, or other recommended treatments. Treatment options may be insufficiently specialized for substance use, addiction, or co-occurring disorders. Waiting lists of two to six months or more are common for psychotherapy or medication assisted treatments (MAT) using methadone, naltrexone, or suboxone. Access to care can be obstructed by providers who are biased against Medicaid or other insurance. Health insurance *ghost networks* hamper access to treatment by providing inaccurate or outdated information about in-network healthcare providers.

Consider this: How often are your well-intended efforts to coordinate mental health treatment thwarted by any of these barriers? We've all been there, whether advocating for a patient's care or for our own. It's easy to become frustrated, and a person's motivation to follow recommended treatment may plummet. Thus, the current recommended terminology for patients who do not follow treatment plans has changed: We use 'treatment non-adherence' in place of the disapproving-sounding 'treatment non-compliance.' Non-adherence shifts the perspective to the patient's experience, contributing to better patient engagement.

LACK OF ACCESS TO PSYCHIATRIC CARE AND TREATMENT FOR PEOPLE WITH MENTAL ILLNESS

Another reason people who suffer from mental illness frequently lack treatment is the shortfall of psychiatric beds, which have steadily decreased in number over recent decades. During the 1950s there were over 500,000 dedicated inpatient state and county psychiatric beds. Deinstitutionalization and closures of psychiatric hospitals in the 1970s reduced bed totals considerably (American Psychiatric Association Presidential Report, 2022). Insurance reimbursement practices led to further program closures, with a 95 percent reduction in beds between 1970 and 2018. Reports from this timeframe show a decrease in beds from 339 per 100,000 persons to 18 (Gao, 2021; Hudson et al., 2021; Lutterman, 2022). Additional factors, like limited funding for lower levels of care, contribute to patients finding few places to obtain interventions.

These factors contribute to length of stay and resource management pressures for case managers. Among emergency departments at 6,000 U.S. hospitals, 70 percent reported holding psychiatric patients for several days, and 10 percent reported boarding patients for several weeks (Simko et al., 2022). Reimbursement for inpatient psychiatric programs in general hospital settings has been inadequate over the past decade. For the few programs maintaining dedicated psychiatric beds, insufficient reimbursement has affected the quality of their treatment programs. For-profit private psychiatric hospitals have reduced administrative costs to match the lower reimbursement rates, and as a result patients experience inadequate staffing, limited treatment interventions, and ineffective psychopharmacological management.

Furthermore, many patients with SMI rely on public insurance such as Medicaid or Medicare Advantage, but many psychiatrists no longer accept these payors. In some states less than 33 percent accept Medicaid managed care plans but 95 percent accept private commercial group insurance plans (Benson et al., 2020). Patient stabilization and prescription management are grossly compromised when individuals can't access medication due to insurance limitations, and patients experience mental health deterioration, regression, and readmission. Case managers must then cope with a vicious cycle of high healthcare utilization and chronic length of stay challenges.

MENTAL HEALTH STIGMAS

Collective negative stereotypes, beliefs, and prejudiced attitudes lead to pervasive damaging views of individuals with mental health conditions. Known as stigmas, these views can yield feelings of shame in patients (and in the professionals rendering care) and discriminatory behaviors from healthcare workers, both of which impede the provision and receipt of healthcare. Four types of mental health stigma appear in the literature: *perceived*, *experienced*, *internalized*, and *anticipated,* displayed in Figure 1.3.

When conscious of stigmas about their condition, patients may delay care or not adhere to their medication or treatments. Those existing feelings of stigma can then be exacerbated by a mental health crisis, as their symptoms become more intense and their perceptions of others' views of them are distorted. From the provider standpoint, patients experiencing a psychotic episode may arrive in the ED in a disheveled state, with poor hygiene. To limit their own contact or other staff contact with the person, clinicians may make hasty evaluations and diagnosis and discharge prematurely. The patient may be readmitted to the ED before long, and the emotions around stigma continue indefinitely on both sides.

Case managers may witness the swift transition of mental health patients through a treatment space. When the bar for patient care quality is unconsciously lowered due to stigmas, it's plain to see that patients with AMI and SMI are subjected to fragmented, reactive, and often emergent care, one of many reasons for their poorer health outcomes and premature mortality rates—10-20 years earlier than the general population (Luciano et al., 2022).

Case managers know that such gaps in care obstruct the industry's patient-centric vision for population health, the quality 'north star' defined by the *Quintuple Aim*: inclusive care rendered at the right cost and the right time by individuals who value the work and account for a whole-person view reflecting health equity (Itchhaporia, 2021).

Figure 1.3: *The four mental health stigmas*

PERCEIVED STIGMA

- Perception of social beliefs (e.g., stereotypes, prejudice, discrimination)
- Can occur on part of the patient or the provider

EXPERIENCED STIGMA

- Perception of being a victim of stereotypes, prejudice, and discrimination
- Occurs on part of the patient

INTERNALIZED STIGMA

- Internalization of stereotypes, prejudice, and social discrimination to self
- Occurs on part of the patient

ANTICIPATED STIGMA

- Expectation of discrimination, often associated with internalized stigma
- Occurs on part of the patient

Adapted from De Oliveira Cardoso et al., 2020

CASE MANAGEMENT'S BEHAVIORAL HEALTH CONVERSATION MAP

Case managers frequently work with patients and their families who present with DSM-diagnoseable anxiety disorders, or history of one. Their patients also often experience health issues that prompt or intensify anxiety, from unplanned hospitalizations or sudden illness onset to insurance authorizations, reimbursement, and other coping challenges. The displaced emotions of patients and families are often directed at healthcare employees. How can case managers approach these individuals and situations more intentionally? Enter *conversation maps*.

Conversation maps are structured frameworks to navigate patient and practitioner interactions. They provide a visual guide to maintain dialogues about a specific condition or illness. The diversity in education, onboarding, and training for case managers highlights the benefit of a template for these conversations. Guideposts assure the conversation maintains a logical flow, and they align with the *Case Management Process* and its six seminal steps (Powell & Tahan, 2019).

Table 1.5 displays a universal conversation map for behavioral health case management, which can be replicated across conditions. The seven phases of the map delineate a clear pathway for case managers to follow, independent of their place of employment. Conversation prompts cue the employee to advance their actions. Particular notice should be placed on Phase 7, *Analyze Actions for Outcomes*. This phase highlights case management's role in quality improvement processes with the interprofessional team, rather than a conversation with the patient, family, or decision-maker. As reviewed in Chapter 3, TQM and CQI are a priority focus for case managers in many organizations and should be on every professional's radar.

Table 1.5: *Case management's behavioral health conversation map*

Conversation Phase	Case Management Process	Conversation Prompts
Phase 1: Advance engagement Introduce case manager role and function Establish rapport to partner with patient (or legal decision-maker)	Identify, select, and engage	Hello, my name is ___, and I'm the case manager. Have you worked with a case manager before? I focus on ___ and partner with my patients on their care. What questions can I answer for you today?
Phase 2: Activate inclusive patient assessment Assess for psychological safety (e.g. screening tools for conditions) and accommodations (e.g., visible and invisible physical, visual, and cognitive disabilities; teletypewriter (TTY) system; language literacy; digital health literacy; etc.) Evaluate clinical capacity Define biopsychosocial needs, including HRSNs Align requisite clinical guidelines (e.g., MCG, InterQual)	Assess and identify patient issues	My role involves working with you (and ___) to develop a treatment plan. (Note: This statement may vary based on practice setting and scope of role.) To accomplish this effort, it would help me to know more about you. Is this a good time to ask you are few questions? We use a questionnaire called ___. This tool helps identity resources you may need. Most patients need something, such as transportation to appointments, guidance on their diet, or a safer place to live. If this moment is not convenient to talk, when might be a good time?
Phase 3: Align interprofessional team Consult with psych/behavioral health for treatment needs Identify needed clinical consultations Coordinate with all parties, including interagency partners (e.g., health plan and community case managers, treatment providers)	Develop and coordinate plan of care	I'll be working with your team of providers to coordinate their assessments and treatment recommendations for you. What questions can I answer for you about that process?
Phase 4: Affirm patient voice (or that of the legal decision-maker) Advocate for patient autonomy Leverage shared decision-making Process patient coping Empower self-efficacy Monitor for ongoing behavioral health intervention	Develop and coordinate plan of care	There can be a lot of moving parts in any treatment plan. I like to check in with my patients to make sure everyone hears the same information. How do you understand what has been presented about your (treatment plan, condition, medication, etc.?) Note: Patient involvement for Phases 4-6 will vary based on: Clinical presentation, clinical capacity, and legal capacity Regulations and expectations specific to practice setting

Conversation Phase	Case Management Process	Conversation Prompts
Phase 5: Arrange treatment plan Reaffirm patient choice Facilitate discharge planning Collaborate and communicate with all parties Complete needed documentation (e.g., PAD, PASRR)	Implement and coordinate plan of care	When we talked last you shared your goal to ___? Is that still your plan? What are your next steps after you (leave the hospital, finish this program)? As we discussed, I called your ___ to discuss your treatment plan.
Phase 6: Assure closed loop referrals Verify patient acceptance Confirm follow-up appointments Terminate with: Patient Family or legal decision-maker Interagency partners	Case closure and termination of CM services	I understand you have questions about your (discharge plan, treatment, next level of programming). Let's talk about those. I have compiled a list of your appointments and follow-up contacts. As we discussed, I have provided your treatment arrangements and contacts to your (family, guardian, or other legal decision-maker, community case manager, etc.).
Phase 7: Analyze actions for outcomes Advance TQM approach aligned with organizational goals Use established CQI tools (e.g., PDSA, Lean) Align outcomes with department/individual performance appraisals	Continuous monitoring, reassessment, and evaluation	Note: Be aware of the scope of your role related to quality improvement projects and know the measures, quality requirements, and standards used in your workplace (e.g., CMS, HEDIS, Joint Commission, NQF, URAC).

CONCLUSION

Care for the mental health population is like a building on an unstable foundation. Cracks emerge in the base, then widen, then weaken the entire structure. The building collapses from the foundation that should have supported it for its lifetime.

This chapter provided a general overview of mental health terms, industry-established diagnostic resources, and ethical realities faced by case management. The knowledge will fuel your journey with this complex population through the case management process.

CONTEMPLATION QUESTIONS

1. Consider your experience(s) with patients or people you know who have been diagnosed with AMI or SMI.
    a) How did the experience impact your view of the person?
    b) How did the experience impact your view of the population(s) he or she belongs to?
    c) Identify one lesson learned from the experience.
    d) How has the experience impacted your work in case management, and how will it moving forward?
2. Reflect on your experiences collaborating with behavioral health professionals from disciplines other than your own.
    a) Identify something you learned from one of those interactions.
    b) If you were to pursue a different behavioral health profession, what would it be, and why?
3. Access the State of Mental Health in America Annual Report from the resources list. Review and compare the following metrics for any two states:
    - General state ranking
    - Access to care
    - Adults with AMI
    - Youth with a major depressive episode who did not receive mental health services
4. Review the four mental health stigmas in Figure 1.3.
    - Which have you experienced, personally or professionally?
    - At the time did you notice how the stigma contributed to the interaction?
    - Should you experience one of these stigmas in the future, how might you address it?
    - Read the following case scenario and answer the questions.

You're an ED case manager. A patient well-known to the staff (and identified as a "frequent flyer"), with a history of substance use, presents with calf pain, rapid pulse, shortness of breath, and elevated blood pressure. You cue the physician to the patient's appearance: He's grabbing his calf in visible pain and presents as agitated. Aware of his previous substance use, staff subconsciously presume his symptoms are caused by current use, even though toxicology and other diagnostics haven't been done. The patient is discharged from the ED without being evaluated. Shortly after, he collapses and dies from a pulmonary embolism.

a) Which of the four mental health stigmas can you identify?
b) What factors contributed to the patient's discharge?
c) What could have happened differently to yield better patient and provider outcomes?

RESOURCES

- **American Academy of Physicians Assistants**
  https://www.aapa.org/career-central/become-a-pa/
- **American Association of Colleges of Nursing**
  https://www.aacnnursing.org/about-aacn
- **American Psychiatric Nurses Association**
  https://www.apna.org

American Psychological Association

- Education and career: https://www.apa.org/education-career/guide

- **American Society of Addiction Medicine**
  https://www.asam.org/
- **Association of Social Work Boards**
  https://www.socialwork.org/license/
- **Behavioral Analyst Certification Board**
  https://www.bacb.com/bcba/
- **Behavioral Risk Factors Surveillance System**
  https://www.cdc.gov/brfss/index.html
- **Centers for Medicare and Medicaid Services: ICD-10 resources**
  https://www.cms.gov/medicare/coding-billing/icd-10-codes
- **Council of Social Work Education**
  https://www.cswe.org/
- **Mental Health America**
  https://www.mhanational.org
- **National Alliance on Mental Illness**
  https://www.nami.org/
- **National Association of Social Workers**
  https://www.socialworkers.org

National Center for Health Statistics

- **Browsing Tool by ICD-10-CM code**
  https://icd10cmtool.cdc.gov/?fy=FY2025
- **National Institute of Mental Health**
  https://www.nimh.nih.gov
- **Social work degrees and licensure scope**
  https://www.socialworkers.org/Careers/Career-Center/Explore-Social-Work/Types-of-Social-Work-Degrees
- **Substance Abuse Counselor Credentialing**
  https://substanceabusecounselor.org/state-and-national-certification/
- **The Diagnostic Statistical Manual of Mental Health Disorders, 5th Edition, Text Revision**
  https://www.psychiatry.org/psychiatrists/practice/dsm/about-dsm

Substance Abuse and Mental Health Services Administration

- **Behavioral Health Workforce Career Navigator by State**
  https://www.samhsa.gov/behavioral-health-careers

REFERENCES

- American Board of Clinical Social Work. (n.d.) What Is Clinical Social Work? Retrieved November 12, 2024, from https://www.abcsw.org/what-is-clinical-social-work
- American Psychiatric Association. (2022). *Diagnostic and Statistical Manual of Mental Disorders* (5th ed., text rev.). https://doi.org/10.1176/appi.books.9780890425787
- American Psychiatric Association Presidential Report on the Assessment of Psychiatric Bed Needs in the United States. (2022). The psychiatric bed crisis in the United States: Understanding the problem and moving toward solutions. *The American Journal of Psychiatry*, *179*(8), 586-588. https://doi.org/10.1176/appi.ajp.22179004
- Benson, N.M., Myong, C., Newhouse, J.P., Fung, V., & Hsu, J. (2020). Psychiatrist participation in private health insurance markets: Paucity in the land of plenty. *Psychiatric Services*, *71*(12), 1232-1238. https://doi.org/10.1176/appi.ps.202000022
- Bolnick, H.J., Bui, A.L., Bulchis, A., Chen, C., Chapin, A., Lomsadze, L., Mokdad, A.H., Millard, F., & Dieleman, J.L. (2020). Health-care spending attributable to modifiable risk factors in the USA: An economic attribution analysis. *The Lancet Public Health*, *5*(10), e525-e535. https://doi.org/10.1016/S2468-2667(20)30203-6
- De Oliveira Cardoso, N., Sanvincente-Vieira, B., De Mattos Vieira Ferracini, I., & Iracema de Lima Argimon, I. (2020). Instruments for measuring perceived and experienced mental illness stigma: A systematic review. *Psychology: Theory and Practice*, *22*(1), 64-88. https://doi.org/10.5935/1980-6906/psicologia.v22n1p64-88

- Crapanzano, K.A., Deweese, S., Pham, D., Le, T., & Hammarlund, R. (2023). The role of bias in clinical decision-making of people with serious mental illness and medical co-morbidities: A scoping review. *The Journal of Behavioral Health Services & Research*, *50*(2), 236-262. https://doi.org/10.1007/s11414-022-09829-w
- Gao, Y.N. (2021). Relationship between psychiatric inpatient beds and jail populations in the United States. *Journal of Psychiatric Practice*, *27*(1), 33-42. https://doi.org/10.1097/PRA.0000000000000524
- Hudson, C.G. (2021). Benchmarks for needed psychiatric beds for the United States: A test of a predictive analytics model. *International Journal of Environmental Research and Public Health*, *18*(22), 12205. https://doi.org/10.3390/ijerph182212205
- Itchhaporia, D. (2021). The evolution of the Quintuple Aim: Health equity, health outcomes, and the economy. *Journal of the American College of Cardiology*, *78*(22), 2262-2264. doi:10.1016/j.jacc.2021.10.018. PMID: 34823665; PMCID: PMC8608191.
- Launders, N., Dotsikas, K., Marston, L., Price, G., Osborn, D.P.J., & Hayes, J.F. (2022). The impact of comorbid severe mental illness and common chronic physical health conditions on hospitalisation: A systematic review and meta-analysis. *PloS One*, *17*(8), e0272498. https://doi.org/10.1371/journal.pone.0272498
- Luciano, M., Pompili, M., Sartorius, N., & Fiorillo, A. (2022). Editorial: Mortality of people with severe mental illness: Causes and ways of its reduction. *Frontiers in Psychiatry*, *13*, 1009772. https://doi.org/10.3389/fpsyt.2022.1009772
- Lutterman, T. (2022). *Trends in Psychiatric Inpatient Capacity, United States and Each State, 1970 to 2018*. Technical Assistance Collaborative Paper No. 2. Alexandria, VA: National Association of State Mental Health Program Directors.
- Mental Health America. (2024). State of Mental Health in America 2024. Retrieved October 22, 2024, from https://mhanational.org/issues/state-mental-health-america
- National Center of Health Statistics. (2024). ICD-10-CM. Retrieved October 21, 2024, from https://www.cdc.gov/nchs/icd/icd-10-cm/index.html
- National Institute of Mental Health. (2024). Mental illness. *Mental Health Information;* Retrieved September 26, 2024, from https://www.nimh.nih.gov/health/statistics/mental-illness
- SubstanceAbuseCounselor.org. (n.d.). How NAADAC and IC&RC Certification Intersect with State-Level Substance Abuse Counselor Credentialing. Retrieved October 23, 2025, from https://substanceabusecounselor.org/state-and-national-certification/
- Seabury, S.A., Axeen, S., Pauley, G., Tysinger, B., Schlosser, D., Hernandez, J.B., Heun-Johnson, H., Zhao, H., & Goldman, D.P. (2019). Measuring the lifetime costs of serious mental illness and the mitigating effects of educational attainment. *Health Affairs*, *38*(4), 652-659. https://doi.org/10.1377/hlthaff.2018.05246
- Shields, M.C., Beaulieu, N.D., Lu, S., Busch, A.B., Cutler, D.M., & Chien, A.T. (2022). Increases in inpatient psychiatry beds operated by systems, for-profits, and chains, 2010-2016. *Psychiatric Services*, *73*(5), 561-564. https://doi.org/10.1176/appi.ps.202100182

- Simko, L., Birgisson, N.E., Pirrotta, E.A., & Wang, E. (2022). Waiting for care: Length of stay for ED mental health patients by disposition, diagnosis, and region (2009-2015). *Cureus, 14*(6), e25604. https://doi.org/10.7759/cureus.25604
- World Health Organization. (2022). Mental Health Fact Sheets. Retrieved September 26, 2024, from https://www.who.int/news-room/fact-sheets/detail/mental-health-strengthening-our-response
- World Health Organization. (2004). ICD-10: *International Statistical Classification of Diseases and Related Health Problems*: 10th revision, 2nd ed. World Health Organization.

CHAPTER 2

REGULATIONS AND REQUIREMENTS

INTRODUCTION

A long-standing foundational pillar in case management is administration of the highest quality of patient-centric care in the least-intensive, least-restrictive setting possible. But what does this mean for behavioral health, a domain of care that has long featured gaps and lapses in care? The pent-up demand for mental healthcare has only worsened this situation.

This chapter will explore how behavioral healthcare has been regulated, managed, and provided across treatment levels and settings. The continuum of care, as defined by health plans, will be presented. Relevant legislation, regulations, and requirements impacting screening, assessment, intervention, and treatment will be reviewed, along with the latest generation of privacy laws. The chapter will also address court-mandated treatment options, age of treatment parameters, and mandatory duty to warn requirements.

BEHAVIORAL LEARNING OBJECTIVES

1. Understand the mental health continuum of care and treatment
2. Define Preadmission Screening and Resident Review requirements (PASRR)
3. Understand Psychiatric Advance Directives (PADs)
4. Identify the age of consent for youth mental health treatment around the U.S.
5. Distinguish between clinical and legal capacity
6. Understand the types of court-mandated treatments
7. Identify relevant regulations and requirements for case managers
8. Understand the impact of the *Tarasoff* Ruling on Mandatory Duty to Warn legislation
9. Apply CMS Conditions of Participation for behavioral health
10. Apply the 21st Century Cures Act
11. Understand the impact of Open Notes for behavioral health
12. Understand 42-CFR Part 2 legislation relevant to substance use treatment

ESSENTIAL TERMS

- 21st Century Cures Act
- Age of majority
- Age of consent
- Clinical capacity
- Clinical guidelines
- Competence
- Community Mental Health Act of 1963
- Crisis intervention
- Day treatment
- Emancipation (emancipated minor)
- Emergency commitment order (ECO)
- Family support services
- Home-based treatment
- Inpatient hospitalization
- Intensive case management
- Intensive outpatient programs (IOP)
- Involuntary admission (civil commitment)
- Legal capacity
- Mandatory duty to warn
- Mature minor doctrine
- Medicare Conditions of Participation (CoPs)
- Minor
- Omnibus Budget Reconciliation Act of 1987 (OBRA)
- Open Notes Rule
- Outpatient treatment
- Part 2 Title 42-CFR
- Partial hospital programs (PHP)
- Preadmission Screening and Resident Review (PASRR)
- Psychiatric advance directive (PAD)
- Residential treatment center (RTC)
- Respite care
- *Tarasoff* Ruling
- Temporary detention order (TDO)

AN OVERVIEW OF THE BEHAVIORAL HEALTHCARE CONTINUUM

The behavioral healthcare continuum is expansive. Programs and services are defined by clinical guidelines and encompass multiple levels of care, as well as opioid treatment. Availability of treatments and programs differs across states and jurisdictions, as does access to them.

LEVELS OF CARE AND SERVICE DEFINITIONS

Mental health treatment services and programs tend to be grouped according to two main life stages: youth and adulthood. Clinical guidelines differentiate treatments, which fall into five levels of care (inpatient, residential, partial hospital, intensive outpatient, or outpatient), as well as crisis intervention, observation, day treatment, and long-term care (MCG, 2025). The behavioral healthcare continuum for adults appears in Table 2.1 and includes a detailing of ambulatory treatment settings.

Table 2.1: *Levels of behavioral healthcare for adults*

Level of Care	Explanation
Hospitalization	• The highest level of skilled psychiatric and substance abuse services provided in a facility • May be a freestanding psychiatric hospital, psychiatric unit of a general hospital, or detoxification unit in a hospital • Settings eligible for this level of care are licensed at the hospital level and provide 24-hour medical and nursing care

Level of Care	Explanation
23-hour observation	• Allows for individuals in crisis to be promptly evaluated and stabilized • Up to 23 hours and 59 minutes of observation and crisis stabilization is provided • A secure and protected environment staffed with medical and clinical personnel, including psychiatric supervision and 24-hour nursing coverage • Includes comprehensive assessment and development and delivery of a treatment plan
Crisis intervention	• Includes services for managing acute care crises
Residential treatment centers (RTC)	• Provides 24-hour care to persons with long-term or severe mental disorders and persons with substance-related disorders • Care is medically monitored, with availability of 24-hour medical and nursing serv ces • Provides less intensive medical monitoring than subacute hospitalization care and includes treatment with a range of diagnostic and therapeutic behavioral health services that are not provided through community programs • Patients receive training in basic skills of living, as necessary • Care includes residential treatment for psychiatric conditions and residential rehabilitation treatment for alcohol and substance abuse
Partial hospitalization (PHP)	• Structured and medically supervised day, evening, and/or night treatment programs • Services include medical and nursing, but at lower intensity than a hospital setting • Care may address mental health and/or substance-related disorders through individualized treatment provided by a coordinated interdisciplinary treatment team
Intensive outpatient (IOP)	• Provides planned, structured services over multiple weeks, which may include weekends • Patient encounters are comprised of coordinated and integrated interdisciplinary services • Care may address mental or substance-related disorders, and potentially group, individual, family, or multi-family group psychotherapy, psychoeducation, and adjunctive services such as medical monitoring

Ambulatory services and outpatient treatment	• Encompasses outpatient treatment services, provided by licensed, credentialed mental health professionals
	• Directed toward reversing symptoms of acute mental health disorders and/or substance use disorders to facilitate improvement, maintain stability, and increase functional autonomy
	• Services target the symptoms or problem being treated
	• Durations span 15 minutes (e.g., medication checks) to 50 minutes (e.g., individual, conjoint, family psychotherapy), or up to 2 hours (e.g., group psychotherapy)
	• **Types of counseling and psychotherapy include:**
	  • individual psychotherapy
	  • behavioral therapy
	  • medication management
	  • shared medical appointments
	  • psychiatric, psychological, and psychosocial assessment
	  • group psychotherapy
	  • conjoint/marital therapy
	  • family therapy
	  • outpatient detox services
	  • medically assisted treatment (e.g., outpatient buprenorphine maintenance services)

Level of Care	Explanation
Day Treatment	• Encompasses a community-based mix of psychosocial treatments, educational, and recreational activities for patients with behavioral health conditions associated with functional impairment, such as inability to maintain full-time engagement in work, school, or home environment • Addresses chronic issues, rather than acute exacerbations or urgent clinical issues • Coordination with school or work schedules is often required • Programs are of longer duration than IOP or PHP

Magellan Healthcare Inc., 2024

BEHAVIORAL HEALTHCARE FOR CHILDREN AND ADOLESCENTS

Though the first screening for mental health intervention would ideally occur in a provider's office, for many patients the first screening happens in an ambulatory or ED setting, or as mandated by a court. For youth, it may first occur in school. The levels of mental healthcare and treatment available for youth are distinct from those offerings for adults. They appear in Table 2.2.

Table 2.2: *Levels of behavioral healthcare for youth*

Level of Care	Explanation
Inpatient hospital	• Comprehensive psychiatric treatment in a hospital, with programs designed for youth; duration of stay depends on patient needs
Residential treatment	• Seriously disturbed patients receive intensive and comprehensive psychiatric treatment in a campus-like setting on a longer-term basis
Crisis residence	• 24-hour supervision during short-term (usually less than 15 days) crisis intervention and treatment
Therapeutic group home	• Serving 6-10 youth for residential treatment; may be linked with all-day treatment or a specialized educational program
Respite care	• Offers patients brief stays with staff trained in the age-appropriate care and mental health management of youth
Emergency services	• 24-hour emergencies services, such as hospital emergency room or mobile crisis team
Partial hospital	• The treatment services of an inpatient psychiatric hospital, with patients spending nights at home
Intensive outpatient	• Outpatient programming that may occur all day in school or after school, often including group therapy, individual therapy, family therapy, and medication management
Day treatment	• Intensive psychiatric treatment with special education, usually 5 days per week
Family support services	• Support for families in caring for their children, including parenting training and support groups
Home-based treatment	• Home visits followed by a treatment program for the child and family

Level of Care	Explanation
Intensive case management	• Psychiatric, financial, legal, and medical services coordinated or provided by a trained clinician so a patient may live successfully at home
Office or outpatient clinic	• Treatments during 30- or 60-minute appointments based on patient need, often 1-2 times weekly

American Academy of Child and Adolescent Psychiatry, 2023

REGULATIONS AND REQUIREMENTS FOR ADULTS

The demand for a quality mental healthcare continuum is not new. A series of regulations and legal landmarks passed over decades have influenced how case management facilitates patient behavioral health treatment.

THE COMMUNITY MENTAL HEALTH ACT OF 1963

In the early 1960s, the federal government strived to decrease the number of people in institutions by shifting care for severe mental illness (SMI) patients from institutions to community mental healthcare centers (CMHC). The Community Mental Health Act was well-intended; three years of federal grant payments totaling $150 million went to the states. Monies were spent on construction and initial staffing of 1,500 CMHCs. Programming established a mental health infrastructure of consultations and education for community and professional organizations, inpatient facilities, outpatient clinics, emergency response, and partial hospitalization (Erikson, 2021).

Unfortunately, the Act experienced problems from its start. The initial funding was insufficient, and only 700 of the 1,500 planned CMHCs were built. States defined their own priorities for CMHCs; in some states only individuals with less serious mental illnesses received care. This lack of standardization meant the National Institute of Mental Health (NIMH) could not evaluate and regulate the CMHCs. The vision for a mental health safety net failed. Instead, a patchwork of outpatient programs and providers emerged but was unable to meet growing need.

PREADMISSION SCREENING AND RESIDENT REVIEW (PASRR)

Through the 1960s and 1970s, a generation of patients with severe psychiatric conditions was aging. That, combined with a deinstitutionalization movement and closure of psychiatric units in the 1980s, contributed to a rising number of psychiatric patients placed in group homes and nursing homes. Many others were homeless: Adults with developmental and intellectual disabilities who had been cared for by elderly parents were abandoned by remaining family upon the death of one or both parents. They were often left to wander the streets. Other patients were veterans of

World War II or the Vietnam War with untreated post-traumatic stress, combat fatigue, or chronic substance use.

These patient populations had high rates of chronic illness and co-occurring disorders that prompted frequent ED visits and hospitalizations. Most required ongoing skilled or custodial care after discharge (Bucy et al., 2022; George et al., 2023) and were inappropriately admitted to nursing home facilities.

The Preadmission Screening and Resident Review (PASRR) program was created by Congress in 1987 to end the inappropriate placement of patients with mental health conditions in nursing homes for long-term care. The PASRR was intended to help states rebalance services *away* from institutions and *toward* supporting people in their homes. The program was a federal requirement under the Omnibus Budget Reconciliation Act (OBRA), also known as the Nursing Home Reform Act (Federal Register, 2024). Box 2.1 lists PASRR facts and requirements.

Box 2.1: 42 CFR Part 483 Subpart C, Preadmission Screening and Resident Admission Review Assessment (November 30, 1992)

§ 483.100 Basis. The requirements of §§ 483.100 through 483.138 governing the State›s responsibility for preadmission screening and annual resident review (PASRR) of individuals with mental illness and intellectual disability are based on section 1919(e)(7) of the [Social Security] Act.

1. Evaluate all applicants for serious mental illness and/or intellectual disability, and
2. Offer all applicants the most appropriate setting for their needs (in the community, a nursing facility, or an acute care setting)

These actions are accomplished by:

- Screening: All applicants to Medicaid-certified nursing facilities must undergo a preliminary assessment, called a "Level I screen." Those who test positive are evaluated in greater depth, called "Level II" PASRR.
- Regulations: The regulations to govern PASRR were written after the Americans with Disabilities Act (ADA) passed in 1990 and reflect the intent of that law. The regulations are found in the Code of Federal Regulations at 42 CFR 483.100-138.
- Compliance: CMS requires all states operate a PASRR program that complies with federal regulations.

Federal Register, 2024

The PASRR program would also later align with the 1999 Supreme Court decision, *Olmstead v. L.C.,* under the Americans with Disabilities Act (ADA). The *Olmstead* case involved two women, Lois Curtis and Elaine Wilson, both diagnosed with mental illnesses and developmental disabilities who were voluntarily admitted to the psychiatric unit at State-run Georgia Regional Hospital. After they received medical treatment, they were cleared by mental health professionals for transfer to a community-based program. However, both women remained confined to the institution for several years after their initial treatment concluded due to a lack of available community settings and services. Consequently, Ms. Curtis and Ms. Wilson filed suit under the ADA for release from the hospital (Justia U.S. Supreme Court, n.d.).

As a result of the *Olmstead* decision, individuals with disabilities cannot be required to be institutionalized to receive public benefits that can be furnished in community-based settings. The U.S. Supreme Court ruled that unjustified segregation of persons with disabilities constitutes discrimination and violates the ADA (Justia U.S. Supreme Court, n.d.). Therefore, public entities must provide community-based services to persons with disabilities when the services are appropriate, the affected persons do not oppose community-based treatment, and the community-based services can be reasonably accommodated, considering the resources available to the public entity and the needs of others who are receiving disability services from the entity (Justia U.S. Supreme Court, n.d.).

The PASRR screen and its accompanying processes safeguard an individual's psychological, psychiatric, and functional needs, along with personal goals and preferences, when planning longer-term care needs, including those in residential settings. All applicants to Medicaid-certified nursing facilities must receive the Level I preliminary assessment to determine if they may have severe mental illness or intellectual disability. Individuals who test positive for SMI or intellectual disability at Level I are evaluated further. Level II testing yields a determination of need, determination of appropriate setting, and a set of recommendations for services to inform the patient's plan of care (Federal Register, 2024).

Despite the implementation of PASRR in all states, the number of adults diagnosed with SMI in nursing homes has continued to rise. They have historically ranged from 10-18 percent of the nursing home population, but adults 50 years old or younger, with a history of SMI, including substance use disorder, are increasingly being placed there (Laws et al., 2022). Over 1.1 million Americans reside in nursing homes and over 300,000 have a psychiatric diagnosis; 150,000 of these persons are diagnosed with SMI (Gerlauch & Maust, 2023).

PSYCHIATRIC ADVANCE DIRECTIVES

In 1990, Congress passed the Patient Self-Determination Act (PSDA), which required all providers receiving Medicare and Medicaid reimbursement to ask patients (or designated family) about advance directives and options to accept or refuse medical treatment. These legal instruments had a ripple effect, as many patients wanted to also delineate their mental health treatment preferences. Psychiatric advance directives (PADs) were the industry response to this desire: a legal instrument to document a competent individual's preferences regarding mental health treatment (National Resource Center on Psychiatric Advance Directives, 2024). Through PADs, a person can share their desires with their primary care provider and their hospital or health system—even police departments. Like advance directives, PADs also allow individuals to appoint a health proxy who will ensure the preferences are followed in the event of an acute medical or psychiatric emergency.

Patients with a mental illness, especially an SMI, frequently fall off loved ones' radar. Through PADs, however, involved family members, guardians, conservators, or other surrogates remain informed about the patient's treatment preferences, and thus, are better advocates for the patient. Through these actions, the patient's autonomy is prioritized, as their wishes for care have been made clear.

Across states there is disparity in PAD language and document scope. In states without a legal provision for PADs, an individual may document his or her desires in general healthcare directives or living wills. Yet the nuances of mental healthcare are complicated when documents are not specific. For example, in some states, generic advance directives may be limited to a certain number or types of mental healthcare decisions. They may also prohibit the health proxy from making mental health treatment decisions (National Resource Center on Psychiatric Advance Directives, 2024).

Some states have hit the quality bar for PADs, however. In 2019 the Colorado General Assembly implemented House Bill 19-1044, Advance Behavioral Health Orders Treatment (Colorado General Assembly, 2024). The legislation created a distinct behavioral health order form allowing adults to communicate their behavioral health history, decisions, and preferences should they lack decisional capacity. The form and law allow patients to provide consent for, withdraw from, or refuse behavioral health treatment or medication. See a summary of HB19-1044 in Box 2.2.

Joint Commission's Behavioral Health Care Accreditation program includes a Care, Treatment, and Services standard, CTS.01.04.01. The standard requires accredited behavioral healthcare organizations that serve adults with SMI to document whether the adult has completed a PAD. In addition, accredited behavioral healthcare organizations must provide resources on creating PADs when requested by patients. The standard also specifies that if an adult possesses a PAD, clinical staff involved in that patient's care, treatment, or services must be aware that the PAD exists and know how to access it (Joint Commission, 2020).

The National Resource Center on Psychiatric Advance Directives (2024) helpfully provides a clearinghouse of federal and state policies, state-specific PAD forms and documentation, educational videos, and other resources. Several states have developed formal online registries for PADs, which provide healthcare workers quick access to documents. Consumers choose whether to participate in the secure online registry. All information entered is confidential protected health information (National Resource Center on Psychiatric Advance Directives, 2024).

Box 2.2: Colorado HB19-1044 Advance Behavioral Health Orders Treatment

The Act:

- Lists the requirements for a behavioral health orders for scope of treatment form;
- Details the duties and immunities of emergency medical services personnel, health care providers, and health care facilities with respect to treating an adult with behavioral health orders for scope of treatment;
- Details how a behavioral health orders for scope of treatment form is executed, amended, or revoked; and
- Prohibits an effect on a health insurance contract, life insurance contract, or annuity, due to executing or failing to execute a behavioral health orders for scope of treatment.

Colorado General Assembly, 2024

CLINICAL CAPACITY, INFORMED CONSENT, AND LEGAL CAPACITY

A case manager's primary obligation is to patient autonomy (CMSA, 2024). This ethical tenet can be tough to heed, however, when a patient's clinical or legal capacities are unclear. This section unravels the complex processes around consent and capacity.

CLINICAL CAPACITY AND INFORMED CONSENT

The starting point for a discussion on legal capacity is *clinical capacity*, or a patient's ability to make informed decisions and provide *informed consent*. Case managers verify whether patients (and those involved in their care) possess clinical capacity to understand and participate in discussions about their care and treatment. It is far more than a box to be checked. Case managers must be sure patients have sufficient information to demonstrate their understanding of:

- The proposed treatment
- Risks and benefits of proposed treatment
- Alternatives to the proposed treatment
- Risks and benefits of the alternative treatments, and
- Risks and benefits of doing nothing

(Shah et al., 2024)

The three elements of clinical capacity are shown in Box 2.3.

Box 2.3: Elements of clinical capacity

Medical factors, such as the patient's medical condition, sensory deficits, drug side effects, and emotional and psychiatric issues

Functional abilities, such as physical, cognitive, or psychological

Environmental factors, such as stressful living conditions, availability of helpers, isolation, and time of day variations caused by medication schedules or fatigue

Pope, 2023

LEGAL CAPACITY

Legal capacity is a step beyond clinical capacity; it is a legal determination of a person's capability to act on his or her own behalf in legal proceedings or transactions, such as business, financial, or medical decisions. A court, not healthcare professionals, renders the decision on a patient's legal capacity following an assessment of mental capacity performed by a psychiatrist or other trained behavioral health professional, as presented in Table 1.4 in Chapter 1. (Note: The industry recently shifted from the term 'competency,' to the term 'legal capacity.')

A court determination of *legal incapacity* means the individual lacks the mental capacities to reason and deliberate, to hold appropriate values and goals, to appreciate his or her circumstances, to understand the information given, and to communicate a choice (Pope, 2023). The requirements defined by the courts appear in Box 2.4.

Box 2.4: Requirements for legal incapacity, as defined by U.S. court of law

A disabling condition (e.g., intellectual disability, mental disorder, dementia or other brain disorder, chronic use of drugs)

A lack of cognitive ability to receive and evaluate information or to make or communicate decisions

An inability to meet essential requirements of physical health, safety, or self-care without protective intervention

A finding that guardianship or conservatorship is the least restrictive alternative for protecting the person

Pope, 2023

AGE OF CONSENT AND ACCESS TO TREATMENT FOR MINORS

Much has been written about the recent increase in youth mental health disorders and the growing need for treatment to address anxiety, eating disorders, depression, and substance use. Smartphones, tablets, and their varied applications have created new options for adolescents to receive mental healthcare. Expanded reimbursement for virtual therapy has further increased access to treatment.

At 18 years old, all mentally competent individuals are permitted by law to consent to or refuse medical treatment. But at what age do *minors* have the legal right to make decisions about their mental healthcare and obtain treatment? The answer to this question is guided by several factors, including the *age of majority,* the *age of consent,* and age at which a minor may access specific treatment within their state or jurisdiction.

A minor is any person who is under the specified age of majority for their state or jurisdiction. The age of majority in the U.S. is traditionally 18, though it varies among states: The age of majority is 19 in Alabama, Colorado, Maryland, and Nebraska, and 21 in Indiana and Mississippi, for example. In contrast, the age of consent is the minimum age within a state or jurisdiction that a person can legally give permission for a specific activity, such as mental health or substance use treatment, or sexual relations (Legal Information Institute, 2023). Table 2.3 provides distinctions between age of majority and age of consent.

The age at which patients may obtain mental health treatment can feel like a moving target. In many states, minors as young as 12 years of age may consent to and participate in mental health treatment with or without parental consent (Kerwin et al., 2015; Naroozi et al., 2018). In this way, the barriers to programs addressing substance use, trauma, or severe emotional distress are removed for vulnerable youth who might be unable or unwilling to involve their parents. Adolescents elsewhere may have their access to mental health limited if lacking parental (or guardian) consent, however. Several states (e.g., Rhode Island, Virginia, West Virginia, Wyoming) may require permission of the minor and parent for inpatient mental health and/or substance use treatment (Kerwin et al., 2015; Hijano & Yaun, 2024; Sharko et al., 2022). Some states, such as New Mexico, maintain separate regulations covering the age at which minors may be prescribed psychotropic and other medications (Sharko et al., 2022). Box 2.5 provides basic summaries of current laws for age of consent and access to mental health treatment by minors across the U.S.

State laws and regulations guiding substance use treatment are particularly complex. Countless clinical, legal, and political factors influence this reality, including age of majority and emancipated minor and mature minor doctrines. The age of consent for addiction or detox treatment may intersect with laws on parental rights and provider recommendations. For example, the age of consent for substance use intervention ranges from 12 years old in Arkansas and California, to 15 in Oregon, and 18 in Alaska and Arizona. In New York state 12-year-olds found to be drug dependent by two or more physicians may access substance abuse treatment without parental permission, except methadone maintenance (National Center for Youth Law, 2024h).

There are legal exceptions to the age of majority. A person under age 18 who lives independently without the support of parents and makes his or her own day-to-day decisions may petition the court for *emancipation;* such a youth is then known as an *emancipated minor.* This term includes minors who are married, serve in the armed forces, or have legally obtained a formal court decree. If granted, the minor is provided the same legal rights as an adult, including the right to consent to and refuse medical treatment (Hijano & Yaun, 2024).

Minors may also become the sole decision-maker about their medical care under the *mature minor doctrine,* a rule that allows mature adolescents to provide consent (Hijano & Yaun, 2024). In jurisdictions where mature minor doctrines exist, a child's age and situation are considered in determinations of maturity. The doctrine has been consistently applied when the minor is at least 16 years old and understands the medical procedure in question, and the procedure is not serious (U.S. Legal, n.d.).

Because of the variations in age of consent, case managers should verify the presence and scope of all laws relevant to the populations they work with. The age of majority for each state is accessible through each state or jurisdiction's official government or legislative website. The Legal Information Institute and the National Center for Youth Law also provide information on the ages at which minors can access mental health and substance use treatment. Both appear in the chapter's resources list. Furthermore, case managers may wish to seek guidance from their organizations' risk management, legal, and ethics representatives.

Table 2.3: *Distinctions between age of majority and age of consent*

Age of majority	Age of consent
Definition: The age at which a person is legally considered an adult, responsible for all their own legal, financial, and medical decisions In most U.S. states the age of majority is 18, but in some states it is 19 or 21	Definition: The minimum age for a person to legally give permission for a specific activity The age varies by state and jurisdiction The age generally ranges from 16 to 18 years old, though can be lower based on the given state/territory and the law For example, Rhode Island and South Carolina permit consent for some activities at age 14, with unrestricted ability to consent at 16. That is, a 14-year-old in Rhode Island can legally consent to sex with someone 16 or 17 years old but cannot consent to sex with someone 18 or older.
Scope of legal abilities: address legal matters (e.g., contracts) make healthcare decisions manage finances vote	Scope Applies to specific activities, most commonly sexual relations

Legal Information Institute, 2023

Box 2.5: State laws for minimum age of consent and access to mental health treatment

Alabama: Minors 16 or older may access outpatient treatment; minors under 16 must have a parent's or legal guardian's written consent for most mental health services (Griffith, 2025)

Alaska: No law in place*

Arizona: No law in place*

Arkansas: Minors 12 years or older may consent to mental health services "if the patient has sufficient maturity to appreciate the consequences" (Arkansas Department of Human Services, 2023)

California: Minors 12 or older may access outpatient treatment without parental consent, "though must be mature enough to participate" (California Department of Healthcare Services, 2024)

Colorado: Minors 12 or older may access outpatient treatment without parental consent (Colorado Behavioral Health Administration, 2025)

Connecticut: Minors may access outpatient treatment; parental consent is required for inpatient treatment (State of Connecticut, 2025)

Delaware: Minors over age 14 may consent to outpatient treatment; parental consent required for inpatient treatment*

District of Columbia: Minors may access outpatient mental health services; parental consent is required for inpatient treatment*

Florida: Minors over 13 may access outpatient treatment; parental consent required for inpatient treatment*

Georgia: Parental consent is required for minors under 18 years old, unless an emancipated minor or a minor parent*

Hawaii: Minors over 14 may consent for outpatient treatment; parental consent is required for inpatient treatment*

Idaho: Minors may consent for outpatient treatment; minors over 14 may consent for inpatient treatment*

Illinois: Minors over age 12 may access outpatient treatment; parents must consent for inpatient treatment (Illinois Legal Aid, 2024)

Indiana: Minors under age 21 may access outpatient treatment*

Iowa: Minors may consent to immediate or short-term treatment if a victim of sexual abuse or assault*

Kansas: Minors 14 and older may consent to treatment*

Kentucky: Minors 16 and older may consent to treatment*

Louisiana: Minors are permitted to access outpatient mental health treatment*

Maine: Minors are permitted to access mental health treatment*

Maryland: Minors 12 or older may consent to outpatient mental health treatment; parental consent is required for minors 16 or younger to use prescription medications to treat a mental or emotional disorder (Maryland People's Law, 2024)

Massachusetts: Parental consent is required for minors 16 or younger to receive inpatient or outpatient treatment (National Center for Youth Law, 2024a)

Michigan: Minors 14 or older may consent to outpatient care, with parental consent required for inpatient care*

Minnesota: Minors 16 or older may access outpatient mental health treatment (Minnesota Department of Health, n.d.)

Mississippi: Minors 15 or older may access outpatient mental health treatment*

Missouri: Parental consent for anyone under age 18 for access to outpatient mental health treatment (National Center for Youth Law, 2024b)

Montana: Minors 16 years or older may access outpatient mental health treatment (National Center for Youth Law, 2024c)

Nebraska: Parental consent is required for any minor under 18 years of age*

Nevada: Parental consent is required for any minor under 18 years of age to access outpatient mental health treatment, unless an emancipated minor (National Center for Youth Law, 2024d)

New Hampshire: Parental consent is required for any minor under 18 years old (National Center for Youth Law, 2024e)

New Jersey: Parental consent is required for any minor under 16 years old for outpatient treatment (National Center for Youth Law, 2024f)

New Mexico: Minors 14 or older may access outpatient mental health treatment (National Center for Youth Law, 2024g)

New York: Minors 16 or older can access inpatient treatment, psychotropic medication (in certain circumstances), and outpatient mental health treatment without parental consent (National Center for Youth Law, 2024h)

North Carolina: Minors may access outpatient therapy and treatment; parental consent is required for inpatient therapy (National Center for Youth Law, 2024i)

North Dakota: Minors are unable to access mental health treatment unless they are "homeless unaccompanied minors" (National Center for Youth Law, 2024j)

Ohio: Minors over 14 years old may access outpatient therapy; parental consent required for inpatient therapy*

Oklahoma: Minors 16 or older may access outpatient therapy or inpatient therapy; parental consent is required for inpatient therapy*

Oregon: Minors over 14 years old may access outpatient therapy; parental consent required for inpatient therapy*

Pennsylvania: Minors over 14 years old may access outpatient therapy; parental consent required for inpatient therapy*

Rhode Island: Minors over 16 years old may access outpatient therapy; parental consent required for inpatient therapy*

South Carolina: Minors over 16 years old can consent to mental health services; parental consent is required for treatment under 16 (National Center for Youth Law, 2024k)

South Dakota: The notarized, written consent of one parent or legal guardian is required for a minor between 16 and 18 years old to receive mental health treatment (National Center for Youth Law, 2024l)

Tennessee: Minors 16 or older may access outpatient treatment; parental consent required for those under 16 years old and for inpatient treatments (National Center for Youth Law, 2024m)

Texas: Minors may consent to counseling for: "(1) suicide prevention; (2) chemical addiction or dependency; or (3) sexual, physical, or emotional abuse" (National Center for Youth Law, 2024n)

Utah: No law in place*

Vermont: Minors may consent to outpatient mental health treatment without parental consent, excluding prescription drugs for which parental consent is required; parental consent is required for inpatient treatment (National Center for Youth Law, 2024o)

Virginia Minors 14 or older can access outpatient treatment; parental consent is required for inpatient treatment (Virginia Law, 2025)

Washington: Minors 13 or older may access outpatient treatment, and they may admit themselves for inpatient evaluation and treatment "if a professional agrees that inpatient care is necessary due to a mental disorder and less restrictive treatment is not feasible" (Washington State Department of Social Services, 2025)

West Virginia: Minors 14 or older may access outpatient treatment*

Wisconsin: Minors 14 or older may access outpatient treatment*

Wyoming: Minors can consent to mental health treatment in specific situations (e.g., being married, active-duty military, emancipated, self-supporting, or at least 12 years old and seeking tobacco cessation services); parental consent required for access to outpatient and inpatient mental health treatment (National Center for Youth Law, 2024p)

**Sourced from iCanNotes, 2022 and National Center for Youth Law, 2024 (other references are noted above)*

COURT-MANDATED TREATMENT

Imagine this case management scenario: A patient presents to an ED or other outpatient setting with suicidal or homicidal ideation. The treatment team has weighed in, and a psychiatric consultation assesses the person is in imminent danger of harming himself or others; personal and public safety are at grave risk. The patient adamantly refuses voluntary admission to psychiatry or another behavioral health unit, though. What happens next?

Case managers experience these situations across every age group and practice setting. Voluntary requests for psychiatric evaluation, treatment, and admission may quickly shift to court-mandated treatment actions. Case managers should be aware of the continuum of these actions, as displayed in Figure 2.1. The requirements and timeframes for each action vary across states and jurisdictions.

EMERGENCY COMMITMENT ORDER

An emergency commitment order (ECO) or involuntary psychiatric hold is a legal process that allows a person to be taken into custody by law enforcement without their consent for the purposes of psychiatric evaluation, or to be held by a psychiatric facility for the purpose of evaluation. The psychiatric evaluation must be completed by a professional skilled in diagnosis and assessment of mental illness (Virginia Department of Behavioral Health & Developmental Services, 2020).

TEMPORARY DETENTION ORDER

A temporary detention order (TDO) is a court order issued by a magistrate, judge, or other judicial authority requiring an individual be held in a psychiatric facility for a designated period. Requirements vary across the states, though the allowed timeframe is typically up to 72 hours, until a commitment hearing is held. The length of time a person is hospitalized before the hearing may increase due to an intervening weekend or legal holiday. While magistrates are generally available every day of the year for 24 hours a day, holidays and high volumes of case may impact the timing of their decisions (Virginia Department of Behavioral Health & Developmental Services, 2020).

INVOLUNTARY ADMISSION (CIVIL COMMITMENT)

Involuntary admission is also referred to as involuntary civil commitment, or simply, commitment. The action refers to a legal process that forces someone to be treated for a mental illness, serious developmental or physical disability, and/or substance abuse, per each state's statues. The typical case for commitment is a patient who poses a danger to self or others; most states also interpret the inability to provide for one's basic needs as reflecting a danger to self. A hearing is scheduled to review the clinical team's formal evaluation and define a treatment plan (Virginia Department of Behavioral Health & Developmental Services, 2020).

Imagine you're standing at a bus stop and observe a person cursing at the sky, yelling obscenities at bystanders, then defecating on the sidewalk. Or perhaps you're at home in your apartment and see an elderly neighbor pacing the parking lot, wearing shorts and a light blouse amid sub-freezing temperatures. The person periodically bends down to dig in the dirt. You venture outside to ask the reason for their actions, and the person says, "I know there's money buried here and I need it to pay my bills." Either individual may be subject to involuntary civil commitment, if they're found to pose a threat or are unable to provide for their basic needs due to mental illness.

MANDATORY OUTPATIENT TREATMENT (COURT-MANDATED TREATMENT)

Due to a court sentence or probation, patients may be legally mandated to undergo treatment for a mental health disorder or addiction. The requirement may specify the duration, frequency, and/or type of treatment (e.g., addiction counseling, anger management). There may be defined documentation or monitoring requirements. As state and local processes vary, case managers are reminded to check with their local jurisdictions for all related requirements.

Figure 2.1: *Continuum of court-mandated mental health treatment*

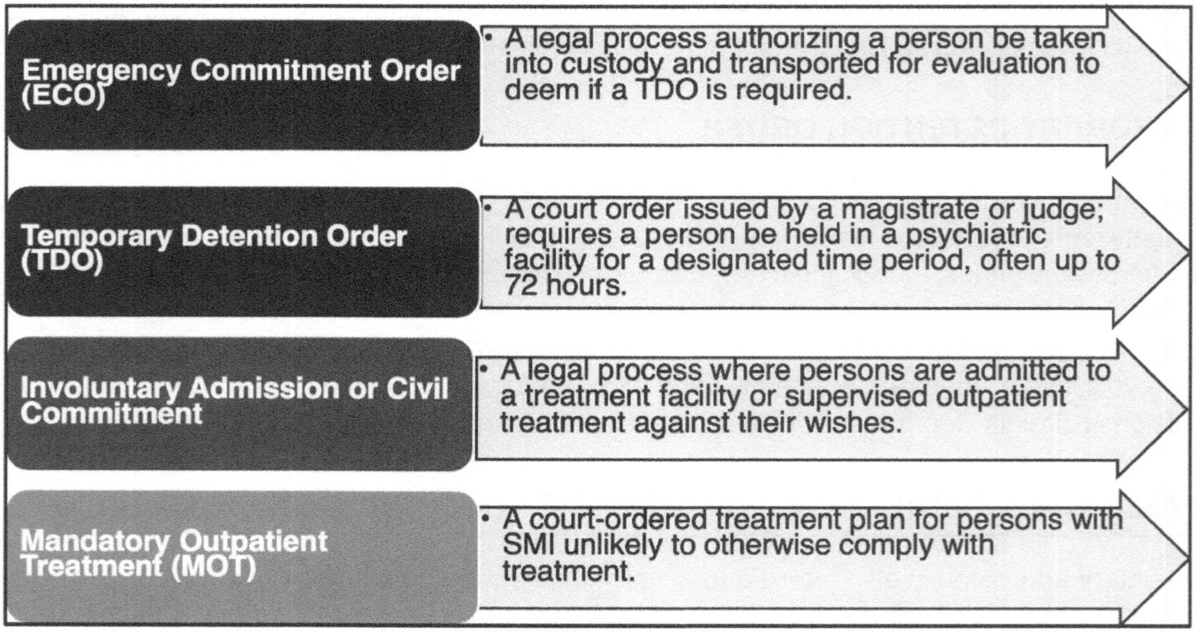

CONSIDERATIONS FOR CASE MANAGERS

Case managers must comply with other important regulations. Exposure to these laws will vary based on practice setting, population, and state or jurisdiction. The Established Resources of Guidance for Case Managers (Fink-Samnick, 2023) explicitly speaks to a professional's primary responsibility to heed all applicable federal, state, and local laws and regulations governing all aspects of case management practice (CMSA, 2024). These seminal resources refer to all professional regulations governing scope of practice and codified ethical standards, organizational accreditation, case management certification, professional association standards of practice, and codes of ethics (Fink-Samnick, 2023).

MANDATORY DUTY TO WARN AND THE TARASOFF RULING

Case managers may believe, falsely, that HIPAA law prevents them from disclosing information about patients to law enforcement, family members, or others. However, just as case managers have legal duty under their scope of practice to report child and adult abuse, neglect, and/or exploitation to law enforcement or appropriate authorities, they are also mandated to disclose a patient's healthcare information when they assess the patient presents a danger to himself or others.

The *Tarasoff* ruling established this duty to warn. The case originated with a 1969 murder. A University of California, Berkeley student was infatuated with a woman, Tatianna Tarasoff, who had rejected his advances. He told his therapist he planned to kill Ms. Tarasoff, and several months later, he carried out his plan. Ms. Tarasoff's parents sued the school and the therapist for not notifying them or Ms. Tarasoff of the danger she was in. The court addressed the issue of when a therapist's duty to uphold a patient's privacy is superseded by a duty to protect members of the public from danger. See Box 2.6 for details of the *Tarasoff* ruling.

Case managers can be confused by inconsistent mandatory duty to warn legislation across the U.S. Some states' mandatory laws require reporting all potential danger. Other states' laws are "permissive," meaning a case manager (or their discipline of origin, such as nurse or social worker) is not *required* by law to report, but is permitted to do so. Other states' mandatory duty to warn laws apply only to some professional disciplines (e.g., mental health practitioners, psychiatrists). Furthermore, practitioners vary in their comfort to exercise professional judgement and contact law enforcement. The answers to the following questions are rarely clear: Was the patient communicating an explicit threat of self-harm, and with a clear plan? Does the person have access to a weapon to accomplish the threat? Did the person express a desire to inflict physical harm or death to a clearly identifiable individual or group of people at a defined location? Is the person able to carry out the threat? Case managers should review the laws in their state or jurisdiction and consult with risk management or other appropriate personnel to define their best course of action. The National Conference of State Legislatures website provides an interactive map and listing of all current mandatory duty to warn laws. A link for the website is found in the chapter resource list.

Box 2.6: Tarasoff v. Regents of the University of California (1976)

Facts and events

- A University of California (UC) Berkeley graduate student, Prosenjit Poddar, became infatuated with another student, Tatianna Tarasoff. She rebuked his advances.
- June 5, 1969: Mr. Poddar sought and received emergency psychological treatment from Dr. Lawrence Moore, a psychologist employed by the Cowell Memorial Hospital at UC Berkeley.
- August 20, 1969: During the seventh therapy session with Dr. Moore, Mr. Poddar confessed his plan to kill Ms. Tarasoff. Dr. Moore diagnosed Poddar as having an acute and severe "paranoid schizophrenic reaction." He and two other doctors determined that Poddar should be committed to a psychiatric hospital for observation, and they contacted the police.
- The police detained Poddar, then released him after he promised to stay away from Tarasoff. Following Poddar's release, Dr. Moore's superior:
  - instructed police to return the letter from Dr. Moore requesting they detain Poddar,
  - ordered the letter and all notes taken on Poddar be destroyed, and
  - instructed Dr. Moore to take no further action in detaining Poddar.
- Dr. Moore and his colleagues did not notify Ms. Tarasoff or her family about the threatening statements. Mr. Poddar did not return to therapy.
- October 27, 1969: Mr. Poddar sought out Ms. Tarasoff while she was alone in her home. He shot her with a pellet gun, chased her into the street, and stabbed her seventeen times with a kitchen knife, causing her death.

COURT FINDINGS AND RULING IMPACT

The Supreme Court of California ruled that mental health professionals have a duty to protect individuals who are threatened with bodily harm by one of their patients. The 1974 decision mandated *warning* the threatened individual, but a 1976 rehearing of the case by the California Supreme Court called for a "duty to protect" the intended victim.

A case manager may execute the duty in several ways, including notifying police, warning the intended victim, and/or other reasonable steps to protect the threatened individual.

Gorshkalova & Munakomi, 2023

MEDICARE CONDITIONS OF PARTICIPATION FOR BEHAVIORAL HEALTH

Case managers might be familiar with *Medicare Conditions of Participation,* or *CoPs.* They are a set of health and safety standards with which all healthcare organizations must comply to participate in Medicare. The CoPs for behavioral health primarily focus on Community Mental Health Centers (CCMCs). CMHCs must meet specific standards to ensure quality and safety of care. The standards encompass staffing qualifications, thorough client assessments upon admission, comprehensive treatment plans, coordinated service delivery, client rights protection, and quality improvement measures. These collective actions assure appropriate care and smooth discharge or transfer processes for patients. Key points about Medicare CoPs for behavioral health are in Box 2.7.

Box 2.7: Medicare Conditions of Participation for behavioral health: Community Mental Health Centers

Department of Health and Human Services Centers for Medicare & Medicaid Services

42 CFR Part 485

[CMS-3202-F]

RIN 0938-AP51

10/29/2013

- Personnel qualifications: All staff providing services must be appropriately licensed and qualified according to state regulations.
- Client rights: Providers must respect and protect client rights, informing them of their options and ensuring their participation in treatment decisions.
- Admission and assessment: A thorough initial evaluation and comprehensive assessment are mandatory upon admission to identify individual needs and create a personalized treatment plan.
- Treatment plan: A person-centered active treatment plan must be developed, including goals, interventions, and coordination with other healthcare providers.
- Discharge planning: A detailed discharge plan outlining post-treatment needs and referrals must be created for each client.

Quality improvement: Providers must have systems in place to monitor and improve the quality of care delivered to clients, including data collection and analysis. Federal Register, 2013

THE 21ST CENTURY CURES ACT AND THE OPEN NOTES RULE

Even as patient privacy and confidentiality remain a concern for healthcare professionals and organizations, transparency of healthcare documentation has also become a priority. The 21st Century Cures Act and its second phase, the Open Notes Rule, have expanded access to electronic health information and reduced information blocking (Sharko et al., 2022).

The Department of Health and Human Services (HHS) Office for Civil Rights diligently regulates privacy, new technology, and consumer protections. The adoption of transparency guidelines by organizations has been a welcome, though sluggish, process. The first phase of the 21st Century Cures Act was passed by Congress in 2016 with the goal of ensuring greater accountability for the safety, quality, and accessibility of client documentation. This phase addressed funding and programming enhancements. Emphasis was on interoperability of electronic health records and greater financial support for all health and human service programs and agencies, including smaller community agencies and safety-net programs.

The second phase of the 21st Century Cures Act—known as the Open Notes Rule—was operationalized in October 2022. With healthcare information more readily shared among providers via web portals and software applications, there was need for greater emphasis on how that information could be shared with patients than was reflected in prior regulations, such as the Health Insurance Portability and Accountability Act (HIPAA). The Open Notes Rules directed that patient documentation should be written in a way that is understandable, addresses a patient's needs and requests, and accounts for health literacy, language proficiency, and patient accommodations. Language should be inclusive and respectful of cultural realities. In addition, the documentation should reflect how patients and their families are engaged in treatment processes and how their care aligns with patient preferences.

The requirements for transparency remind case managers to be mindful of documentation (Coyle, 2022). Open Notes provides an exclusion for psychotherapy notes if the documentation meets the criteria defined by HIPAA. Details of the 21st Century Cures Act appear in Box 2.8. More information is available through the Federal Register with links in the chapter resources list.

Box 2.8: The 21st Century Cures Act: Summary and key points

Department of Health and Human Services

Office of the Secretary

45 CFR Parts 170 and 171

RIN 0955-AA01

Signed into effect in December 2016, the Act:

- Promotes and funds the acceleration of research into preventing and curing serious illnesses
- Accelerates drug and medical device development
- Attempts to address the opioid abuse crisis
- Improves mental health services delivery
- Includes provisions that foster interoperability, adoption of electronic health records (EHRs), and support for human services programs

Specialized programming:

- Funds precision medicine initiatives
- Improves healthcare information technology, most notably in relation to nationwide interoperability and information blocking
- Improves quality of care for patients through interoperability
- Emphasizes patient access to personal electronic health information that is easy to understand, secure, and updated automatically

The Open Notes Rule, effective October 2022, details that:

- Patients must have immediate, direct, and free access to their records, including:
  - Consultation notes
  - Discharge summary notes (may also include closing summary)
  - History and physical (including the psychosocial assessment and plan of care)
  - Procedure notes (description of interventions used)
  - Progress notes (summary of each interview, goals, and progress)
  - Imaging, lab, and pathology reports
- Records specific to behavioral health settings:

- Counseling session start/stop times
- Modalities and frequencies of treatment furnished
- Results of clinical tests
- Summary of diagnosis, functional status, treatment plan, symptoms, prognosis, and progress to date

Note: Psychotherapy notes may be excluded from the Open Notes Rule under the HIPAA definition:

"Psychotherapy notes are recorded (in any medium) by a health care provider who is a mental health professional documenting or analyzing the contents of conversation during a private counseling session or a group, joint, or family counseling session and that are separated from the rest of the individual's medical record."

To be excluded, psychotherapy notes must be stored separately in a designated "psychotherapy notes" section of an electronic health record, or physically apart from the rest of a medical/clinical record.

Federal Register, 2020

42 CFR PART 2

The 42 CFR Part 2 regulations protect patient records generated in federally-assisted programs for substance use disorder treatment. Confidentiality is of vital importance for persons receiving substance use disorder treatment, and it is legally protected through HIPAA. Part 2 means individuals can share information about their drug use history without worrying it will be used against them by employers, landlords, law enforcement, or social workers. The law was revised in 2024 to enhance care coordination related to the opioid epidemic, while maintaining protections against unauthorized disclosure by Part 2 Federal Programs, as shown in Box 2.9. The final rule includes modifications to Part 2, which were proposed in the Notice of Proposed Rule Making, as shown in Box 2.10.

Box 2.9: Part 2 Programs Under 42 CFR Part 2

A program is considered federally assisted if it is:

(1) Conducted in whole or in part, whether directly or by contract or otherwise, by any department or agency of the United States

(2) Being carried out under a license, certification, registration, or other authorization granted by any department or agency of the United States including but not limited to:

(i) Participating provider in the Medicare program;
(ii) Authorization to conduct maintenance treatment or withdrawal management;
(iii) Registration to dispense a substance under the Controlled Substances Act to the extent the controlled substance is used in the treatment of substance use disorders.

(3) Supported by funds provided by any department or agency of the United States by being:

(i) A recipient of federal financial assistance in any form, including financial assistance which does not directly pay for the substance use disorder diagnosis, treatment, or referral for treatment;

(ii) Conducted by a state or local government unit which, through general or special revenue sharing or other forms of assistance, receives federal funds which could be (but are not necessarily) spent for the substance use disorder program

(4) Assisted by the Internal Revenue Service of the Department of the Treasury through the allowance of income tax deductions for contributions to the program or through the granting of tax-exempt status to the program.

Federal Register, 2024

Box 2.10: Modifications to 42 CFR Part 2 (February 8, 2024)

Patient consent

- Allows a single consent for all future uses and disclosures for treatment, payment, and health care operations.
- Allows HIPAA covered entities and business associates that receive records under this consent to redisclose the records in accordance with HIPAA regulations.

Other uses and disclosures

- Permits disclosure of records without patient consent to public health authorities, provided that the records disclosed are de-identified per the standards established in the HIPAA Privacy Rule.
- Restricts the use of records and testimony in civil, criminal, administrative, and legislative proceedings against patients, absent patient consent or a court order.

Penalties: Aligns Part 2 penalties with HIPAA by replacing criminal penalties currently in Part 2 with civil and criminal enforcement authorities that also apply to any HIPAA violations.

Breach notification: Applies the same requirements of the HIPAA Breach Notification Rule to breaches of records under Part 2.

Patient notice: Aligns Part 2 Patient Notice requirements with the requirements of the HIPAA Notice of Privacy Practices.

Safe harbor: Creates a limit on civil or criminal liability for investigative agencies that act with reasonable diligence to determine if a provider is subject to Part 2 before making a demand for records in the course of an investigation. Safe harbor requires investigative agencies take certain steps should they discover that Part 2 records were received without having first obtained the requisite court order.

U.S. Department of Health and Human Services, 2024

CONCLUSION

This concludes our travels down the road of behavioral health regulations and requirements for case managers. This road is ongoing, with continuous updates and new legislation. You've gained a foundation to continue life-long learning.

Next on the docket is Chapter 3 and material on core quality measures, value-based care models, and reimbursement for behavioral health.

CONTEMPLATION QUESTIONS

1. Review the levels of behavioral healthcare for youth and adults presented in Tables 2.1 and 2.2. Which levels of care are you familiar with?
    a) Discuss your experiences with any of the care levels identified, and whether the patient outcomes were successful.
2. Review the content on clinical and legal capacity.
    a) Reflect on situations you have been involved in or case managed where a patient's clinical or legal capacity was questioned by the care team.
    b) What was the outcome of the situation?

Read the case scenario, then answer questions 3-5.

A patient is brought to the ED by a friend after she makes comments about "getting back at everyone," and "running those mindless colleagues over with a car." The patient knows the weekly schedule of specific work colleagues, including when they arrive and leave the workplace. After finishing the assessment, the patient turns to you, smiles, and says: "Oh, I may be pissed off about the way these idiots treated me but wouldn't do anything to harm anyone."

1. Which law(s) in Chapter 2 apply to this situation and a case manager's mandatory duty to report?
2. On a scale of 1-10, with 1 being the least comfortable and 10 being the most, define your comfort level in reporting this situation to local authorities.
    a) Reflect on your concerns about reporting (or not) and why you feel this way.
3. Go to the website for the National Conference of State Legislatures in the resource list and review the map for State Duty to Protect/Warn Laws. Identify the Mandatory Duty to Warn legislation for state(s) you practice in.
    a) Is the law mandatory or permissive?
    b) What are your views on the scope of laws relevant to your practice (e.g., identified professionals, scope of practice)?
    c) Reflect on the experience of a time you invoked your Mandatory Duty to Warn.

RESOURCES

- Federal Register
- 21st Century Cures Act
- 42 CFR Parts 414, 425, and 495
- 45 CFR Part 171

- **RIN 0955-AA05**
  https://www.federalregister.gov/documents/2024/07/01/2024-13793/21st-century-cures-act-establishment-of-disincentives-for-health-care-providers-that-have-committed
- **Medicare Program: Conditions of Participation (CoPs) for Community Mental Health Centers: Published Document: 2013-24056 (78 FR 64604)**
  https://www.federalregister.gov/documents/2013/10/29/2013-24056/medicare-program-conditions-of-participation-cops-for-community-mental-health-centers
- **Preadmission Screening and Annual Review of Mentally Ill and Mentally Retarded Individuals. 42 CFR Part 483; 57 FR 56506, Nov. 30, 1992**
  https://www.ecfr.gov/current/title-42/chapter-IV/subchapter-G/part-483/subpart-C
- **42 CFR Part 2, Final Rule: Confidentiality of Substance Use Disorder (SUD) Patient Records**
  https://www.federalregister.gov/documents/2024/02/16/2024-02544/confidentiality-of-substance-use-disorder-sud-patient-records
- **Legal Information Institute**
  https://www.law.cornell.edu
- **National Center for Youth Law**
  https://youthlaw.org/
- **National Conference of State Legislatures**
  https://www.ncsl.org/health/mental-health-professionals-duty-to-warn
- **National Resource Center on Psychiatric Advance Directives: State by State listing**
  https://nrc-pad.org/states/

REFERENCES

- American Academy of Child and Adolescent Psychiatry. (2023). Continuum of Mental Health Care. Retrieved November 23, 2024, from https://www.aacap.org/AACAP/Families_and_Youth/Facts_for_Families/FFF-Guide/The-Continuum-Of-Care-For-Children-And-Adolescents-042.aspx
- Arkansas Department of Human Services. (2023). Division of Youth Services. Retrieved October 29, 2025, from https://humanservices.arkansas.gov/wp-content/uploads/710-23-0006-Attachment-DD-DYS-Secure-Care-Standards.pdf
- Bucy, T., Moeller, K., Bowblis, J.R., Shippee, N., Fashaw-Walters, S., Winkelman, T., & Shippee, T. (2022). Serious mental illness in the nursing home literature: A scoping review. *Gerontology & Geriatric Medicine*, *8*, 23337214221101260. https://doi.org/10.1177/23337214221101260
- California Department of Healthcare Services. (2024, December 30). Behavioral Health Information Notice No: 24-046. Retrieved October 29, 2025, from https://www.dhcs.ca.gov/Documents/BHIN-24-046-Minor-Consent-to-Outpatient-Mental-Health-Treatment-or-Counseling.pdf
- Case Management Society of America. (2024). *Standards of Practice for Case Management*, revised.
- Colorada Behavioral Health Administration. (2025). Children, Youth, and Families. Retrieved October 29, 2025, from https://bha.colorado.gov/about/programs-we-fund/children-youth-and-families
- Colorado General Assembly. (2024). HB19-104; Advance Behavioral Health Orders Treatment. Retrieved November 16, 2024, from https://leg.colorado.gov/bills/hb19-1044
- Coyle, S. (2022). The Cures Act looks to remedy records access. *Social Work Today, 22*(1), 22. https://www.socialworktoday.com/archive/Winter22p22.shtml
- English, A. & Gudeman, R. (2024). *Minor Consent and Confidentiality: A Compendium of State and Federal Laws*. National Center for Youth Law. Retrieved October 25, 2025, from https://youthlaw.org/sites/default/files/2024-10/NCYLMinorConsentCompendium2024.pdf
- Erickson, B. (2021). Deinstitutionalization through optimism: The Community Mental Health Act of 1963. *The American Journal of Psychiatry Residents' Journal*, *16*(4), 6-7. https://doi.org/10.1176/appi.ajp-rj.2021.160404
- Federal Register. (2013). Medicare Program: Conditions of Participation (CoPs) for Community Mental Health Centers: Published Document: 2013-24056 (78 FR 64604). Retrieved November 18, 2024, from https://www.federalregister.gov/documents/2013/10/29/2013-24056/medicare-program-conditions-of-participation-cops-for-community-mental-health-centers
- Federal Register. (2020). 21st Century Cures Act: Interoperability, Information Blocking, and the ONC Health IT Certification Program: 2020-07419 (85 FR 25642). Retrieved November 18, 2024, from https://www.federalregister.gov/documents/2020/05/01/2020-07419/21st-century-cures-act-interoperability-information-blocking-and-the-onc-health-it-certification

- Federal Register. (2024). Subpart C—Preadmission Screening and Annual Review of Mentally Ill and Mentally Retarded Individuals. 42 CFR Part 483; 57 FR 56506, Nov. 30, 1992. Retrieved November 19, 2024, from https://www.ecfr.gov/current/title-42/chapter-IV/subchapter-G/part-483/subpart-C
- Fink-Samnick, E. (2023). *The Ethical Case Manager: Tools and Tactics*. Blue Bayou Press.
- George, P., Jones, N., Goldman, H., & Rosenblatt, A. (2023). Cycles of reform in the history of psychosis treatment in the United States. *SSM - Mental Health*, *3*, 100205. https://doi.org/10.1016/j.ssmmh.2023.100205
- Gerlach, L.B., & Maust, D.T. (2023). Falling off a cliff: Psychiatric care of nursing home residents. *Journal of the American Geriatrics Society*, *71*(4), 1014-1016. https://doi.org/10.1111/jgs.18249
- Gorshkalova, O. & Munakomi, S. (2023). Duty to Warn. [Updated 2023 Aug 28]. StatPearls Publishing: Treasure Island, FL. Available from: https://www.ncbi.nlm.nih.gov/books/NBK542236/
- Giffith, K. (2025). New Alabama Law Raises Age of Medical Consent from 14 to 16. Burr & Forman, reprinted with permission from Birmingham Medical News. Retrieved October 29, 2025, from https://www.burr.com/newsroom/articles/new-alabama-law-raises-age-of-medical-consent-from-14-to-16
- HealthIT.gov. (n.d.). Overview: State laws expressly granting minors the right to consent to healthcare without parental permission and addressing disclosure of related information to parents—Outpatient alcohol and substance abuse. Appendix A-8c. Retrieved November 23, 2024, from https://www.healthit.gov/sites/default/files/appa8-1.pdf
- Hijano, D.R., & Yaun, J.A. (2024). Mature minor doctrine clarification act: A setback in pediatric immunizations. *Journal of the Pediatric Infectious Diseases Society*, *13*(2), 155-158. https://doi.org/10.1093/jpids/piae006
- ICANotes. (2022). The Age of Consent for Mental Health Treatment by State. Retrieved November 18, 2024, from https://www.icanotes.com/2022/12/23/age-of-consent-mental-health-treatment/
- Illinois Legal Aid. (2024, November 19). Mental Health Treatment for Children. Retrieved October 29, 2025, from https://www.illinoislegalaid.org/legal-information/children-and-mental-health-facilities
- Joint Commission. (2020). Improving care with psychiatric advance directives. *Quick Safety*, Issue 53. Retrieved November 2020, from https://www.jointcommission.org/en-us/knowledge-library/newsletters/quick-safety/issue-53
- Justia U.S. Supreme Court. (n.d.). *Olmstead v. L. C.*, 527 U.S. 581 (1999). Retrieved November 24, 2024, from https://supreme.justia.com/cases/federal/us/527/581/
- Kerwin, M.E., Kirby, K.C., Speziali, D., Duggan, M., Mellitz, C., Versek, B., & McNamara, A. (2015). What can parents do? A review of state laws regarding decision making for adolescent drug abuse and mental health treatment. *Journal of Child & Adolescent Substance Abuse*, *24*(3), 166-176. https://doi.org/10.1080/1067828X.2013.777380

- Laws, M.B., Beeman, A., Haigh, S., Wilson, I.B., & Shield, R.R. (2022). Changes in nursing home populations challenge practice and policy. *Policy, Politics & Nursing Practice*, *23*(4), 238-248. https://doi.org/10.1177/15271544221118315
- Legal Information Institute. (2023). Minor, defined. Cornell Law School. Retrieved October 24, 2025, from https://www.law.cornell.edu/wex/minor
- Magellan Healthcare Inc. (2024). 2024-2025 Magellan Care Guidelines, Revised July 2024. Retrieved November 23, 2024, from https://www.magellanprovider.com/media/45694/mcg.pdf
- MCG. (2025). Behavioral Health Clinical Guidelines. Retrieved August 27, 2025, from https://www.mcg.com/care-guidelines/behavioral-healthcare/
- Maryland Peoples' Law. (2024). Youth Mental Health. Retrieved October 29, 2025, from https://www.peoples-law.org/youth-health-law
- Minnesota Department of Health. (n.d.). Adolescents and confidential health care. Retrieved October 29, 2025, from https://www.health.state.mn.us/people/adolescent/youth/minorconsent.pdf
- National Center for Youth Law. (2024a). Massachusetts: Minor Consent and Confidentiality. Retrieved October 29, 2025, https://youthlaw.org/sites/default/files/2024-10/NCYLMinorConsentCompendium2024-Massachusetts.pdf
- National Center for Youth Law. (2024b). Missouri: Minor Consent and Confidentiality. Retrieved October 29, 2025, from https://youthlaw.org/sites/default/files/2024-10/NCYLMinorConsentCompendium2024-Missouri.pdf
- National Center for Youth Law. (2024c). Montana: Minor Consent and Confidentiality. Retrieved October 29, 2025, from https://youthlaw.org/sites/default/files/2024-10/NCYLMinorConsentCompendium2024-Montana.pdf
- National Center for Youth Law. (2024d). Nevada: Minor Consent and Confidentiality. Retrieved October 29, 2025, from https://youthlaw.org/sites/default/files/2024-10/NCYLMinorConsentCompendium2024-Nevada.pdf
- National Center for Youth Law. (2024e). New Hampshire: Minor Consent and Confidentiality. Retrieved October 29, 2025, from https://youthlaw.org/sites/default/files/2024-10/NCYLMinorConsentCompendium2024-NewHampshire.pdf
- National Center for Youth Law. (2024f). New Jersey: Minor Consent and Confidentiality. Retrieved October 29, 2025, from https://youthlaw.org/sites/default/files/2024-10/NCYLMinorConsentCompendium2024-NewJersey.pdf
- National Center for Youth Law. (2024g). New Mexico: Minor Consent and Confidentiality. Retrieved October 29, 2025, from https://youthlaw.org/sites/default/files/2024-10/NCYLMinorConsentCompendium2024-NewMexico.pdf
- National Center for Youth Law. (2024h). New York: Minor Consent and Confidentiality. Retrieved October 29, 2025, from https://youthlaw.org/sites/default/files/2024-10/NCYLMinorConsentCompendium2024-NewYork.pdf

- National Center for Youth Law. (2024i). North Carolina: Minor Consent and Confidentiality. Retrieved October 29, 2025, from https://youthlaw.org/sites/default/files/2024-10/NCYLMinorConsentCompendium2024-NorthCarolina.pdf
- National Center for Youth Law. (2024j). North Dakota: Minor Consent and Confidentiality. Retrieved October 29, 2025, from https://youthlaw.org/sites/default/files/2024-10/NCYLMinorConsentCompendium2024-NorthDakota.pdf
- National Center for Youth Law. (2024k). South Carolina: Minor Consent and Confidentiality. Retrieved October 29, 2025, from https://youthlaw.org/sites/default/files/2024-10/NCYLMinorConsentCompendium2024-SouthCarolina.pdf
- National Center for Youth Law. (2024l). South Dakota: Minor Consent and Confidentiality. Retrieved October 29, 2025, from https://youthlaw.org/sites/default/files/2024-10/NCYLMinorConsentCompendium2024-SouthDakota.pdf
- National Center for Youth Law. (2024m). Tennessee: Minor Consent and Confidentiality. Retrieved October 29, 2025, from https://youthlaw.org/sites/default/files/2024-10/NCYLMinorConsentCompendium2024-Tennessee.pdf
- National Center for Youth Law. (2024n). Texas: Minor Consent and Confidentiality. Retrieved October 29, 2025, from https://youthlaw.org/sites/default/files/2024-10/NCYLMinorConsentCompendium2024-Texas.pdf
- National Center for Youth Law. (2024o). Vermont: Minor Consent and Confidentiality. Retrieved October 29, 2025, from https://youthlaw.org/sites/default/files/2024-10/NCYLMinorConsentCompendium2024-Vermont.pdf
- National Center for Youth Law. (2024p). Wyoming: Minor Consent and Confidentiality. Retrieved October 29, 2025, from https://youthlaw.org/sites/default/files/2024-10/NCYLMinorConsentCompendium2024-Wyoming.pdf
- National Council of State Legislatures. (2022). Mental Health Professionals' Duty to Warn. Retrieved November 18, 2024, from https://www.ncsl.org/health/mental-health-professionals-duty-to-warn
- National Resource Center on Psychiatric Advance Directives. (2024). Psychiatric Advance Directives: Getting Started. Retrieved October 9, 2025, from https://nrc-pad.org/getting-started/
- Noroozi, M., Singh, I., & Fazel, M. (2018). Evaluation of the minimum age for consent to mental health treatment with the minimum age of criminal responsibility in children and adolescents: A global comparison. *Evidence Based Mental Health*, *21*(3), 82-86. https://doi.org/10.1136/ebmental-2018-300032
- Pope, M.T. (2023). Capacity (competence) and incapacity. *Merck Manual Professional Version.* Retrieved November 16, 2024, from https://www.merckmanuals.com/professional/special-subjects/medicolegal-issues/capacity-competence-and-incapacity
- Shah, P., Thornton, I., Turrin, D., Kopitnik, N. L., & Hipskind, J.E. (2024). Informed Consent. [Updated 2024 Oct 15]. StatPearls Publishing: Treasure Island, FL. Available from: https://www.ncbi.nlm.nih.gov/books/NBK430827/

- Sharko, M., Jameson, R., Ancker, J.S., Krams, L., Webber, E.C., & Rosenbloom, S.T. (2022). State-by-state variability in adolescent privacy laws. *Pediatrics, 149*(6): e2021053458. https://doi.org/10.1542/peds.2021-053458
- State of Connecticut Judicial Branch. (2025). Access to Information in Juvenile Court Proceedings: Legal Guide – Medical Treatment of Minors. Retrieved October 29, 2025, from https://www.jud.ct.gov/juv_infoguide/IJCP_MedicalTreatmentMinors.html
- U.S. Legal. (n.d.). The Mature Minor Doctrine. Retrieved November 18, 2024, from https://healthcare.uslegal.com/treatment-of-minors/the-mature-minor-doctrine/
- U.S. Department of Health and Human Services. (2024). Fact Sheet 42 CFR Part 2, Final Rule. Retrieved November 23, 2024, from https://www.hhs.gov/hipaa/for-professionals/regulatory-initiatives/fact-sheet-42-cfr-part-2-final-rule/index.html
- Virginia Department of Behavioral Health & Developmental Services. (2020, October 29). Medical Temporary Detention Orders: DBHDS Policies and Procedures. Retrieved November 24, 2024, from https://dbhds.virginia.gov/assets/doc/ei/medical-tdo-policy-and-procedures.pdf
- Virginia Law. (2025). Code of Virginia; Article 16. Psychiatric Treatment of Minors Act. Retrieved October 29, 2025, from https://law.lis.virginia.gov/vacodefull/title16.1/chapter11/article16/
- Washington State Department of Social and Health Service. (2025). How Can Minors Admit Themselves to Inpatient Mental Health Treatment? Retrieved October 29, 2025, from https://www.dshs.wa.gov/faq/how-can-minors-admit-themselves-inpatient-mental-health-treatment

CHAPTER 3

CORE QUALITY MEASURES, VALUE-BASED CARE MODELS, AND REIMBURSEMENT

INTRODUCTION

In the past 30 years we have witnessed a revolution in quality core measures, value-based care models, and incentives for reimbursement. Most of these changes occurred after 1990, roughly 20 years after Joint Commission established its Behavioral Health Care Accreditation Program. It would be easy to just list here the many quality endeavors, but for case managers to serve as true stewards of quality, they must *understand* them. Quality is at the heart of healthcare and case management, and successful outcomes owing to strong quality management processes reinforce case management's importance.

A disclaimer: Chapter 3 is not meant to provide step-by-step instructions for implementing quality improvement. The chapter resources list provides links to many existing resources to adhere to compliance requirements. Instead, Chapter 3 provides a 30,000-foot view of quality definitions, measures, and value-based programs, from a historical perspective. Case managers will learn how core measures drive and sustain quality management in behavioral health.

BEHAVIORAL LEARNING OBJECTIVES

1. Define terms related to quality, quality improvement, and quality management
2. Distinguish between total quality management (TQM) and continuous quality improvement (CQI)
3. Explain the historical timeline for behavioral health quality
4. Recognize core measures for behavioral health
5. Describe the role of the Mental Health Parity and Addiction Equity Act (MHPAEA) in advancing quality
6. Distinguish among the entities with quality oversight for the industry

7. Explain the goals of the Hospital Consumer Assessment of Healthcare Provider and Systems (HCAHPS) Survey
8. Describe the impact of Meaningful Use for behavioral health providers
9. Explain how the Affordable Care Act (ACA) advanced quality measures
10. Identify Value-based Payment Models for behavioral health
11. Explain the role of CMS's Innovation Center (CMMI)
12. Recognize the value of Patient-Reported Outcomes Measures (PROMs)
13. Identify behavioral health quality requirements for Medicare Advantage
14. Explain the focus of Joint Commission's National Patient Safety Goals for Behavioral Health

ESSENTIAL TERMS

- Alternative Payment Models (APM)
- Benchmarking
- Certified community behavioral health clinics (CCBHC)
- Community Health Centers (CHC)
- Consumer Assessment of Healthcare Providers and Systems (CAHPS)
- Continuous quality improvement (CQI)
- Core measures
- Critical access
- Federally Qualified Health Centers (FQHC)
- Healthcare Effectiveness Data and Information Set (HEDIS)
- Hospital Consumer Assessment of Healthcare Providers and Systems (HCAHPS)
- Lean Six Sigma
- Medicare Access and CHIP Reauthorization Act of 2015 (MACRA)
- Meaningful Use
- Mental Health Parity Act
- Mental Health Parity
- Mental Health Parity and Addiction Equity Act (MHPAEA)
- Merit-based Incentive Payment System (MIPS)
- National Patient Safety Goals for behavioral health
- National Quality Forum (NQF)
- Patient-Reported Outcomes Measures (PROMs)
- Quality
- Quality management
- Quality Payment Program (QPP)
- Safety net
- Total quality management (TQM)
- Value-based care (VBC)

QUALITY, QUALITY IMPROVEMENT, AND QUALITY MANAGEMENT

Every product is measured against a certain level of excellence, or *quality*. For example, coffee aficionados savor distinct beans and roasts. Croissant lovers long for a light, flaky, buttery pastry sheltered under a crispy external layer. Though consumers vary in likes and dislikes for a product, their expectation are based on a minimum standard defined by evidence.

The quality concept is similarly applied to healthcare: It is the degree to which healthcare services increase the likelihood of desired health outcomes and are consistent with current professional knowledge (Institute of Medicine, 1990). This seminal definition was written in 1990, at the start of the quality era. Pursuing quality is challenging because it's not a static concept; it depends on contextual influences over time, such as industry advancements, changes in funding streams, and consumer demands.

Six elements at the center of healthcare quality discussions appear in Table 3.1. These seminal domains are often referred to by the acronym STEEEP. They were first presented in *Crossing the Quality Chasm* (Institute of Medicine, 2001). This bold text was written as the 21st century began. Imagine the promises and pitfalls of the sudden emergence of electronic health records, online order entry, and expedited diagnostics. These products enhanced access to care and treatment options for patients but also sped up the rate at which care was rendered. Medical errors and other safety issues rose drastically. The workforce could not keep up with the ripple-effect of innovation on products, treatments, and models of care. Medical errors, risk management missteps, workforce burnout, and other staffing challenges became chronic occurrences.

A call to arms echoed across the industry. The hope was that addressing these six domains would bridge the growing quality gap—or rather, chasm—between the existing state of poor-quality of care and a future state defined by improved health outcomes, fewer medical errors, and a patient-centered approach to care delivery and treatment.

Table 3.1: *Six domains of healthcare quality (STEEEP)*

Quality healthcare is...	Definition	Explanation
Safe	Care that protects patients from harm and medical errors	Safe care reduces medical errors, adverse events, and unnecessary risks of harm to patients.
Timely	Care that reduces waits and delays for both patients and caregivers	Timely order entry, lab draws, and other diagnostic tests enhance patient satisfaction and reduce risk of infection or other patient harms.
Effective	Care based on scientific knowledge and evidence-based practices that provides results	Effective care reduces the likelihood of unnecessary healthcare utilization, readmission, and costs.
Efficient	Care that avoids waste of resources, such as equipment, supplies, and energies	Efficient systems use resources effectively, reducing waste and controlling costs, while maintaining excellent patient care.
Equitable	Care that is consistent in quality and does not vary based on personal characteristics like gender, ethnicity, or socioeconomic status	Equitable care is accessible to all individuals; everyone receives the same high standard of care, regardless of socioeconomic, cultural, or demographic factors.
Patient-centered	Care that is responsive to a patient's needs, values, and preferences	Patient-centric care is associated with higher levels of patient satisfaction and builds greater patient trust and increased treatment adherence.

Adapted from Institute of Medicine (US) Committee on Quality of Health Care in America, 2001

QUALITY IMPROVEMENT

Orgrinc et al. (2022) identify *quality improvement* as a shared and intentional responsibility marked by ongoing and consistent efforts by employees. There is clear accountability by departments or designated individuals. Even though commitment to enhancing the quality of clinical, fiscal, and administrative operations is vital to long-term success, quality improvement initiatives easily fall by the wayside, replaced by more pressing obligations. Thus, the main goal of quality improvement is to create sustainable changes that drive three critical areas: better patient outcomes, better system performance, and better professional development. See Figure 3.1.

Figure 3.1: *Goals of quality improvement*

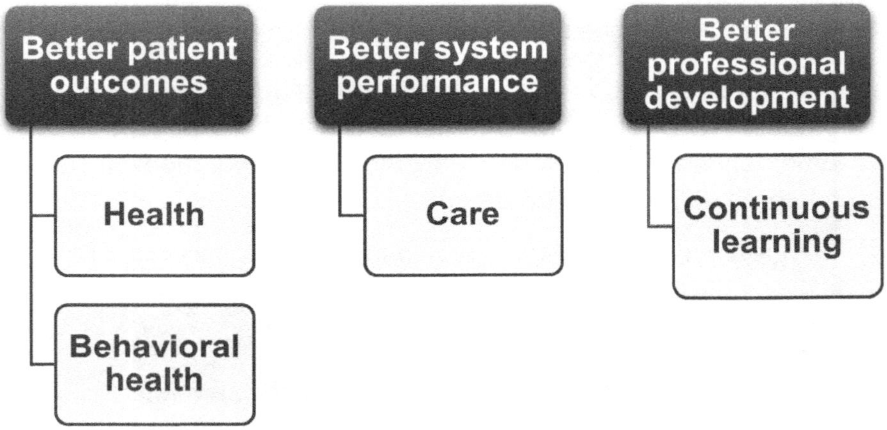

QUALITY MANAGEMENT

In contrast, *quality management* refers to a system for implementing a quality agenda. Two approaches are often married to attain this goal: *total quality management* (TQM) and *continuous quality improvement* (CQI).

TQM is a management philosophy to guide a concerted effort to improve care outcomes; it encompasses all employees, structures, and procedures in an organization. Under TQM, customer satisfaction is prioritized, and there is collective commitment to solve problems or delays in the care process. Planning and development actions are scrutinized for how they will affect care outcomes. A strong TQM focus relies on methodical analysis by employees, metrics- and data-driven decision-making (aka *benchmarking),* and compliance with regulatory standards.

Case managers might be familiar with the TQM focus on measuring and reducing healthcare utilization. This effort includes monitoring unnecessary costs of care, such as ED mental health evaluations or extra unnecessary inpatient days awaiting a PASRR. Eight principles of TQM are shown in Figure 3.2.

TQM is sustained by CQI, which encompasses tools to proactively identify and analyze strengths and barriers to quality care. The goal for CQI is to avoid reactive responses by continually testing ways to improve outcomes. Examples of CQI models include Lean Six Sigma, Plan-Do-Study-Act (PDSA), and Kaizen, among others.

Figure 3.2: *Principles of TQM*

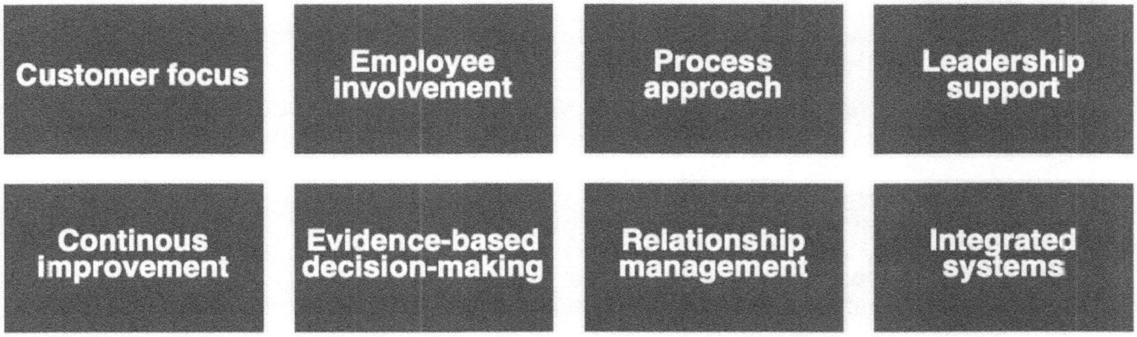

Aichouni et al., 2023

THE BEHAVIORAL HEALTH QUALITY TIMELINE

The timeline of behavioral health quality measures spans over 30 years. Critical milestones appear in Figure 3.3. The pathway has been grounded in new legislation, development of industry standards, and establishment of organizations to oversee TQM and CQI. Each action has contributed to improving treatment of mental health and substance use disorders.

Figure 3.3: *Behavioral health quality timeline*

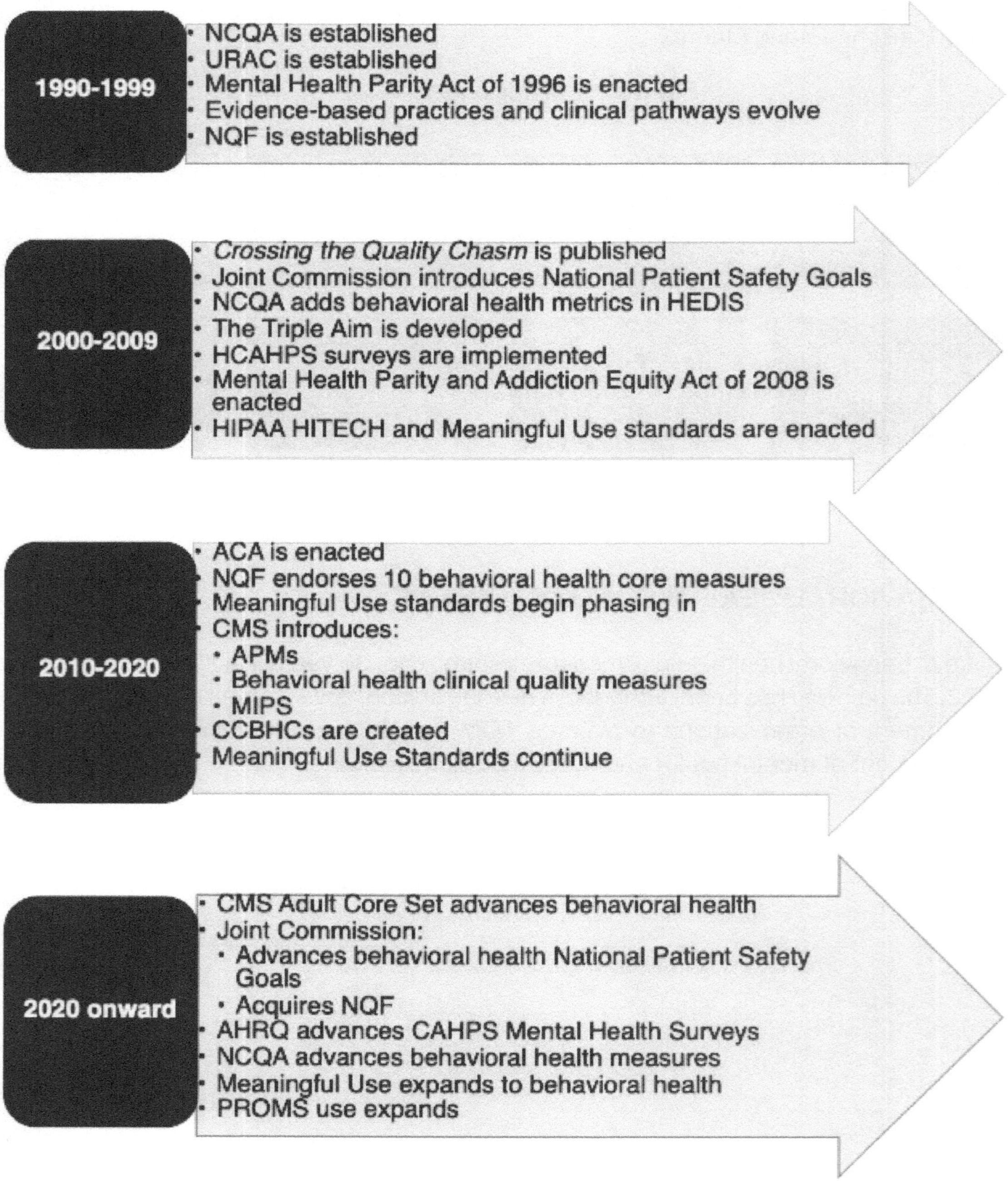

THE 1990S: INCREASING OVERSIGHT AND A FIRST ATTEMPT AT PARITY

At the start of the quality revolution, concern for quality of care was not limited to inpatient settings. The revolution was underway in managed care and commercial health plans, too. Increasing occurrence of complex, costly chronic illnesses required new oversight of disease-specific care and treatment. Targeted quality programs had met success during prior decades, such as when nurses and social workers worked as catastrophic case managers and collaborated with their hospital-based inpatient counterparts on utilization review, discharge planning, and social work. Over time, this collaboration between multiple departments became more consolidated, and a single case manager in each unit often covered the functions that had been managed by several roles and individuals (Treiger & Fink-Samnick, 2016).

Team case management models were quickly advancing within hospitals and other settings. They were often staffed by nurses, social workers, or other professionals. These facility-based case managers spoke the same language as their counterparts at health plans and the growing number employed for workers' compensation and other case management companies. Their shared understanding of the scope of a case manager's role allowed them to partner on all aspects of care coordination, from assessment and approval of clinical treatment, to defining care plans, and authorization of timeframes for that care.

The Utilization Review Accreditation Commission

Simultaneously, the lack of care standards was causing headaches for those tasked with oversight¾and often that was case managers. By the 1990s the issue demanded attention, and the *Utilization Review Accreditation Commission* (URAC) was formed in 1990 in direct response. The primary function of URAC was to assure consistent care delivery across the industry though establishment of national standards. National standards would also allow healthcare organizations¾health plans, hospitals, pharmacies, case management, utilization management, and disease management, for example¾to demonstrate their commitment to quality care by opening themselves to external reviews. Over time URAC has developed a range of accreditation programs and standards, which can be viewed on their website. Box 3.1 displays URAC's accreditation programs specific to mental health.

Box 3.1: URAC accreditation programs for mental health

Mental Health at Work Accreditation

- Recognizes organizations that prioritize mental health at work
- Promotes growth in mental health awareness and strategies within the employer space

Mental Health Parity Accreditation (Mental Health and Substance Use Disorder & Parity Program)

- URAC's mental health/substance use disorder parity accreditation standards track to the federal MHPAEA Final Rules and align with state mental health parity laws
- The accreditation:

  - Promotes national consistency
  - Supplies a proactive roadmap for health plans, issuers, and third-party administrators
  - Recognizes organizational parity excellence
  - Promotes risk mitigation
  - Establishes dynamic thresholds

Utilization Review Accreditation Commission, 2024

The National Committee for Quality Assurance

The *National Committee for Quality Assurance* (NCQA) was also formed in 1990. Like URAC, NCQA is a nonprofit tasked with accrediting healthcare organizations, but the organizations' scope and focus differ. In fact, as a pair they create a comprehensive quality landscape. URAC has traditionally addressed consumer protection and quality improvement, while NCQA concentrates on care coordination and population health. NCQA also assesses health organization performance using report cards and star ratings. These products communicate assessment outcomes to consumers and the industry.

By 2001 NCQA crafted a set of rigorous standardized measures to evaluate health plans, providers, and other healthcare entities, called HEDIS, the *Health Effectiveness Data and Information Set.* HEDIS computes the quality of care across 90 measures covering six domains of care. The six domains appear in Box 3.2.

Over 90 percent of health plans in the U.S. use HEDIS data. Data is collected via a questionnaire submitted by healthcare organizations. Submission formats are defined for each type of health plan (e.g., commercial, Medicare, Medicaid) and data provider group. To maintain integrity and transparency, schedules for data submission, analysis, and release of ratings are displayed on the HEDIS website, which also appears in the chapter resources list.

NCQA's foray into mental health has been recent. It started working on behavioral health measures in 2018 and began offering accreditation to behavioral health organizations in January 2024. Behavioral health measures will be fully implemented in HEDIS by the start of 2026.

Box 3.2: HEDIS domains

1. Effectiveness of care
2. Access/availability of care
3. Experience of care
4. Utilization and risk-adjusted utilization
5. Health plan descriptive information
6. Measures reported using electronic clinical data systems

The Mental Health Parity Act of 1996

For years practitioners viewed utilization management as a rigid preauthorization hoop they had to jump through before they could evaluate and treat behavioral health, both inpatient and outpatient. Appealing the decisions was frustrating and time-consuming for practitioners. *The Mental Health Parity Act of 1996* was passed to mitigate these preauthorization and appeal challenges. It laid the groundwork for quality measurement by established parity standards for mental health and medical benefits—that is, large group health plans with at least 50 employees were required under the law to apply the same annual and lifetime dollar limits to mental health benefits as to medical and surgical benefits. The law also prohibited group health plans from applying a mental health limit if they didn't apply a medical or surgical limit (Barry et al., 2010).

However, the law was doomed from the start. The law's authority was diminished by being passed as an attachment to yet another appropriations bill; we could say it was "lost in the sauce." As a result, health plans dodged the law when they could, and mental health benefits overall were *tightened* after the law was passed. Submitting clinical justification and getting approval for acute inpatient psychiatry, substance abuse treatment, or outpatient mental health treatment became excessively difficult.

THE 21ST CENTURY AND A NEW ERA OF QUALITY

The 21st Century started on a firm foundation for quality. *Crossing the Quality Chasm* by the Institute of Medicine's Committee on Quality of Health Care in America (2001) was among the most popular reads for healthcare leaders and case managers. New case managers learned evidence-based protocols for intervention. Defined clinical pathways and care templates were embedded into mental health treatment programs. Implementation of standardized, data-driven approaches led to better evaluations of intervention efficacy. Emphasis was on increasing quality measures for the burgeoning behavioral health market.

Joint Commission's National Patient Safety Goals

Joint Commission released its first set of *National Patient Safety Goals* (NPSGs) in 2003 to help accredited organizations address specific patient safety concerns. Goals and standards were developed for the continuum of care: laboratory services; ambulatory, acute, and post-acute settings; homecare; critical access; and rural health. These items were selected based on input from practitioners, healthcare organizations, health plans, and healthcare consumers. NPSGs for Behavioral Health and Human Services were included early on and are updated annually. The 2025 goals, standards, and elements of performance are viewable on the Joint Commission website, linked in the chapter resources list.

The National Quality Forum

The *National Quality Forum* (NQF) was created in 1999 by a coalition of public- and private-sector leaders after the President's Advisory Commission on Consumer Protection and Quality in the Healthcare Industry concluded that the United States needed an organization to ensure patient protections and promote healthcare quality. The NQF would do so by publicly reporting healthcare metrics, similar to NCQA and URAC. The NQF and CMS together recommend measures for federal programs and set the national framework (National Quality Forum, n.d.).

NQF originally endorsed 45 behavioral health quality measures spanning hospital psychiatric services, mental illness, and substance abuse treatment. By 2012 it focused the list to 10 behavioral health *core measures,* with oversight by established entities. Table 3.2 displays the behavioral health core measures and the entities assigned stewardship.

National Quality Forum (2023) continues to enhance the measures, addressing care delivery for:

- Alcohol and drug use
- Care coordination
- Depression
- Medication use
- Experience of care
- Tobacco use
- Physical health

NQF was acquired by Joint Commission in 2023. Together the organizations emphasize quality practices for high-performing healthcare organizations. At the core of their work is development of evidence-based performance metrics, implementation of dedicated standards, and monitoring and evaluating results.

Table 3.2: *The NQF's initial 10 behavioral health core measures*

Behavioral health core measure	Steward	Years in Place
Follow-up care for children prescribed attention-deficit/hyperactivity disorder (ADHD) medications	NCQA	2010-2025
Screening for depression and follow-up plan: ages 12-17	CMS	2018-2025
Follow-up post hospitalization for mental illness	NCQA	2010-2025
Child and adolescent major depressive disorder/suicide risk assessment	PCPI*	2015-2017
Metabolic monitoring for children and adolescents on antipsychotics	NCQA	2019-2025
Use of first-line psychosocial care for children and adolescents on antipsychotics	NCQA	2017-2025
Follow-up post-ED-visit for substance use: ages 13-17	NCQA	2022-2025
Follow-up post-ED-visit for mental illness: ages 6-17	NCQA	2022-2025
Use of multiple concurrent anti-psychotics in children and adolescents	NCQA	2016-2019
Post-partum depression screening and follow-up: under age 21	NCQA	Pending 2025

**Physician Consortium for Process Improvement Information adapted from Medicaid.gov, 2024*

The Triple Aim

In 2007, the Institute for Healthcare Improvement (IHI) published population health's quality north star, known as the *Triple Aim*: rendering the right patient-centered care at the right time and for the right cost. Through the Triple Aim, IHI sought to enhance the patient care experience while reducing per capita costs of care and optimizing overall health system performance (Whittington et al., 2015). The Triple Aim became part of the national strategy for addressing healthcare quality.

The Triple Aim has subsequently been updated, as displayed in Figure 3.4. The Quadruple Aim addressed workforce wellness and retention, and the Quintuple Aim is dedicated to health equity (Itchhaporia, 2021), as discussed in Chapter 1.

Figure 3.4: *The Quintuple Aim*

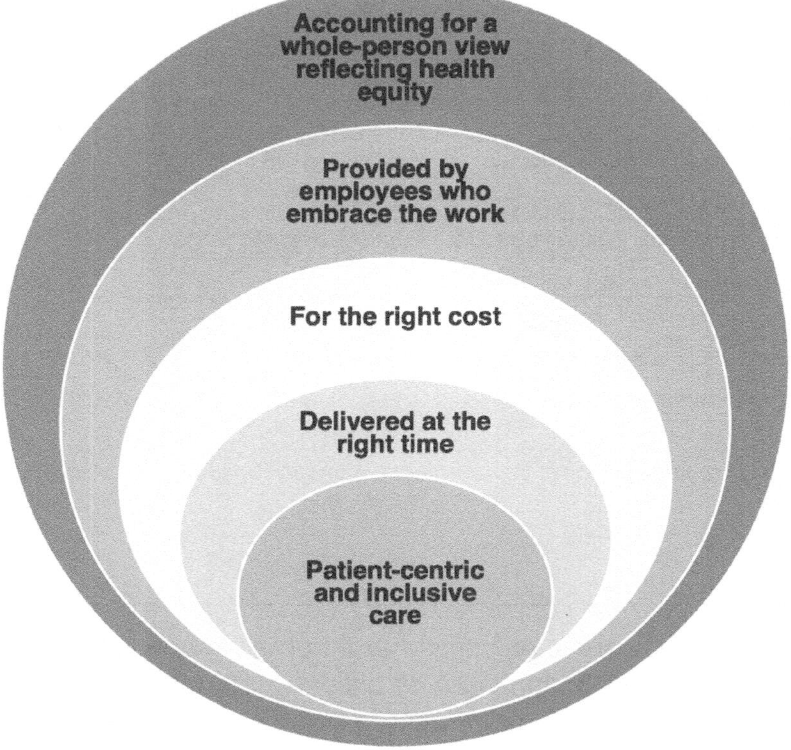

AHRQ's Consumer Assessment of Healthcare Providers and Systems (CAHPS) Survey

In 2005, the NQF endorsed the *Hospital Consumer Assessment of Healthcare Providers and Systems* (HCAHPS), as did other entities. This hospital-focused survey ultimately became part of the broader *Consumer Assessment of Healthcare Providers and System* (CAHPS). The survey focused on three critical goals: objective data comparison, incentives for quality enhancement, and accountability for transparency. The goals are described in Figure 3.5.

The first survey was completed in 2006, with the data publicly reported in March 2008. Since 2007 all facilities have been required to complete the HCAHPS survey to receive their full annual CMS payments, as directed by the Inpatient Prospective Payment System (IPPS).

In 2024 CAHPS expanded to behavioral health, mental health, and substance use disorder services in a separate survey called the Outpatient Mental Health Survey. The standardized instrument is given to adults who have received mental health or substance use disorder services in the previous six months. Information on the surveys are available on the HCAHPS website, linked in the chapter resources list.

Figure 3.5: *HCAPHS/CAHPS goals*

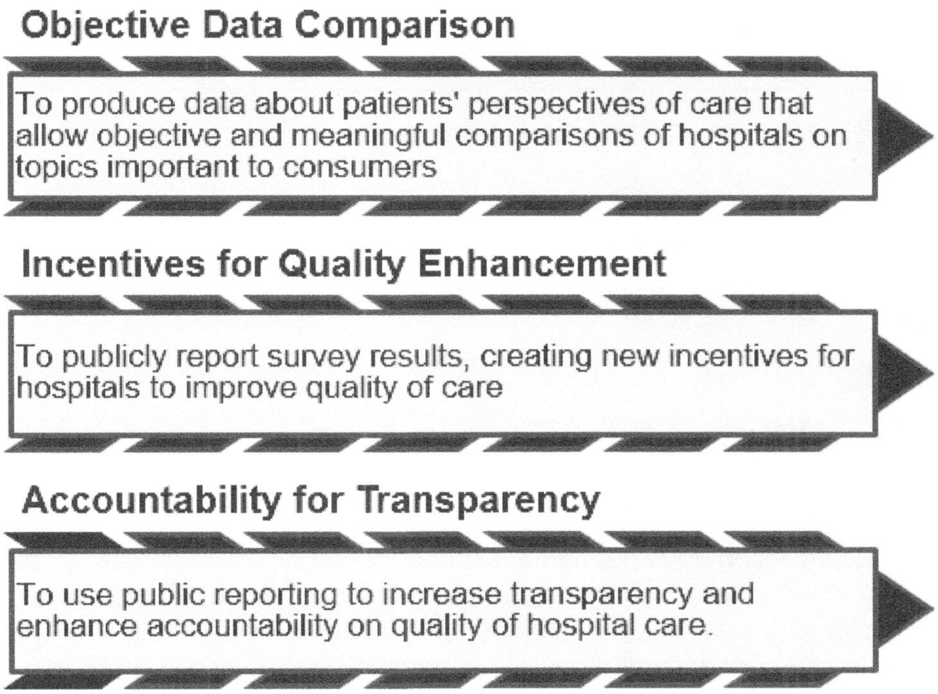

Adapted from CMS.gov, 2024

The Mental Health Parity and Addiction Equity Act (MHPAEA)

In the late 2000s, there was growing attention to behavioral health. Legislators pushed for a more comprehensive law, and the Paul Wellstone and Pete Domenici *Mental Health Parity and Addiction Equity Act of 2008* (MHPAEA) was passed. The law improved on the Mental Health Parity Act of 1996 by requiring the same standards for mental health and substance use disorder as for physical health. The MHPAEA required clearer and more intentional behavioral metrics. For many in healthcare, it stands to reason that depression or SMI treatments should be paid as readily as cardiac issues. Even still, the MHPAEA has received considerable pushback across the industry. The conundrum continues amid the passage of another law, in 2024, which will be discussed at the end of this chapter.

THE 2010S: A DECADE OF DISRUPTION

The 2010s saw dramatic disruption and transformation at the federal level, with domino effects in state and local governments. At the core of these changes were requirements for interoperability—of technology devices and the prodigious data collected for quality initiatives.

Meaningful Use (but not for behavioral health)

As the 2000s ended, the safety and security of electronic health records (EHR) garnered attention. A 2009 law, the Health Information Technology for Economic and Clinical Health (HITECH) Act, included programs to define best practices for EHR security. Among these programs was Meaningful Use. HITECH provided financial and technical support to extend EHR implementation at eligible providers, hospitals, and critical access (safety net) facilities. These efforts were to be phased in over three stages:

Stage 1 (2011-2012): Data capture and sharing

Stage 2 (2014): Advanced clinical processes

Stage 3 (2016): Improved outcomes

By supporting the costly technology needed to expand EHR use, the three phases of Meaningful Use would enhance data collection, analysis, care coordination, and patient engagement. These were necessary actions to attain high quality performance metrics. Yet only a few groups were eligible to receive the support: doctors, dentists, podiatrists, optometrists, and chiropractors. Most behavioral health and substance use treatment providers and programs did not qualify for incentives to cover the technology upgrades. It would take another decade to pass legislation expanding Meaningful Use to behavioral health.

The Affordable Care Act

The Affordable Care Act (ACA) was enacted in 2010. It was a game changer for healthcare, particularly healthcare quality. The ACA expanded health coverage and protected people with preexisting conditions from being denied coverage. States were allowed to expand Medicaid eligibility up to 138 percent of the federal poverty level, which enabled more low-income people to enroll. Behavioral health was woven into essential health benefits. The ACA's meaningful behavioral health benefits appear in Figure 3.6.

Figure 3.6: *ACA behavioral health enhancements*

Expanded coverage

- Classified behavioral health services as essential health benefits, ensuring most health plans would cover mental health and substance abuse treatment

Medicaid expansion

- Expanded Medicaid gave low-income individuals greater access to behavioral health services

Parity protections

- Strengthened enforcement of MHPAEA, requiring insurers to provide equal coverage for mental health services and medical services

Reduced financial barriers

- Enhanced access to affordable insurance coverage, which reduced the number of people who delayed mental healthcare or went without due to cost

Improved access to preventive services

- Coverage mandates for preventive mental health services (e.g., depression screenings) promoted early intervention and treatment

The Center for Medicare & Medicaid Innovation and Value-based Payment Models

Following passage of the ACA, the Center for Medicare & Medicaid Innovation (CMMI) was launched in 2010 to pilot new payment and service delivery models for Medicare, Medicaid, and the Children's Health Insurance Program (CHIP). The goals were simple: improve patient care, lower costs, and promote patient-centric practice.

The CMMI, in partnership with the federal and state governments, piloted value-based payment models. A *value-based payment model* in behavioral health means the same as it does in medical healthcare: that the *value* of care is prioritized over the *volume* of care, such that providers are reimbursed for positive outcomes rather than the quantity of services delivered. Essentially, providers and their organizations are financially incentivized to focus on quality care and successful patient outcomes. Payments are tied to such metrics as reduced hospitalizations and readmissions, high patient engagement, improved patient satisfaction, and decreased mortality.

Most value-based payment models have been extended pilot programs, which take an integrated care approach, rendering physical, behavioral, and psychosocial health together. Box 3.3 offers a snapshot of current offerings. Several are operational, and others were due for activation in 2025. Detailed information is on the CMMI website.

Box 3.3: CMMI value-based payment models

Innovations in Behavioral Health Model

- **Focus**: Deliver person-centered, integrated care to Medicaid and Medicare populations: dual eligibles, with moderate to severe mental health conditions, substance use disorder, or both
- **Goals**: Care integration, care management, health equity, health information technology
- **Participants***: Specialty behavioral health practices (e.g., community mental health centers, opioid treatment programs, public or private practices, and safety-net providers)
- **Number of participants**: Determined once the NOFO (Notice of Funding Opportunity) period has ended; up to eight states eligible
- **Authority**: Section 1115A of the Social Security Act

Transforming Maternal Health Model

- **Focus**: Reduce disparities in access and treatment and improve maternal health care for people enrolled in Medicaid and CHIP. Support from participating state Medicaid agencies.
- **Goals**: Access to care, infrastructure, quality improvement and safety, whole-person approach to pregnancy, childbirth, and postpartum care addressing physical health, mental health, and social needs
- **Participants***: State Medicaid agencies, along with managed care organizations (MCOs), perinatal quality collaboratives, hospitals, birth centers, health centers, rural health clinics, maternity care providers, and community-based organizations
- **Number of participants**: Cooperative agreements signed with up to 15 state Medicaid agencies
- **Program duration**:
  - Three-year pre-implementation period for states to receive targeted technical assistance to advance model elements and achieve required pre-implementation milestones;
  - Then seven-year implementation period for model execution
- **Authority**: Section 1115A of the Social Security Act

GUIDE Model

- **Focus**: Deliver comprehensive, coordinated dementia care and improve quality of life for impacted persons, reduce strain on unpaid caregivers, and allow patients to stay at home and in their communities
- **Goals**: Care coordination, caregiver education and support, respite
- **Participants***: Medicare Part B enrolled providers/suppliers
- **Number of participants**: 390 across the U.S.

- **Program duration**: Beginning July 1, 2024, followed by eight years of executing the model
- **Authority**: Section 1115A of the Social Security Act

Integrated Care for Kids Model

- **Focus**: A child-centered local service delivery and state payment model to reduce expenditures and improve the quality of care for children <21 years old, covered by Medicaid through prevention, early identification, and treatment of behavioral and physical health needs
- Some programs include CHIP beneficiaries and pregnant woman >21 covered by Medicaid
- **Goals**: Care coordination and integration, prevention
- **Participants***: the state Medicaid agency, a defined local leader organization, and a partnership council
- **Number of participants**: Eight cooperative agreements among seven states and organizations
- **Program duration**: January 2, 2022, through December 31, 2026
- **Authority**: Section 1115A of the Social Security Act

Value in Opioid Use Disorder Treatment Program

- **Focus**: Four-year demonstration project to increase access of applicable beneficiaries to opioid use disorder treatment, improve physical and mental health outcomes, and reduce Medicare expenditures
- **Goals**: Care integration, care management, health equity, health information technology
- **Participants***:
  - Dual-eligibles who are:
    - entitled to or enrolled for benefits under Medicare Part A and Medicare Part B
    - not enrolled in a Medicare Advantage plan under Medicare Part C
    - Have a current diagnosis for opioid use disorder (OUD), and
    - Establish an OUD care team and use the team to furnish or arrange for OUD treatment services in the outpatient setting under the demonstration
- **Number of participants**: 53
- **Program duration**: April 1, 2021, through April 1, 2025

Authority: Section 6042 of the Substance Use-Disorder Prevention that Promotes Opioid Recovery and Treatment for Patients and Communities Act (SUPPORT Act)

**CMS defines participants as healthcare providers and organizations that have formally agreed to take part and bear financial risk in particular programs*

CMS Innovation Center, 2024

Quality Payment Program

The Medicare Access and CHIP Reauthorization Act of 2015 introduced the Quality Payment Program (QPP) to transition Medicare from its volume-based payment model to a value-based payment model. The QPP included two payment pathways: Merit-based Incentive Payment System (MIPS) and Advanced Alternative Payment Models (APMs). APMs gave incentive payments to providers based on patient and treatment risk or complexity. MIPS accomplishes a similar aim, though evaluates the quality of clinician intervention spanning four domains: quality, cost, improvement activities, and promoting interoperability. APMs apply to specific clinical conditions, care episodes, or populations. Box 3.4 displays the current popular APM quality measures, which may be familiar to many case managers.

Box 3.4: Examples of APMs

Hospital-wide, 30-day, all-cause unplanned readmission rate for MIPS-eligible clinician groups

Clinician and group risk-standardized hospital admission rates for patients with multiple chronic conditions

Diabetes: Hemoglobin A1c poor control

Preventive care and screening: Screening for depression and follow-up plan

Controlling high blood pressure

Consumer Assessment of Healthcare Providers and Systems for MIPS

CMS.gov, 2024

The Child and Adult Core Quality Measures

ACA coverage mandates have given rise to a plethora of quality metrics under Medicaid, CHIP, and Medicare. By 2012 the Agency for Health Care Research and Quality (AHRQ) and CMS developed Adult Core Quality Measurements; voluntary reporting of these measures began in 2014. The Child Core set became supported in 2018. In August 2023, CMS released a final rule requiring states report standardized behavioral health quality measures starting in 2024.

Growth of certified community behavioral health clinics

Plans for the next generation of community-based programming, *Certified Community Behavioral Health Clinics* (CCBHCs), were federally defined in 2014. CCBHCs met a critical need for outpatient mental health and substance use care and crisis services, regardless of a patient's' ability to pay. The first CCBHCs opened in October 2016.

CCBHCs typically developed out of community mental health centers that offered outpatient behavioral healthcare. But other types of facilities achieve CCBHC designation, too, such as hospitals, *community health centers*, *federally qualified health centers,* and *rural health clinics*. CCBHCs are required to follow the full scope of CMS Child and Adult Core Quality Measurements, as well as those from NCQA defined specifically for behavioral health. The set of quality measures required for CCBHCs appears in Box 3.5. Box 3.6 provides required behavioral health clinic state-collected measures (Substance Abuse and Mental Health Services Administration, 2024).

Box 3.5: Required behavioral health quality measures for CCBHCs

Measure	Measure Steward
Time to services	Substance Abuse and Mental Health Services Administration (SAMHSA)
Depression remission at 6 months	Minnesota Community Measurement
Preventative care and screening:	NCQA
Unhealthy alcohol use: Screening	
and brief counseling	
Screening for social drivers of health	CMS
Screening for clinical depression and follow-up plan	CMS

Substance Abuse and Mental Health Services Administration, 2023

Box 3.6: Required state-collected measures for CCBHCs

Measure	Measure Steward
Patient experience of care survey	SAMHSA
Youth/family experience of care survey	SAMHSA
Antidepressant medication management	SAMHSA
Use of pharmacotherapy for opioid use disorder	CMS
Adherence to antipsychotic medications for individuals with schizophrenia	CMS
Plan all-cause readmissions rate	NCQA
Follow-up care for children prescribed attention-deficit/hyperactivity disorder medications	NCQA
Hemoglobin A1c control for patients with diabetes	NCQA
Initiation and engagement of alcohol and other drug dependence treatment	NCQA
Follow-up post-hospitalization for mental illness	NCQA
Follow-up after emergency department visit for mental illness	NCQA
Follow-up after emergency department visit for alcohol and other drug dependence	NCQA

Substance Abuse and Mental Health Services Administration, 2024

THE FUTURE OF QUALITY MEASURES IN BEHAVIORAL HEALTH

Behavioral healthcare legislation and standards continue to evolve in response to societal demand for a robust mental health treatment continuum, advances in artificial intelligence, and changing federal, state, and local funding priorities. While my crystal ball is on the fritz due to backordered replacement parts, the material in this section highlights areas of anticipated attention relevant to case managers.

TELEHEALTH

Exciting opportunities (and uncertainties) lie ahead for quality improvements in behavioral health. One of the greatest uncertainties is telehealth. Advancements in virtual patient interaction intersect with quality of care concerns. As of this writing, there are no standardized quality measures specifically for behavioral telehealth. But as reimbursement and regulatory guidance shifts, we can expect performance metrics specific to this platform.

THE SOCIAL DETERMINANTS OF HEALTH, PATIENT EXPERIENCE, AND PROMS

The focus on whole-person health in value-based care models means keen attention to behavioral, physical, *and* psychosocial health, such as social determinants of health (SDoH), health-related social needs, and social risks. Regarding the full triad of behavioral, physical, and psychosocial health is critical to successful patient outcomes, which suggests increasing provider screenings and assessments for SDoH, plus prioritizing the patient's voice and experience of care through expansion of *patient reported outcomes measures* (PROMs). Case managers may be familiar with some common PROMs, such as health-related quality of life, functional status, symptoms and symptom burden for the patient and caregiver, health behaviors (as discussed in Chapter 1), and the patient's healthcare experience (e.g., CAHPS).

CMS and Joint Commission have added psychosocial health screening requirements. CMS mandated social risk screening under the In-patient Prospective Payment System (IPPS) beginning in January 2024 and the Out-Patient Prospective Payment System (OPPS) in January 2025. Joint Commission implemented voluntary screening for social drivers of health starting in January 2023, followed by mandatory reporting in 2024.

AHRQ's CAHPS program added an Outpatient Mental Health Survey in June 2024, with particular focus on mental health providers, primary and specialty medical care groups, hospitals, health systems, health plans, healthcare monitoring organizations, and community health centers. The standardized Outpatient Mental Health Survey asks adult patients about their experiences in receiving mental health and substance abuse services in any outpatient setting over the past six months. Detailed information about the survey results are available on the CAHPS Mental Health Surveys website.

MENTAL HEALTH PARITY

Challenges to mental health parity laws continue. In fall 2024, 45 CFR Parts 146 and 147 was passed by Congress. The law prohibits group health insurance from using non-quantitative treatment limits (NQTLs), as they're typically used for stringent behavioral health preauthorization requirements or denials of care. The law places tighter restrictions on mental health and substance use disorder benefits compared to medical/surgical benefits, however (Federal Register, 2024).

Advocacy groups continue to push for mental health parity, including the National Alliance for Mental Illness (NAMI) and the Kennedy Forum. The latter provides legal updates and public policy advocacy. Both entities have written position papers to inform the public and lawmakers on mental health treatment parity. Further information on these position papers is in the chapter resources list.

MEDICARE ADVANTAGE AND BEHAVIORAL HEALTH

CMS has proposed limiting copayments to 20 percent for mental health specialty services, partial hospitalization, intensive outpatient, and outpatient substance use treatment. Current regulations allow for 30 percent to 50 percent copayments for these services. Proposed rules would also require insurance to cover opioid treatment programs with no copayment, whereas plans can currently require up to 50 percent copayment. Public comment was accepted on the proposed regulations until January 27, 2025. The federal government applied a transition period on new regulations to avoid disruptions for patients and providers.

There was concern in the industry that Medicare Advantage plans offered limited options for behavioral healthcare providers—as few as a handful of providers per 1,000 beneficiaries (CMS, 2024). In April 2024 CMS finalized rules requiring Medicare Advantage plans to offer adequate in-network outpatient behavioral health providers. Low reimbursement rates have been among the challenges in effecting this change. Medicare Advantage expansion to telehealth is also on the horizon.

CONCLUSION

You have now completed Section 1, and three of your five critical knowledge pillars are now solidified: foundational concepts, regulations and requirements, and core measures and reimbursements. We move on to Section 2, understanding behavioral health conditions, incidence of impact, and strategic management considerations.

CONTEMPLATION QUESTIONS

1. Review the Six Domains of Quality in Table 3.1.
    a) Identify the domains you have experienced personally or professionally.
    b) Identify information in this chapter that would have helped you navigate the situation.
2. Explore the CMMI value-based programs in Box 3.3.
    a) Which program holds greatest relevance for you and your patient populations?
    b) Review information on that program on the CMMI website (see the chapter resources list), and reflect on how the offering may benefit your patients.
3. Reflect on the ACA information in the chapter.
    a) Which of the ACA enhancements in Figure 3.6 impact your patient populations most?
    b) How have your patients benefitted from the ACA?
    c) How has the ACA not benefitted your patients?
        i. Identify strategies to mitigate these situations.
4. Review the NQF's Initial 10 Behavioral Health Core Measures in Table 3.2. As you reflect on the measures shown, consider:
    a) What measures not currently addressed would you like to see in the future?
    b) How do these measures meet the Quintuple Aim?
5. Review the material on mental health parity laws. Consider:
    a) How would you describe the concept of mental health parity?
    b) Why has it been difficulty to attain?
    c) The latest law, 45 CFR Parts 146 and 147, was passed in fall 2024. How is it shifting the mental health parity landscape?

RESOURCES

- **Agency for Healthcare Research and Quality (AHRQ): Consumer Assessment of Healthcare Providers and Systems (CAHPS) Mental Health Surveys**
  https://www.ahrq.gov/cahps/surveys-guidance/mental-health/index.html

CMS

- Hospital Consumer Assessment of Healthcare Providers and Systems Survey (HCAHPS) https://www.cms.gov/medicare/quality/initiatives/hospital-quality-initiative/hcahps-patients-perspectives-care-survey
- The Mental Health Parity and Addiction Equity Act (MHPAEA) https://www.cms.gov/marketplace/private-health-insurance/mental-health-parity-addiction-equity
- **CMS Innovation Center: Value-based Care Models**
  https://www.cms.gov/priorities/innovation/models

- Innovations in Behavioral Health Model https://www.cms.gov/priorities/innovation/innovation-models/innovation-behavioral-health-ibh-model
- **Transforming Maternal Health Model**
  https://www.cms.gov/priorities/innovation/innovation-models/transforming-maternal-health-tmah-model
- **GUIDE**
  https://www.cms.gov/priorities/innovation/innovation-models/guide
- **Integrated Care for Kids Model**
  https://www.cms.gov/priorities/innovation/innovation-models/integrated-care-for-kids-model
- Value in Opioid Use Disorder Treatment Program https://www.cms.gov/priorities/innovation/innovation-models/value-in-treatment-demonstration
- **Congress.gov: Excellence in Mental Health Act**
  https://www.congress.gov/bill/113th-congress/senate-bill/264
- **Institute of Healthcare Improvement**
  https://www.ihi.org/

Joint Commission

- **Behavioral Health Care**
  https://www.jointcommission.org/what-we-offer/accreditation/health-care-settings/behavioral-health-care/
- **National Patient Safety Goals for Behavioral Health Care 2025**
  https://www.jointcommission.org/standards/national-patient-safety-goals/behavioral-health-care-national-patient-safety-goals/
- **The Kennedy Forum**
  https://www.thekennedyforum.org
- **National Commission of Quality Assurance (NCQA): HEDIS and Performance Measurement**
  https://www.ncqa.org/hedis/
- **National Quality Forum**
  https://www.qualityforum.org/Home.aspx
- **Utilization Review Accreditation Commission (URAC)**
  https://www.urac.org

REFERENCES

- Aichouni, M., Touahmia, M., Alshammari, S., Said, M.A., Aichouni, A.B.E., Almudayries, M., & Aljohani, H. (2023). An empirical study of the contribution of total quality management to occupational safety and health performance in Saudi organizations. *International Journal of Environmental Research and Public Health, 20*(2), 1495. https://doi.org/10.3390/ijerph20021495
- Barry, C.L., Huskamp, H.A., & Goldman, H.H. (2010). A political history of federal mental health and addiction insurance parity. *The Milbank Quarterly, 88*(3), 404-433. https://doi.org/10.1111/j.1468-0009.2010.00605.x
- Consumer Assessment of Healthcare Providers and Services. (2024). CAHPS. Retrieved December 8, 2024, from https://www.ahrq.gov/cahps/index.html
- CMS.gov. (2024). Contract year policy and technical changes to the Medicare Advantage Program, Medicare Prescription Drug Benefit Program, Medicare Cost Plan Program, and Programs of All-inclusive Care for the Elderly (CMS-4208-P); CMS Newsroom. Retrieved December 8, 2024, from https://www.cms.gov/newsroom/fact-sheets/contract-year-2026-policy-and-technical-changes-medicare-advantage-program-medicare-prescription
- CMS Innovation Center. (2024). Innovation Models. Retrieved December 6, 2024, from https://www.cms.gov/priorities/innovation/models
- Federal Register. (2024). 2024-20612 (89 FR 77586), Requirements Related to the Mental Health Parity and Addiction Equity Act. Retrieved December 4, 2024, from https://www.federalregister.gov/documents/2024/09/23/2024-20612/requirements-related-to-the-mental-health-parity-and-addiction-equity-act
- Institute of Medicine (US) Committee to Design a Strategy for Quality Review and Assurance in Medicare. (1990). *Medicare: A Strategy for Quality Assurance*: *Volume 1*. Lohr K.N., Ed. National Academies Press: Washington, D.C. PMID: 25144047.
- Institute of Medicine (US) Committee on Quality of Health Care in America. (2001). *Crossing the Quality Chasm: A New Health System for the 21st Century*. National Academies Press: Washington, D.C.
- Itchhaporia, D. (2021). The evolution of the Quintuple Aim: Health equity, health outcomes, and the economy. *Journal of the American College of Cardiology, 78*(22), 2262-2264. doi: 10.1016/j.jacc.2021.10.018. PMID: 34823665; PMCID: PMC8608191.
- Joint Commission. (2024). Behavioral Health Care and Human Services: 2025 National Patient Safety Goals. Retrieved December 8, 2024, from https://www.jointcommission.org/standards/national-patient-safety-goals/behavioral-health-care-national-patient-safety-goals/
- Medicaid.gov. (2024). 2025 core set of behavioral health measures for Medicaid and CHIP (Behavioral Health Core Set). Retrieved October 9, 2025, from https://www.medicaid.gov/medicaid/quality-of-care/downloads/2025-bh-core-set.pdf
- National Commission for Quality Assurance. (2024). Healthcare Effectiveness Data and Information Set (HEDIS) and Performance Management. Retrieved December 5, 2024, from https://www.ncqa.org/hedis/

- National Quality Forum. (2023). *Behavioral Health and Substance Use, Spring 2022 Cycle: CDP Report.* Retrieved October 17, 2025, from https://cms.qualityforum.org/Publications/2023/01/Behavioral Health Final Report - Spring 2022 Cycle.aspx
- National Quality Forum. (n.d.). NQF's History. Retrieved December 8, 2024, from https://www.qualityforum.org/about_nqf/history/
- Orgrinc, G.S., Headrick, L.A., Barton, A.J., Dolansky, M.A., Madigosky, W.S., Miltner, R.S., Hall, A.G. (2022). *Fundamentals of Health Care Improvement: A Guide to Improving Your Patients' Care, 4th Edition*; Institute for Healthcare Improvement, Joint Commission Resources.
- Substance Abuse and Mental Health Services Administration. (2023). Quality Measures Guidance and Webinar Series. Retrieved October 9, 2025 from https://www.samhsa.gov/communities/certified-community-behavioral-health-clinics/guidance-and-webinars
- Substance Abuse and Mental Health Services Administration. (2024). Quality Measures for Behavioral Health Clinics: Technical Specifications and Resource Manual. Retrieved October 9, 2025, https://www.samhsa.gov/sites/default/files/ccbhc-quality-measures-technical-specifications-manual.pdf
- Treiger, T.M. & Fink-Samnick, E. (2016). *COLLABORATE for Professional Case Management: A Universal Competency-Based Paradigm.* Wolters Kluwer Health, Philadelphia, PA.
- Utilization Review Accreditation Commission. (2024). Mental health/substance abuse accreditation and parity. Retrieved October 9, 2025, from https://www.urac.org/accrediations-certification/programs/mental-health-substance-use-disorder-parity
- Whittington, J.W., Nolan, K., Lewis, N., & Torres, T. (2015). Pursuing the Triple Aim: The first 7 years. *The Milbank Quarterly*, *93*(2), 263-300. https://doi.org/10.1111/1468-0009.12122

SECTION 2

BEHAVIORAL HEALTH CONDITIONS AND MANAGEMENT

CHAPTER 8

SUBSTANCE USE AND MISUSE

CHAPTER 9

SUICIDAL IDEATION

CHAPTER 10

TRAUMA EXPOSURE

INTRODUCTION TO SECTION 2

While crafting Section 2 of this book, I thought of the countless conversations I have had with fellow case managers about their wish lists for the book's content. My colleagues span many disciplines, though a majority are not trained in, or licensed as, behavioral health professionals. Yet they face increasing manifestations of psychopathology in interactions with patients, their families, and other consumers of care. Many colleagues are health profession educators who teach students best practices in these situations. Even still, these colleagues requested the book address common questions, like:

- What are the most common mental health conditions I will face?
- Which diagnoses are most prevalent?
- How do I approach patients with mild, moderate, or severe symptoms?
- What is the prevalence of these conditions across youth, adults, and older adults?
- How will symptoms present across each age group?
- What are population-related considerations for unique groups, such as military members, veterans, and their families; persons who identify as LGBTQIA+; persons with cognitive, developmental, or physical disabilities; and women?
- What are the primary screening tools for each condition?
- Can you provide a conversation map to address each condition?
- What are some counseling interventions and techniques for non-therapists?
- What must I really know so I won't crash and burn when faced with patients experiencing anxiety, depression, stress, trauma, or something else?

The seven chapters in Section 2, arranged alphabetically, address these prompts and much more. I have chosen the most common mental health conditions and behavioral health manifestations encountered by case managers. Boxes, tables, and figures provide a snapshot of associated diagnoses and general treatment recommendations. While specific counseling interventions and techniques are noted for each disorder, more detailed information on short-term and other interventions appear in Section 3.

CHAPTER 4

ANXIETY

INTRODUCTION

Chapter 4 is about all things anxiety. This diagnosis has long been identified as the most prevalent behavioral health condition worldwide, across every age group. The condition affects the overall clinical and cost burden of disease, which is among the primary reasons it is on case management's radar.

BEHAVIORAL LEARNING OBJECTIVES

1. Identify the levels of anxiety
2. Distinguish among common presentations of anxiety
3. Relate symptoms and treatment recommendations for common DSM diagnoses
4. Understand how anxiety appears across developmental life stages
5. Analyze the incidence of anxiety across life stages and populations
6. Identify screening tools to assess for anxiety
7. Apply Case Management's Behavioral Health Conversation Map to patients and families living with anxiety disorders

ESSENTIAL TERMS

- Agitation
- Agoraphobia
- Anxiety
- Anxiety continuum
- Case management process
- Cisgender
-
- Dissociation
- Gender diverse
- Generalized anxiety disorder
- Neurodiversity
- Other specified anxiety disorder
- Panic attacks
- Perseveration
- Phobias
- Phobia-related disorders
- Social anxiety disorder
- Somatic complaints
- Unspecified anxiety disorder

TERMS AND FEATURES OF ANXIETY

Momentary fear and worry are normal responses to life experienced by all human beings. Yet many individuals live with constant, inescapable feelings of fear and worry known as *anxiety*. Let's explore the continuum of anxiety and how it can be incapacitating for some people.

THE ANXIETY CONTINUUM

Everyone experiences occasional stress and anxiety. But challenges affect people differently; it is normal to see varying levels and types of anxiety in response to similar stressors. People worry about job stability, or whether retirement will be realistic at the age they want, or the quality of platonic and intimate relationships. Working people stress over time for parenting, sick days, vacation, and other personal activities. For caregivers, life requires constant juggling to coordinate a loved one's care with other daily responsibilities. Appointments with physicians and specialists must sync with the caregiver's work or class schedules. Reliable transportation must be arranged. The pressure to manage it all prompts stress for even the most organized person.

Even good stress affects us. Before my husband and I adopted two kittens last year, we were excited and anxious about whether our 5-year-old twin cats would accept their new baby "brothers." Here's another example. Imagine you're planning a party—a birthday, a graduation, or a wedding. Underlying the joy of the event is dread. Will the event be a success or an epic failure? Does the seating account for relatives who don't like each other? Are dietary or other preferences addressed? We can see that stress and anxiety are a reality for everyone, but at varying degrees. The *Anxiety Continuum* appears in Figure 4.1.

Figure 4.1: *The anxiety continuum*

Mild

- Minor worry and feelings of restlessness and agitation
- Individual may fidget, sweat, or have heightened senses
- Usually able to continue day-to-day activities

Moderate

- Increased heart rate, persistent apprehension, and difficulty concentrating
- May feel on edge or unable to stop worrying or perseverating
- Experience somatic complaints (e.g., stomach pains, body aches) or rapid speech

Severe

- Debilitating fear and avoidance behaviors
- Frequent somatic complaints and physical symptoms, overwhelmed by worry, difficulty making decisions, scattered thoughts
- Intense physical symptoms of vomiting, chest pain, or diarrhea

Panic

- Recurrent panic attacks and intense physical symptoms
- Profound fear of repeated panic attacks

The continuum of anxiety begins when a person has momentary or mild concern about a situation. Emotions may escalate to periods of restlessness or *agitation*, when a person is quick to frustration, anger, or more disruptive aggressive behaviors. This phase is followed by a consistent and moderate pattern of *perseveration* over one or more concerns, where constant and chronic worry is the norm. Perseveration may intensify to such a degree that a person is unable to socialize or to complete routine activities because hesitation and overthinking accompany every step of a task. The most severe level of anxiety reflects panic about unrealistic consequences for the person's actions. The person may experience a panic attack, obstructing social, academic, or occupational functioning.

How do the specifiers discussed in Chapter 1 apply to anxiety disorders? Do DSM-5-TR anxiety diagnoses always include specifiers? The short answer is no, because the symptoms for anxiety disorders often overlap, making specifiers less clinically distinct and diminishing their purpose. However, DSM-5-TR uses specifiers for some anxiety disorders. For example, social anxiety disorder includes one specifier, for "performance only." And substance/medication-induced anxiety disorder includes distinct ICD-10-CM clinical codes for each substance used and for the level of substance use (e.g., mild, moderate, severe, without use disorder).

COMMON ANXIETY DISORDERS

When does a normal stress response become a diagnoseable mental illness? This is where clinical acumen and established resources for diagnosis come in. The DMS-5-TR's dedicated category for anxiety disorders is an expansive listing; diagnoses appear in Table 4.1. Depending on a case manager's practice setting and population, he or she may encounter certain diagnoses more than others. For example, people who work in pediatrics or elementary schools may encounter patients diagnosed with separation anxiety disorder more often than those who work in adult settings. Case managers in acute care hospitals may interact often with patients with panic disorders or unspecified anxiety disorder. Focus for this chapter is on the disorders most seen by case managers in healthcare settings. The chapter resource list provides websites with detailed information on all diagnoses, including a link to the DSM-5-TR.

Table 4.1: *DSM-5-TR anxiety disorders*

DSM-5-TR Diagnosis	Code
Separation anxiety disorder	F93
Selective mutism	F94
Specific phobias Animal National environment Blood-injection-injury (e.g., needles, invasive procedures) Situational (e.g., buses, planes, subways, enclosed spaces) Other	 F40.218 F40.228 F40.23X* F40.248 F40.298 Select specific ICD-10-CM code for fear of blood, fear of injections, transfusions, other medical care
Social anxiety disorder	F40.10
Panic disorders	F41.10
Agoraphobia	F40.00
Generalized anxiety disorder	F41.1
Substance/medication-induced anxiety disorder • Alcohol • Caffeine • Cannabis • Phencyclidine • Another hallucinogen • Inhalant • Opioid • Sedative, hypnotic, or anxiolytic • Amphetamine-type substance or another stimulant • Cocaine • Another unknown substance	Codes span F10 through F19 A distinct diagnostic code exists for each substance and severity of the disorder (mild, moderate, or severe), as well as "without Use Disorder" *(p. 256) *A substance-induced anxiety disorder is coded "without Use Disorder" when anxiety symptoms are directly linked to the use of a psychoactive substance, but the individual does not meet the diagnostic criteria for a substance use disorder itself.

DSM-5-TR Diagnosis	Code
Anxiety disorder due to another medical condition	F06.4
Other specified anxiety disorder	F41.8
Unspecified anxiety disorder	F41.9

Adapted from American Psychiatric Association, 2022, pp. 215-261

GENERALIZED ANXIETY DISORDER

People with symptoms of *generalized anxiety disorder* chronically experience feelings of dismay that impede their ability to get through the day. Imagine: You try to leave home for work but sense something bad will happen. You can't put your finger on it but feel surrounded by worry. You are tense, irritable, and unable to concentrate. Physical symptoms and *somatic complaints* may occur: generic body aches, headaches, stomach pain, or other unexplained discomfort. Exhaustion is your norm because it's difficult for you to fall asleep or sleep soundly through the night. These are the day-to-day realities of generalized anxiety disorder, as explained further in Box 4.1.

Box 4.1: Signs, symptoms, and treatment of generalized anxiety disorder (GAD)

DSM-5-TR criteria:

Patients must have excessive anxiety and worry about activities or events (e.g., work and school performance), occurring more days than not for ≥ 6 months

The worries are difficult to control and must be associated with ≥ 3 of the following:

- Restlessness or a keyed-up or on-edge feeling
- Easy fatigability
- Difficulty concentrating
- Irritability
- Muscle tension
- Disturbed sleep

Symptoms cause significant distress or significantly impair social or occupational functioning.

The anxiety/worry are not accounted for by substance use, a general medical disorder, or other mental disorder.

Treatments:

- Antidepressants such as selective serotonin reuptake inhibitors (SSRIs) or serotonin-norepinephrine reuptake inhibitors (SNRIs)
- Anxiolytic medications such as benzodiazepines or buspirone
- Beta-blockers
- Homeopathic and medicinal herb use is increasingly common (e.g., ashwagandha, chamomile, kava kava, lavender, passionflower, omega-3 fatty acids, St. John's wort), though should be openly reviewed with prescribing practitioners to ensure safety. Careful monitoring and mitigation with other current prescriptions, over-the-counter medications, and other substances should be discussed prior to initiating use to avoid interactions, complications, etc.

- Monitoring diet, exercise, and activity is recommended

Psychotherapy: Cognitive behavioral therapy (CBT), exposure therapies, eye-movement desensitization and reprocessing (EMDR), psychodynamic therapy, relaxation strategies (e.g. box or 4-7-8 breathing), sleep hygiene

Adapted from American Psychiatric Association, 2022, pp. 250-254; Merck Manual, 2024; Zhang et al., 2022

PANIC ATTACKS AND PANIC DISORDER

Consider this: You're thinking about department budget cuts and suddenly feel warm to the point of perspiring. You can't settle your nerves, and dread overwhelms you. Your chest feels tight and your breathing rapid; it's like your body has a mind of its own. You are having a *panic attack,* an abrupt onset of distinct, and usually brief, intense discomfort, anxiety, or fear with somatic or cognitive symptoms (Merck Manual, 2023a).

People experiencing panic attacks may present with *dissociation*, appearing disconnected from reality. On 9/11/2001, I worked at the hospital closest to the Pentagon. As the facility's disaster alarms were going off, I was running down the stairs and smacked into a colleague. The person stood frozen in the stairwell, their eyes wide open and their breathing rapid. They did not respond to my voice. This was an example of dissociation. After several minutes, I got my colleague's attention by gently touching their arm and cueing them to mimic my breath pattern.

When a person experiences panic attacks frequently, he or she may be diagnosed with a *panic disorder*. The person typically worries incessantly about when the next panic attack will occur. Common signs, symptoms, and treatments for panic disorder are in Box 4.2.

Case managers may experience patients or their family members having panic attacks. A hospitalization or sudden health episode can trigger feelings of loss of control, which may set in motion a vicious cycle of perseveration about impending doom or demise. Furthermore, patients or family members can panic when pushed to make a decision despite feeling they don't fully understand their choices or feel otherwise unprepared to commit to one option. These decisions might include treatment options, discharge planning alternatives, or acceptance of referrals and resources. Meanwhile, case managers also face pressure to facilitate timely patient-care processes. But moving through processes will be tense and often unsuccessful if the patient is anxious and, thus, unable to engage in objective decision-making.

Remember one vital aspect of anxiety disorders: No event is experienced the same way by every patient; anxiety and stress are relative. Patients and their families process information in distinct ways. How they cope is affected by cultural elements, timing, and many other factors.

Box 4.2: Signs, symptoms, and treatment of panic disorder

DSM-5-TR criteria:

- Patients have recurrent panic attacks (unspecified frequency) where ≥ 1 attack is followed by one or both of the following for ≥ 1 month:
- Persistent worry about having another panic attack or worry about the consequences of a panic attack (e.g., losing control, going crazy)
- Maladaptive behavioral response to the panic attacks, as in avoiding routine or common activities (e.g., exercise, use of public transportation, routine commutes, social outings) with the goal to prevent further attacks
- The disturbance is not due to physiological effects of a substance, a medical condition, or a mental disorder.

Panic attack symptoms may include, but are not limited to:

1. Palpitations
2. Sweating
3. Trembling or shaking
4. Shortness of breath or feeling like one has difficulty breathing
5. Chest discomfort or pain
6. Gastrointestinal or abdominal discomfort or pain (e.g., nausea, diarrhea)
7. Feeling dizzy or light-headed
8. Feeling that body parts are numb
9. Derealization (feelings of unreality) or dissociation (feeling detached from events)
10. Fear of going crazy, losing control, or dying

- Treatments:
- Antidepressants, benzodiazepines, or both
- Beta-blockers
- Homeopathic and medicinal herb use is increasingly common (e.g., ashwagandha, chamomile, kava kava, lavender, passionflower, omega-3 fatty acids, St. John's wort), though should be openly reviewed with prescribing practitioners to ensure safety. Careful monitoring and mitigation with other current prescriptions, over-the-counter medications, and other substances should be discussed prior to initiating use to avoid interactions, complications, etc.
- Psychotherapy: Cognitive behavioral therapy (CBT), eye-movement desensitization and reprocessing (EMDR), relaxation strategies (e.g., box or 4-7-8 breathing)

Adapted from American Psychiatric Association, 2022, pp. 235-250; Merck Manual, 2023a; Zhang et al., 2022

PHOBIA-RELATED DISORDERS AND AGORAPHOBIA

A *phobia* is an intense fear or aversion to specific objects or situations. Patients who present with intense fear of two or more situations are diagnosed with *agoraphobia*. People with phobias express emotions out of proportion to actual danger. Situations that commonly cause phobias include:

- Traveling by certain means (e.g., airplanes, buses, commuter trains, ships)
- Heights or staying in hotels on high floors
- Certain animals (e.g., spiders, cats, dogs, snakes)

- Diagnostic tests (e.g., MRIs)
- Needles (e.g., lab draws, medical treatments)

Symptoms of a dog phobia might include worrying about encountering dogs on a walk, avoiding certain streets because there may be dogs, or perspiring or hyperventilating when encountering a dog. Box 4.3 displays the signs and symptoms of phobia-related disorders.

Box 4.3: Signs, symptoms, and treatment of phobia-related disorders

DSM-5-TR criteria:

- Marked, persistent (≥ 6 months) fear of or anxiety about a specific situation or object In addition, patients have all the following:
- The situation or object nearly always triggers immediate fear or anxiety.
- Patients actively avoid the situation or object.
- Fear or anxiety is out of proportion to the actual danger (considering sociocultural norms).
- Fear, anxiety, and avoidance cause major distress or significantly impact social or occupational functioning.

The diagnosis of a specific phobia should not be made if the clinical situation is better described by another diagnosis.

Treatments:

- Trial/limited use of benzodiazepines or beta-blockers
- Homeopathic and medicinal herb use is increasingly common (e.g., ashwagandha, chamomile, kava kava, lavender, passionflower, omega-3 fatty acids, St. John's wort), though should be openly reviewed with prescribing practitioners to ensure safety. Careful monitoring and mitigation with other current prescriptions, over-the-counter medications, and other substances should be discussed prior to initiating use to avoid interactions, complications, etc.
- Psychotherapy: Exposure therapy, relaxation techniques (e.g., box or 4-7-8 breathing, guided imagery), hypnosis

Adapted from American Psychiatric Association, 2022, pp. 224-229; Merck Manual, 2023b; Zhao, et al., 2022

SOCIAL ANXIETY DISORDER

As you enter care coordination rounds prepared to discuss your long-stay patients, you have a series of thoughts: *I know the obstacles to discharge, but will they be seen as excuses? Will the physician challenge me? Will my voice crack when I speak? My director and physician advisor are fierce case management champions. What if I embarrass them?* Your throat tightens and you feel flushed. While any case manager can experience routine thoughts like these, a scenario like this usually would not meet the DSM threshold for social anxiety disorder.

People affected by *social anxiety disorder* obsess about being humiliated or embarrassed in front of others. The person may stop going to work or socializing due to their angst, or they may perseverate that certain expectations others have of them can't be met, or that their actions will be subject to extreme scrutiny. Some individuals experience intense worry at the thought of engaging in public activities, from giving presentations to using a communal restroom at work. If invited to brainstorm with colleagues, the person may fear being judged for suggesting the wrong option. These internalized fears obstruct social, academic, and occupational functioning.

Like other anxiety disorders, the presentation and severity of social anxiety disorder varies. Rather than seek formal treatment, many persons find ways to manage their symptoms, such as avoiding social situations or self-medicating with alcohol, nicotine, or other substances. The signs and symptoms of social anxiety disorder appear in Box 4.4.

Box 4.4: Signs, symptoms, and treatment of social anxiety disorder

DSM-5-TR criteria:

- Marked, persistent (≥ 6 months) fear of or anxiety about one or more social situations where a person may be scrutinized by others

Fear must involve a negative evaluation by others (e.g., person may be subject to humiliation, embarrassment or rejection, or will somehow offend others). All the following symptoms should be present:

- The same social situations nearly always trigger fear or anxiety.
- Patient actively avoids the situation.
- Fear or anxiety are out of proportion to an actual threat (considering sociocultural norms).
- Fear or anxiety and/or avoidance cause major distress or significantly impair social or occupational functioning.

Reactions by the patient include, but are not limited to:

- Blushing, sweating, or trembling
- Pounding or racing heart
- Stomach aches
- Rigid body posture
- Speaking with a soft voice
- Inability or difficulty to make eye contact
- Feelings of self-consciousness or worry other people will judge them negatively

The fear and anxiety cannot be more correctly characterized as a different mental disorder.

Treatments:

- Selective serotonin reuptake inhibitors (SSRIs)
- Homeopathic and medicinal herb use is increasingly common (e.g., ashwagandha, chamomile, kava kava, lavender, passionflower, omega-3 fatty acids, St. John's wort), though should be openly reviewed with prescribing practitioners to ensure safety. Careful monitoring and mitigation with other current prescriptions, over-the-counter medications, and other substances should be discussed prior to initiating use to avoid interactions, complications, etc.
- Psychotherapy: Cognitive behavioral therapy (CBT), exposure therapies, eye-movement desensitization and reprocessing (EMDR)
- Relaxation techniques (e.g., box or 4-7-8 breathing, guided imagery)

Adapted from American Psychiatric Association, 2022, pp. 229-235; Merck Manual, 2023c; Yan et al., 2022

OTHER SPECIFIED ANXIETY DISORDER AND UNSPECIFIED ANXIETY DISORDER

Imagine a patient who is frazzled and tense. Their symptoms impact social, occupational, or other areas of functioning but do not meet the full DSM criteria for any anxiety or other disorders. The person has limited symptoms that occur less frequently than the criteria require. There may be a blend of symptoms across various disorders, so one diagnosis does not apply. For example, the patient may be worried about a work situation, but not to the extent of a generalized anxiety disorder or panic disorder. A patient like this may be diagnosed with *other specified anxiety disorder*.

There are times when symptoms are debilitating and notable to the assessing practitioner. *Unspecified anxiety disorder* is a common diagnosis for patients who present to the ED with a vague fear that something will happen, but they can't put their finger on it. The person is agitated, though not due to use of a substance or medication. The patient may be unable to provide an accurate history or specific details about their concerns. Further information about other specified anxiety disorder and unspecified anxiety disorder appear in Box 4.5.

Box 4.5: Signs, symptoms, and treatment of other anxiety disorder (specified and unspecified)

Other Specified Anxiety Disorder

Symptoms reflecting an anxiety disorder cause clinically significant distress or impairment in social, occupational, or other areas of functioning but do not meet the full criteria for disorders in the anxiety disorders diagnostic class, for an adjustment disorder with anxiety, or for an adjustment disorder with mixed anxiety and depressed mood. A clinician records the reason the patient does not meet the criteria, whether:

- Limited symptom attached

  Generalized anxiety occurring less often than not, or
  Other cultural factors (e.g., attack of nerves)

Unspecified Anxiety Disorder

Symptoms reflect an anxiety disorder that causes clinically significant distress or impairment in social, occupational, or other areas of functioning but do not meet the full criteria for any of the following: disorders in the anxiety disorders diagnostic class, an adjustment disorder with anxiety, or an adjustment disorder with mixed anxiety and depressed mood. The clinician specifies the reason the criteria is not met, such as:

- Having insufficient information to make a diagnosis
- Patient is unable to self-report

Treatments:

- Homeopathic and medicinal herb use is increasingly common (e.g., ashwagandha, chamomile, kava kava, lavender, passionflower, omega-3 fatty acids, St. John's wort), though should be openly reviewed with prescribing practitioners to ensure safety. Careful monitoring and mitigation with other current prescriptions, over-the-counter medications, and other substances should be discussed prior to initiating use to avoid interactions, complications, etc.

- Psychotherapies: Cognitive behavioral therapy (CBT), exposure therapy, psychoeducation

Treatment Considerations

- Antidepressants, benzodiazepines, or both
- Psychotherapy: Cognitive behavioral therapy, EMDR, Relaxation strategies

Adapted from American Psychiatric Association, 2022, p. 162; Zhao et al., 2022

DATA AND DEMOGRAPHICS

Anxiety is the most common behavioral health disorder and impacts more than 300 million people around the globe. Roughly 25 percent of the population receive some type of treatment, whether psychotherapy and/or medication management (World Health Organization, 2023).

GENERAL RISK FACTORS

Several factors across Engel's (1977) biological, psychological, and social domains contribute to a person's risk of developing an anxiety disorder. General risk factors for anxiety disorders are:

- A tendency toward shyness, or feeling nervous or uneasy in new situations during childhood
- Exposure to stressful, negative, or traumatic life or environmental events
- A history of anxiety, any mental illness, or severe mental illness in biological relatives

Symptoms of anxiety can be triggered by many causes, including but not limited to:

- Physical health conditions or genetic predisposition
- Prescribed medications or their side effects
- Over-the-counter medications and supplements
- Foods, drinks, or substances including caffeine, spices, and seasonings
- Environmental factors, such as extremes in humidity or temperature

Patients with greater health-related social needs (HRSNs) are more vulnerable to anxiety, as are persons of traditionally marginalized and minoritized populations (Alegría et al., 2022). This is an important consideration for case managers, given recent regulatory requirements from CMS and Joint Commission to screen patients for HRSNs and SDoH. During any patient assessment, there must also be accounting for ways anxiety may be affected by the cultural construct: the socio-political atmosphere, the economy, systemic racism, migrant status, sexual orientation, socioeconomic status, religion, spirituality, and family structures.

Accepting treatment for a mental health disorder is also subject to individual and societal beliefs that should be acknowledged by healthcare workers. Denial or rejection of treatment recommendations does not equate to non-adherence. Instead, it may reflect personal or cultural understanding of mental health (Ahad et al., 2023). Gender and racial bias may also lead to overdiagnosis or misdiagnosis, such as higher rates of anxiety disorder diagnosis in women and members of the LGBTQIA+ community (Garb, 2021).

DEVELOPMENTAL LIFE STAGE

Anxiety presents differently for each person and age group. This section provides a brief review of the clinical presentation of anxiety across the lifespan.

Youth

The onset of symptoms for anxiety disorders occurs primarily in children, but not always. Symptoms are often identified when a child first interacts with other children and adults outside the home. Childcare providers, preschool and kindergarten teachers, and elementary school staff may be the first to point out symptoms to parents. Pediatricians may be consulted about other signs of anxiety, such as irritability, frustration intolerance, somatic complaints, insomnia, or regressive behaviors such as thumb sucking or bedwetting. Anxious children may be reluctant to socialize or engage in other activities. They may isolate from classmates, have difficulty making friends, or be prone to fights and other altercations (Centers for Disease Control and Prevention, 2024).

Early identification and assessment of anxiety is dependent on access to screening, access to and trust in providers, and traditional beliefs regarding mental health (World Health Organization, 2022). Over 36 percent of children and almost 32 percent of adolescents have been diagnosed with some type of anxiety (Bie et al. 2024; U.S. Preventative Services Task Force et al., 2022).

Adults

Over 44 percent of adults aged 18 and older experience symptoms of anxiety during their lives. Kavelaars et al. (2023) found that 32.5 percent of adults self-reported anxiety, and another 11.5 percent admitted to mild to severe anxiety symptoms but did not self-identify with anxiety. Figure 4.2 displays the percent of adults experiencing mild, moderate, and severe anxiety. Along with the diagnostic-specific symptoms identified earlier in this chapter, common behavioral presentations of anxiety include fatigue, impatience, insomnia, lack of or increased appetite, and poor concentration or distractibility.

Figure 4.2: *Levels of anxiety in U.S. adults*

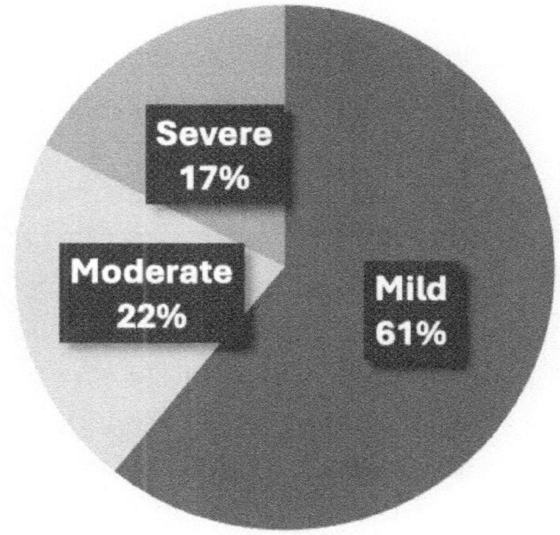

Adapted from O'Connor et al., 2023

Older adults

Anxiety impacts more than 20 percent of older adults, though most aren't formally diagnosed (National Council on Aging, 2024). Fears around loss of mobility and independence are common triggers, as are increased illness and death of friends and family. The onset of a chronic illness, unexpected hospitalization, new medication prescription, or lapses in memory can evoke panic, as they may be perceived as threats to a person's independence.

Certain complexities exist for diagnosing anxiety in this population. Physical symptoms of anxiety, like chest pain, severe headaches, or nausea, are often associated with more serious cardiac or neurological conditions. Frequent urination, insomnia, dry mouth, or cold or sweaty hands are common in the population (National Council on Aging, 2024), confusing an anxiety diagnosis. Patients may perseverate over symptoms of a heart attack, stroke, or other serious medical event, and self-medication for anxiety by substance use is prevalent. Furthermore, stress over life events may contribute to hormonal or other chemical imbalances in older adults. Gastrointestinal and other disorders related to inflammation and auto-immune disorders, such as irritable bowel syndrome, lupus, psoriasis, and rheumatoid arthritis, also commonly present (Zheng et al., 2023). Any of these diagnoses can exacerbate anxiety, which may then warrant further treatment.

POPULATION-FOCUSED MONITORING

This section is divided into two content areas: First, a review of general risk factors for anxiety, and second, content boxes on how anxiety manifests for several traditionally marginalized and at-risk groups: LGBTQIA+, members of the military and veterans, persons with disabilities, and women.

LGBTQIA+

LGBTQIA+ communities have long been understood to experience worse mental health outcomes than people who are *cisgender* (those whose gender identity aligns with their sex at birth). The LGBTQIA+ population contends with stigma and with life stressors over employment stability, finances, housing, and persistent discrimination, which contribute to higher levels of anxiety and higher rates of DSM-diagnosable anxiety disorders (Petruzzella et al., 2020). Moreover, concealment of one's sexual identity from family and friends can add to angst (Cohen et al., 2016). Fear of rejection by healthcare providers and other barriers to care also affect the community, especially transgender and nonbinary youth (Sileo et al., 2022; Tordoff et al., 2022).

Box 4.6 details diagnostic considerations for case managers working with the population. Additional resources for LGBTQIA+ friendly providers appear in the chapter resources list.

Box 4.6: Anxiety and LGBTQIA+

High incidence for:

- Generalized anxiety disorder
- Social phobias
- Panic disorders

Distinct considerations:

- Concealment of sexual identity, especially for youth and young adults
- Worry about rejection by family members and friends
- Fear of inability to access care, especially gender-affirming intervention
- Worry over quality of life and ability to live an authentic life

Feeling guarded with healthcare professionals due to a history of bias, stigma, and discrimination

Access to concordant care providers who respect their autonomy

- Contribution of HRSNs to high incidence of anxiety (e.g., employment, housing, or financial instability)

Military members and veterans

Anxiety is common among military personnel, their families, and veterans. The demands of military service take a toll: sudden deployments, repeated separations from family, combat exposure, moral and ethical conflicts, and high accountability to self and country, among others. Reintegration into civilian life can be difficult, as can a loss of identity and purpose as military members transition into veteran status and the private work sector.

Approximately 8 percent of veterans screened positive on the GAD-7 for mild anxiety and probable generalized anxiety disorder (MacDonald-Gagnon et al., 2024). Upwards of 24 percent of veterans had moderate to severe anxiety (Wounded Warrior Project, 2022). Trauma disorders are also common among military members and veterans. The DSM-5 moved trauma and stressor-related disorders—such as post-traumatic stress disorder, acute stress disorder, and adjustment disorders—out of the anxiety disorders category and into their own. Trauma disorders are addressed in Chapter 10. Box 4.7 summarizes key areas of focus for these populations.

Box 4.7: Anxiety and military members and veterans

High incidence for:

- Comorbid substance use
  - Generalized anxiety disorder
  - Panic disorder
  - Panic attacks

Distinct considerations:

- Worries about reintegrating into family life or a personal role after deployment, retirement, or other separation
  - Isolation
  - For veterans, loss of connection to military, including access to basic allowance for housing and other needs
  - Loss of identity, purpose, and value
  - Perfectionism; use of strict discipline with family, friends, and at work
  - Physical complaints that mask anxiety (e.g., sleep issues, fatigue, racing heartbeat)
  - Reconciling moral and ethical dilemmas from service

Persons with disabilities

Individuals with visible and invisible disabilities have higher rates of mental health conditions, particularly anxiety, than people who aren't disabled. More than the physical or mental impairment itself, the failure of society to ensure appropriate accommodations can trigger anxiety (Koenig et al., 2024). Healthcare providers inadvertently devalue their symptoms or decision-making capacity. Another barrier to care may be ineffective care coordination among multiple specialists. Difficulty coordinating care only adds to the population's anxiety about quality healthcare (Dong et al., 2020).

A person with a functional disability (e.g., vision, hearing, mobility, communicating, concentrating) is 552 percent more likely to be diagnosed with anxiety than someone without, and the population displays higher rates of psychological distress over a 30-day period. Persons with disabilities may face multiple HRSNs, especially unemployment, low socioeconomic status, and housing instability (Lindsay et al., 2024). They also have higher rates of comorbid anxiety and chronic illness (e.g., thyroid, respiratory, and gastrointestinal diseases; migraines; systemic allergies) and higher incidence of mild, moderate, and severe anxiety (Dong et al., 2020; Sereen et al., 2006). Box 4.8 provides a comprehensive view of key areas for case managers.

Box 4.8: Anxiety and persons with disabilities

High incidence for:

- Mild, moderate, and severe anxiety
- Generalized anxiety disorder
- Anxiety due to another medical condition
- Unspecified anxiety disorder
- Comorbid chronic illnesses

Distinct considerations:

- Worry about medical invalidation by providers
- Stress over obstacles to care coordination
- HRSNs
- Being disempowered by others

Women's health

Women experience anxiety disorders more than men, with the highest incidence for generalized anxiety disorder, panic disorder, and specific phobias. Hantsoo and Epperson (2017) found that the lifetime prevalence of a specific phobia is double for women (12-27 percent) what it is for men (6-12 percent). Generalized anxiety disorder rates are similarly doubled—6 percent for women, 3 percent for men. For social anxiety, the prevalence is marginally higher among women (5 percent) than among men (4 percent). Women diagnosed with premenstrual dysphoric disorder (PMDD) experience comorbid generalized anxiety disorder at rates up to 40 percent, panic disorder at 25 percent, and social anxiety disorder at approximately 20 percent (Hantsoo & Epperson, 2017).

Gender-specific factors have long been identified as drivers of anxiety in women. These factors include menstrual cycles, position on the menopause continuum, and hormonal imbalances due to, for example, endocrine-disrupting chemicals, air pollution, or lifestyle factors such as chronic stress or lack of sleep (Rannaud-Bartaire et al., 2024). They are far from the only factors, however. In fact, the understanding of cause is shifting away from gender-specific factors to other reasons, such as neurodiversity. Emerging research demonstrates that executive and cognitive functioning (e.g., intellectual operations, sensory processing), environmental stressors (e.g., socioeconomics, sociopolitics, trauma), and comorbidities influence how anxiety presents (Mendoza et al., 2024). For example, enhanced understanding of *neurodiversity*—variations in how each brain processes information, sustains attention, and manages impulsivity—is forging new views on how each person handles their anxiety (Otu & Sefotho, 2024). These perspectives are shifting the diagnosis and treatment of anxiety and other mental health disorders.

The literature has traditionally attached "women" and "women's health" to people born as biological females. But anxiety is also more prevalent in transgender and *gender diverse* individuals (those outside the gender norm of male or female). Kattari et al. (2020) found that 68.8 percent of transgender and gender diverse people present with anxiety symptoms and potential anxiety disorders, compared with 32.8 percent of cisgender persons. Upwards of 80 percent of trans individuals have symptoms of moderate to severe anxiety (Restar et al., 2024). Increasing political discourse around transgender rights, along with new legislation limiting their healthcare access, may be contributing factors to the population's increased prevalence of anxiety. Box 4.9 presents a comprehensive view of this multifaceted diagnostic area.

Box 4.9: Anxiety and women's health

High incidence of:

- o Generalized anxiety disorder
- o Panic disorder
- o Social anxiety disorder
- o Specific phobia

Distinct considerations:

- o Cognitive functioning (e.g., neurocognitive disorders, neurodiversity)
- o Executive functioning
- o Gender-typical stereotypes about who is defined as "female," which doesn't account for trans and gender-diverse individuals
- o Hormonal imbalances and shifts
- o Presence of premenstrual dysphoric disorder (PMDD)
- o Menopause continuum (perimenopause, menopause, and post-menopause)

SCREENING AND ASSESSMENT TOOLS FOR ANXIETY

Behavioral health screening instruments are so valuable the list of choices keeps expanding. The most popular evidence-based tools are provided here, though case managers and their teams may use others. The American Psychological Association provides a list of screening options for mental health conditions. The website is provided in the chapter resources list.

A variety of standardized screening tools assess anxiety. Their use varies by profession and practice setting. Many settings prefer brief and comprehensive screening tools, such as the GAD-7, while others choose robust tools that give a detailed picture of clinical manifestations for anxiety and other disorders (e.g., depression, stress), such as the DASS-21. Table 4.2 displays several current options.

Table 4.2: *Screening tools for anxiety*

Instrument	Focus	Source
Beck Anxiety Inventory (BAI)	21-item self-report questionnaire measuring the intensity of physical and cognitive anxiety symptoms	Beck, A.T. & Steer, R.A. (1993). *Beck Anxiety Inventory Manual.* San Antonio, TX: Psychological Corporation.
Depression, Anxiety, Stress Scale (DASS-21)	21-item self-report instrument to measure the related emotional states of depression, anxiety, and tension/stress	Lovibond, S.H. & Lovibond, P.F. (1995). *Depression Anxiety Stress Scales (DASS-21, DASS-42)* [Database record]. APA PsycTests. https://doi.org/10.1037/t01004-000
Generalized Anxiety Disorder (GAD-7 and GAD-2)	7-item (or 2-item short version) self-report questionnaire to assess the likelihood of Generalized Anxiety Disorder (GAD) based on DSM criteria	Spitzer, R.L., Kroenke, K., Williams, J.B.W. & Löwe, B. (2006). *Generalized Anxiety Disorder 7 (GAD-7)* [Database record]. APA PsycTests. https://doi.org/10.1037/t02591-000
Geriatric Anxiety Scale	30-item (or 10-item short version) self-report measure to assess and quantify anxiety symptoms in older adults	Segal, D.L., June, A., Payne, M., Coolidge, F.L. & Yochim, B. (2010). Development and initial validation of a self-report assessment tool for anxiety among older adults: The Geriatric Anxiety Scale. *Journal of Anxiety Disorders, 24*, 709-714.
Hamilton Anxiety Rating Scale	14-item clinician-administered scale that provides a detailed assessment of anxiety symptoms	Hamilton, M. (1959). The assessment of anxiety states by rating. *British Journal of Medical Psychology, 32*, 50-55.
Screen for Child Anxiety Related Disorders (SCARED)	41-item self-report questionnaire, covering 5 factors, to measure symptoms of DSM anxiety disorders in children	Muris, P., Merckelbach, H., Mayer, B., van Brakel, A., Thissen, S., Moulaert, V. & Gadet, B. (1998). The Screen for Child Anxiety Related Emotional Disorders (SCARED) and traditional childhood anxiety measures. *Journal of Behavior Therapy and Experimental Psychiatry, 29*(4), 327-339. https://doi.org/10.1016/s0005-7916(98)00023-8
Social Phobia Inventory Scale (SPIN) or Mini-SPIN	17-item (or 3-item short version) self-administered tool to evaluate fear, avoidance, and physiology	Connor, K.M., Davidson, J.R., Churchill, L.E., Sherwood, A., Foa, E. & Weisler, R.H. (2000). Psychometric properties of the Social Phobia Inventory (SPIN). New self-rating scale. *The British Journal of Psychiatry, 176*, 379-386. https://doi.org/10.1192/bjp.176.4.379

CONCLUSION

We've wrapped up our content on anxiety disorders. Anxiety is a complex behavioral health condition with a variety of manifestations. The range of symptoms and DSM-5-TR diagnoses present differently across populations.

Let us now move on to the curious and complex domain of chronic illness and chronic pain. These conditions have unique considerations and intersect with a number of behavioral health manifestations and mental illnesses.

CONTEMPLATION QUESTIONS

1. Consider a situation where you experienced anxiety, then answer the following prompts:
   a) Identify where your symptoms fell on the anxiety continuum.
   b) How did the symptoms impact your social, occupational, or academic functioning?
   c) What did you do to resolve the anxiety?
   d) What did you learn about yourself as you moved through the process?
2. Access the GAD-7 from the MD+CALC website in the chapter resources list.
   a) Review the screening tool.
   b) Complete it for yourself, then total your score.
   c) Reflect on how a standardized tool for anxiety will inform your work.
3. Review the anxiety disorders in Table 4.1.
   a) Which diagnoses are you most familiar with, personally or professionally?
   b) Reflect on your professional experiences with patients diagnosed with anxiety disorders.

Use the following case scenario and the Behavioral Health Conversation Map in Table 1.4 to respond to questions 4 and 5.

Mia, a case manager, is assigned to follow patients who are discharged from the inpatient behavioral health unit and who will attend the hospital's intensive out-patient program. The patients' cases were previously opened by the inpatient case manager, who interacted with the patients and their family/legal decision-makers to varying degrees.

1. Which phase of the conversation map should Mia start at, and why?
2. Reflect on how use of the behavioral health conversation map supports Mia's case management intervention.

RESOURCES

- **American Psychiatric Association:**
  Diagnostic and Statistical Manual of Mental Disorders, DSM-5-TR
  https://www.psychiatry.org/psychiatrists/practice/dsm
- **American Psychological Association: Measurement-based care and suggested measures**
  https://www.apaservices.org/practice/measurement-based-care/suggested-measures
- **Anxiety and Depression Association of America**
  https://www.ncoa.org/older-adults/health/behavioral-health/depression-anxiety/
- **Centers for Disease Control and Prevention: Children's Mental Health**
  https://www.cdc.gov/children-mental-health/about/about-anxiety-and-depression-in-children.html
- **MD+CALC**
  https://www.mdcalc.com/calc/1727/gad7-general-anxiety-disorder7
- **National Council on Aging**
  https://www.ncoa.org/
- **Outcare Health LGBTQIA+ friendly providers and resources**
  https://www.outcarehealth.org/
- **World Health Organization: Anxiety Key Facts**
  https://www.who.int/news-room/fact-sheets/detail/anxiety-disorders
- **Wounded Warrior Project**
  https://newsroom.woundedwarriorproject.org

REFERENCES

- Ahad, A.A., Sanchez-Gonzalez, M., & Junquera, P. (2023). Understanding and addressing mental health stigma across cultures for improving psychiatric care: A narrative review. *Cureus*, *15*(5), e39549. https://doi.org/10.7759/cureus.39549
- Alegría, M., Cruz-Gonzalez, M., O'Malley, I.S., Alvarez, K., Stein, G.L., Fuentes, L., Eddington, K., Poindexter, C., Markle, S.L., & Thorndike, A.N. et al. (2022). Role of social determinants in anxiety and depression symptoms during COVID-19: A longitudinal study of adults in North Carolina and Massachusetts. *Behaviour Research and Therapy*, *154*, 104102. https://doi.org/10.1016/j.brat.2022.104102
- American Psychiatric Association. (2022). *Diagnostic and Statistical Manual of Mental Disorders* (5th ed., text rev.). https://doi.org/10.1176/appi.books.9780890425787
- Bie, F., Yan, X., Xing, J., Wang, L., Xu, Y., Wang, G., Wang, Q., Guo, J., Qiao, J., & Rao, Z. (2024). Rising global burden of anxiety disorders among adolescents and young adults: Trends,

risk factors, and the impact of socioeconomic disparities and COVID-19 from 1990 to 2021. *Frontiers in Psychiatry, 15*, 1489427. https://doi.org/10.3389/fpsyt.2024.1489427

- Centers for Disease Control and Prevention. (2024). Anxiety and Depression in Children: Children's Mental Health. Retrieved December 17, 2024, from https://www.cdc.gov/children-mental-health/about/about-anxiety-and-depression-in-children.html
- Cohen, J.M., Blasey, C., Barr Taylor, C., Weiss, B.J., & Newman, M.G. (2016). Anxiety and related disorders and concealment in sexual minority young adults. *Behavior Therapy*, *47*(1), 91-101. https://doi.org/10.1016/j.beth.2015.09.006
- Dong, L., Freedman, V.A., & Mendes de Leon, C.F. (2020). The association of comorbid depression and anxiety symptoms with disability onset in older adults. *Psychosomatic Medicine*, *82*(2), 158-164. https://doi.org/10.1097/PSY.0000000000000763
- Engel, G.L. (1977). The need for a new medical model: A challenge for biomedicine. *Science, 196*(4286), 129-136. https://doi.org/10.1126/science.847460
- Garb, H.N. (2021). Race bias and gender bias in the diagnosis of psychological disorders. *Clinical Psychology Review*, *90*, 102087. https://doi.org/10.1016/j.cpr.2021.102087
- Hantsoo, L. & Epperson, C.N. (2017). Anxiety disorders among women: A female lifespan approach. *Focus*, *15*(2), 162-172. https://doi.org/10.1176/appi.focus.20160042
- Kattari, S.K., Kattari, L., Johnson, I., Lacombe-Duncan, A., & Misiolek, B.A. (2020). Differential experiences of mental health among trans/gender diverse adults in Michigan. *International Journal of Environmental Research and Public Health*, *17*(18), 6805. https://doi.org/10.3390/ijerph17186805
- Kavelaars, R., Ward, H., Mackie, D.S., Modi, K.M., & Mohandas, A. (2023). The burden of anxiety among a nationally representative U.S. adult population. *Journal of Affective Disorders*, *336*, 81-91. https://doi.org/10.1016/j.jad.2023.04.069
- Koenig, J., McLean, K.J., & Bishop, L. (2024). Psychological distress and mental health diagnoses in adults by disability and functional difficulty status: Findings from the 2021 national health interview survey. *Disability and Health Journal*, *17*(4), 101641. https://doi.org/10.1016/j.dhjo.2024.101641
- Lindsay, S., Fuentes, K., Ragunathan, S., Li, Y., & Ross, T. (2024). Accessible independent housing for people with disabilities: A scoping review of promising practices, policies and interventions. *PloS One*, *19*(1), e0291228. https://doi.org/10.1371/journal.pone.0291228
- Macdonald-Gagnon, G., Stefanovics, E.A., Potenza, M.N., & Pietrzak, R.H. (2024). Generalized anxiety and mild anxiety symptoms in U.S. military veterans: Prevalence, characteristics, and functioning. *Journal of Psychiatric Research*, *171*, 263-270. https://doi.org/10.1016/j.jpsychires.2024.02.013
- Mendoza, L.S.M., Trujillo-Güiza, M., Forero, D.A. *et al.* (2024). Health, psychosocial and cognitive factors associated with anxiety symptoms. *Current Psychology, 43*, 22376-22388. https://doi.org/10.1007/s12144-024-05998-3

- Merck Manual. (2024). *Treatment of Generalized Anxiety Disorder*, Professional version. Retrieved December 14, 2024, from https://www.merckmanuals.com/professional/psychiatric-disorders/anxiety-and-stressor-related-disorders/generalized-anxiety-disorder
- Merck Manual. (2023a). *Panic Attacks and Panic Disorder,* Professional version. Retrieved December 15, 2024, from https://www.merckmanuals.com/professional/psychiatric-disorders/anxiety-and-stressor-related-disorders/panic-attacks-and-panic-disorder
- Merck Manual. (2023b). *Specific Phobias,* Professional version. Retrieved December 15, 2024, from https://www.merckmanuals.com/professional/psychiatric-disorders/anxiety-and-stressor-related-disorders/specific-phobias
- Merck Manual. (2023c). *Social Anxiety Disorder,* Professional version. Retrieved December 15, 2024, from https://www.merckmanuals.com/professional/psychiatric-disorders/anxiety-and-stressor-related-disorders/social-anxiety-disorder
- National Council on Aging. (2024). *Anxiety and Older Adults: A Guide to Getting the Relief You Need.* Retrieved December 17, 2024, from https://www.ncoa.org/article/anxiety-and-older-adults-a-guide-to-getting-the-relief-you-need/
- O'Connor, E.A., Henninger, M.L., Perdue, L.A., Coppola, E.L., Thomas, R.G., & Gaynes, B.N. (2023). Anxiety screening: Evidence report and systematic review for the U.S. Preventive Services Task Force. *JAMA*, *329*(24), 2171-2184. https://doi.org/10.1001/jama.2023.6369
- Otu, M.S., & Sefotho, M.M. (2024). Examination of emotional distress, depression, and anxiety in neurodiverse students: A cross-sectional study. *World Journal of Psychiatry*, *14*(11), 1681-1695. https://doi.org/10.5498/wjp.v14.i11.1681
- Petruzzella, A., Feinstein, B.A., Davila, J., & Lavner, J.A. (2020). Gay-specific and general stressors predict gay men's psychological functioning over time. *Archives of Sexual Behavior*, *49*(5), 1755-1767. https://doi.org/10.1007/s10508-020-01672-4
- Powell, S.K. & Tahan, H.M. (2019). *Case Management: A Practical Guide for Education and Practice*, 4th ed. Wolters Kluwer: Philadelphia, PA.
- Rannaud-Bartaire, P., Demeneix, B.A., & Fini, J.B. (2024). Pressures of the urban environment on the endocrine system: Adverse effects and adaptation. *Molecular and Cellular Endocrinology, 583,* 112125. https://doi.org/10.1016/j.mce.2023.112125
- Restar, A., Layland, E.K., Hughes, L., Dusic, E., Lucas, R., Bambilla, A.J.K., Martin, A., & Shook, A. et al. (2024). Antitrans policy environment and depression and anxiety symptoms in transgender and nonbinary adults. *JAMA Network Open*, *7*(8), e2431306. https://doi.org/10.1001/jamanetworkopen.2024.31306
- Sileo, K.M., Baldwin, A., Huynh, T.A., Olfers, A., Woo, J., Greene, S.L., Casillas, G.L., & Taylor, B.S. (2022). Assessing LGBTQ+ stigma among healthcare professionals: An application of the health stigma and discrimination framework in a qualitative, community-based participatory research study. *Journal of Health Psychology*, *27*(9), 2181-2196. https://doi.org/10.1177/13591053211027652

- Tordoff, D.M., Wanta, J.W., Collin, A., Stepney, C., Inwards-Breland, D.J., & Ahrens, K. (2022). Mental health outcomes in transgender and nonbinary youths receiving gender-affirming care. *JAMA Network Open*, *5*(2), e220978. https://doi.org/10.1001/jamanetworkopen.2022.0978
- U.S. Preventive Services Task Force, Mangione, C.M., Barry, M.J., Nicholson, W.K., Cabana, M., Coker, T.R., Davidson, K.W., Davis, E.M., & Donahue, K.E. et al. (2022). Screening for anxiety in children and adolescents: U.S. Preventive Services Task Force recommendation statement. *JAMA*, *328*(14), 1438-1444. https://doi.org/10.1001/jama.2022.16936
- World Health Organization. (2023). Anxiety Disorders: Key Facts. Retrieved December 16, 2024, from https://www.who.int/news-room/fact-sheets/detail/anxiety-disorders
- Wounded Warrior Project. (2022). *Gaining Control Over Anxiety;* Newsroom. Retrieved December 18, 2024, from https://newsroom.woundedwarriorproject.org/Gaining-Control-Over-Anxiety
- Yan, D., Zheng, G., Wang, C., Chen, Z., Mao, T., Gao, J., Yan, Y., Chen, X., Ji, X., & Yu, J. et al. (2022). HIT 2.0: An enhanced platform for Herbal Ingredients' Targets. *Nucleic Acids Research*, *50*(D1), D1238-D1243. https://doi.org/10.1093/nar/gkab1011
- Zhang, W., Yan, Y., Wu, Y., Yang, H., Zhu, P., Yan, F., Zhao, R., Tian, P., Wang, T., Fan, Q., & Su, Z. (2022). Medicinal herbs for the treatment of anxiety: A systematic review and network meta-analysis. *Pharmacological Research*, *179*, 106204. https://doi.org/10.1016/j.phrs.2022.106204
- Zheng, Y., Liu, Q., Goronzy, J.J., & Weyand, C.M. (2023). Immune aging – A mechanism in autoimmune disease. *Seminars in Immunology*, *69*, 101814. https://doi.org/10.1016/j.smim.2023.101814

CHAPTER 5

CHRONIC ILLNESS

INTRODUCTION

Chronic pain and chronic illness are indelibly connected, and case managers must wrestle with behavioral health manifestations for both conditions. This chapter addresses the intersection of these chronic conditions with behavioral health. We explore the perspective shift away from chronic disease toward chronic illness, the subjective experiences of pain, and DSM-5-TR diagnoses aligned with chronic conditions. The incidence, prevalence, and manifestations of chronic conditions among age groups and populations will also be presented.

BEHAVIORAL LEARNING OBJECTIVES

1. Define chronic pain
2. Understand the different uses of the terms 'chronic illness' and 'chronic disease'
3. Understand the intersection of chronic illness, chronic pain, and mental health
4. Identify signs, symptoms, and treatment recommendations for common DSM diagnoses associated with chronic illness and chronic pain
5. Analyze the incidence of chronic illness and chronic pain across life stages and populations
6. Identify the implications of chronic illness and chronic pain in behavioral health across marginalized and minoritized populations
7. Understand malingering and manipulating
8. Cite how concordant care enhances treatment outcomes
9. Identify how medical gaslighting factors into chronic pain assessment
10. Define screening tools used to assess chronic pain
11. Apply Case Management's Behavioral Health Conversation Map to patients and families living with chronic illness and chronic pain

ESSENTIAL TERMS

- Chronic disease
- Chronic illness
- Chronic pain
- Chronic primary pain
- Chronic secondary pain
- Conversion disorder
- Factitious disorder imposed on another
- Factitious disorder imposed on self
- Functional neurological symptom disorder
- High impact chronic pain
- Illness anxiety disorder
- Labile mood
- Malingering
- Manipulation
- Neuropathic pain
- Somatic symptom disorder
- Psychogenic pain
- Psychological factors impacting other medical conditions

TERMS AND FEATURES OF CHRONIC ILLNESS AND CHRONIC PAIN

Let's start with a common question on this topic: Why the term 'chronic illness' instead of 'chronic disease'? The latter term is used in research and scholarly publications, as a biomedical disease classification. This conventional view of disease categorizes illnesses based on three assumptions (Wade & Halligan, 2004):

1. All illness has one underlying cause,
2. Disease (pathology) is always the single cause, and
3. Removal of the disease will restore health.

Yet the healthcare industry is moving away from viewing chronic disease via a single lens, instead transitioning to a more progressive panoramic view under the term *chronic illness*.

CHRONIC ILLNESS

Case managers know the reality of what drives health outcomes, and it is quite different from the outdated notion of simple biomedical disease classification. It is now common knowledge in healthcare that 80 percent of a person's health is driven by factors outside of biology, such as socioeconomic status, exposure to adverse childhood experiences, employment, housing sufficiency, nutritional sufficiency, and the quality of and access to education and healthcare. Whether you know them as the SDoH, HRSNs, social drivers, influencers of health, or another name, these issues impact illness onset, morbidity, and mortality.

The term *chronic illness*, then, implies a wider perspective that encompasses a person's lived experiences, as well as the medical presentation of his or her chronic disease. The chronic illness framing presumes a biopsychosocial approach to care, accounting for the entirety of the human condition and a whole-person view. The approach also aligns with the latest generation of patient-reported outcomes measures (PROMs) discussed in Chapter 3.

There is no single definition for chronic illness. The construct is broadly defined as a group of conditions that last a minimum of one year and require ongoing medical care or limit daily activities, or both (Centers for Disease Control and Prevention, 2024a). Chronic conditions challenge a person's independence and self-sufficiency and disrupt quality of life. People's sense of self and well-being are undermined by functional limitations, which can lead to isolation from family, friends, and communities. Independent of the primary diagnosis, a person with chronic illness can experience an array of behavioral health manifestations, from anxiety and agitation to *a labile mood* characterized by rapid and sudden shifts in their presentation. These shifts in mood are also caused by unpredictable symptom presentation and the challenge of managing pain medication dosing.

Imagine you are working with a new patient who has been diagnosed with chronic obstructive pulmonary disease (COPD). She experiences worsening respiratory compromise and decreased endurance and appetite. The symptoms interfere with her ability to engage in work, even part-time. Her role as family breadwinner has been drastically altered, and her self-esteem drops. This loss of control of physical functioning takes a toll on a person's mental health as other psychosocial stressors pile on, such as need for a caregiver, reduced income, and weakened family infrastructure.

Not all patients diagnosed with chronic illness develop mental health conditions, but they're at greater risk of co-aligned conditions, compared to the general population. More than 50 percent of persons diagnosed with mental disorders also live with a chronic medical condition (Wan et al., 2021). This fusion of health concerns appears in Figure 5.1. The combination can complicate diagnosis and treatment, but it also emphasizes the value of whole-person care.

Figure 5.1: *Interplay between chronic illness, chronic pain, and mental health*

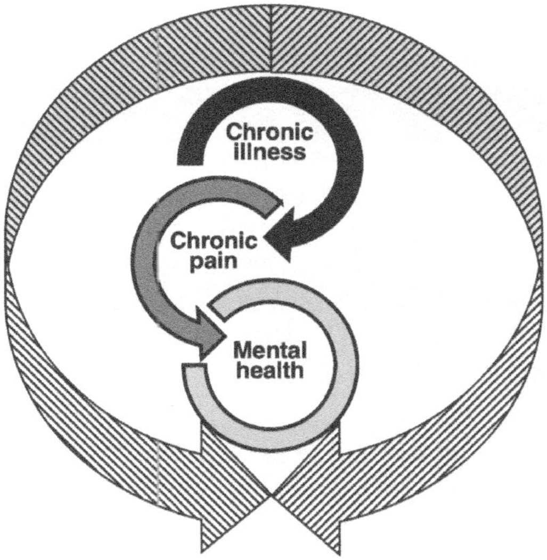

CHRONIC PAIN

There is no standardized consensus of the pain experience, as sensations of pain and discomfort are relative to each person. T*he diagnostic parameters for chronic pain are also far from defined, but it is traditionally* considered pain persisting beyond three months (Dydyk & Conerman, 2024). The International Association for the Study of Pain (IASP) offers an equally subjective definition: an "unpleasant sensory and emotional experience associated with, or resembling that associated with, actual or potential tissue damage" (2020). Figure 5.2 displays the four types of pain and their identified etiology.

The *ICD Official Guidelines* (Centers for Disease Control and Prevention, 2024b) do not define the length of time when pain becomes "chronic," so practitioners make subjective determinations. "R5: Pain, unspecified" is the ICD-10 code typically used when the exact location or cause of pain is not documented. For accurate diagnosis and treatment, however, coding the severity and duration of the pain and associated factors, such as "M54.5: lumbar region pain" or "G89.3: Neoplasm related pain (acute or chronic)" is important. ICD-10 provides 162 distinct codes for pain. The most used codes are shown in Box 5.1.

Figure 5.2: *Four categories of pain*

Acute

- A normal temporary response to injury (e.g., broken bone, cuts, surgical intervention)

Chronic Pain

- Discomfot that lasts more than 6 months
- Caused by a variety of health conditions

Neuropathic Pain

- Caused by nerve damange or dysfunction of the nervous system (e.g., cancer, diabetic neuropathy, stroke)
- Sensations: burning, shooting, stabbing discomfort

Nociceptive Pain

- Caused by tissue damage (e.g., burns, cuts, inflammation, injuries)
- Sensations: throbbing, sharp, aches

Information from Armstrong, S.A. & Herr, M.J., 2023

Box 5.1: Most common ICD-10 codes for pain

- R52.2: Other chronic pain
- M54.5: Low back pain
- M79.6: Pain in limb

Zinboonyahgoon et al., 2021

CULTURAL PERSPECTIVES AND PRESENTATIONS OF PAIN

The ICD-11 Shift

ICD-11 treats chronic pain with a wider lens, providing a diagnostic code, MG30.0, for chronic primary pain, which will no longer only be viewed as a symptom of another condition. There will be differentiation between chronic primary pain, or pain not directly attributable to another disease, and chronic secondary pain, pain arising from a known underlying medical condition (Dohenny, 2022; Treede et al., 2019). These revisions are expected to shift assessment and treatment of chronic pain and reduce the stigma associated with chronic pain diagnosis.

Since pain is a subjective and relative construct, the perception of its severity is unique to each patient. Cultural perspectives of pain demonstrate how the pain experience can present differently. Some populations show extravagant emotional reaction, while others are stoic and restrict visible displays of discomfort (Rogger et al., 2023). *Think about your cultural experiences of pain. Did you grow up with the prevailing U.S. cultural view that showing pain reflects weakness? Did you learn that pain is a test of moral character? Were you told to "grin and bear it" or "just deal with it"? The disparities in presentation of pain by race, ethnicity, and gender have led researchers and practitioners to create multiple pain scales, in attempt to standardize pain measurement. But cultural nuances still complicate assessment of chronic pain, making it among the most challenging behavioral health conditions to address.*

Misconceptions about the pain response contribute to treatment inequities. Mende-Siedlecki et al. (2019) explored the high prevalence for mistreatment of pain across racial groups due to stereotypes and prejudices, including status judgements. Providers' racial biases about pain may lead to biases in treatment decisions. For example, some people endorse the incorrect notion that biological differences provide Black patients higher pain tolerance than other races (Hoffman et al., 2016). Another incorrect idea is that White people display more frequent and visible expressions of pain than do Blacks or other ethnic and racial groups (Mende-Siedlecki et al., 2019). These faulty perspectives invalidate the individual patient's experience and lead to dismissed symptoms, depression due to unresolved symptoms, and ultimately, higher mortality rates (Coady et al., 2024). *It becomes critical for* case managers to rely on their individual assessment of a patient's pain experience, rather than the opinions of colleagues or consultants.

Box 5.2 shows common cultural considerations regarding pain.

The presence of a mental health condition may alter a person's perception of pain. For example, depression or anxiety can exacerbate a person's discomfort, as can stress—consider how your own neck and back respond to emotional distress. Pain may be felt as a somatic, or physical, expression, as in aches, muscle tension, headaches, nausea, or stomach upset. Physical pain also influences mood lability and intense expressions, such as the emotional release of crying, screaming, or groaning. There may be displays of displaced anger or aggression, such as throwing things, lashing out at caregivers, or breaking objects.

Box 5.2: Common cultural considerations of pain

General U.S. beliefs

- The presence of pain is a sign of progress toward recovery
- Pain is a test of religious or spiritual faith or a penance for past sins

Persons of Asian descent

- Pain results from an imbalance between yin and yang

Persons of Hispanic descent

- Pain and illness signify disharmony with or punishment from God
- Pain should be endured bravely, and people—particularly those born as males— who can endure high intensity pain are admired as role models

Persons of Asian, Hispanic, and Indigenous descent

- Stoic or neutral expressions should be displayed, regardless of pain intensity
- Reduced emotional response to pain enhances a person's standing in the afterlife

Hollingshead et al., 2016; Rogger et al., 2023

COMMON BEHAVIORAL HEALTH DISORDERS ASSOCIATED WITH CHRONIC ILLNESS AND CHRONIC PAIN

DSM-5-TR placed somatic symptoms of chronic pain and related disorders in a distinct category, per Table 5.1. The new category replaces the section in prior versions that encompassed all pain-related diagnoses (e.g., somatization disorder, pain disorder, undifferentiated somatoform disorder). Hypochondriasis was reconfigured as somatic symptom disorder. This revised framing can minimize practitioner bias. As with most categories for *other mental illnesses*, 'unspecified' refers to when a patient has some symptoms of a disorder but does not meet the full diagnostic criteria.

Table 5.1: *DSM-5-TR diagnoses associated with chronic pain and chronic illness*

DSM-5-TR Diagnosis	Code
Factitious disorder imposed on another (formerly factitious disorder by proxy or Munchausen syndrome by proxy)	F68.A
Factitious disorder imposed on self	F68.10
• Unspecified	F68.10
• With predominantly psychological signs and symptoms	F68.11
• With predominantly physical signs and symptoms	F68.12
• With combined psychological and physical signs and symptoms	F68.13
Functional neurological symptom disorder (formerly conversion disorder	F44
Illness anxiety disorder	F45.21
Psychological factors affecting other medical conditions	F54
Somatic symptom disorder	F45.1
Other specific somatic symptom and related disorder	F45.8
Unspecified somatic symptom and related disorder	F45.9

Adapted from American Psychiatric Association, 2022

FACTITIOUS DISORDER IMPOSED ON ANOTHER (FORMERLY MUNCHAUSEN SYNDROME BY PROXY) AND FACTITIOUS DISORDER IMPOSED ON SELF

Imagine that a parent brings his child to a pediatrician for symptoms whose etiology can't be defined. There are complaints of chronic nausea, abdominal pain, and lack of appetite, with a 102.5-degree fever. The patient is pale upon examination but displays no other symptoms. When the provider asks the child about the symptoms, the parent interjects, "My daughter needs an upper and lower endoscopy and potentially a colonoscopy." He requests prescription medication to treat his child's discomfort. The clinician is dubious about the child's condition, but the child is rubbing her abdomen. At the parent's insistence, orders are given for routine labs and follow-up with a pediatric gastroenterologist.

As the case manager, embedded in the pediatrician's office or conducting utilization review for an MCO, you wonder what could be contributing to this conflicting presentation of symptoms. Is there a physiological explanation for the symptoms—irritable bowel syndrome, celiac disease, or another condition? Is there medical cause for invasive diagnostics? Movie plots come to mind, where a parent gives a child over-the-counter treatments, from enemas to syrup of ipecac, to induce ailments. Then you wonder if you're overthinking this. The answer is you're most likely not overthinking it, as a case manager's clinical gut instincts appropriately contribute to assessments. You could be seeing a case of factitious disorder imposed on another.

Factitious disorder imposed on another, and its counterpart, *factitious disorder imposed on self,* can be difficult to diagnose, in part due to the high degree of denial by those afflicted. Another reason involves the extent individuals go to convince others of their illness. They may rub thermometers in their hands to display a higher temperature, or they may intentionally ingest substances or foods that induce physical illness. Other common tactics are tampering with bodily fluids for labs, cultures, and toxicology screens.

Another challenge for diagnosing factitious disorders comes from their inconsistent symptoms. A patient may present with sudden and uncontrolled swelling in the limbs during one ED or primary care visit (brought on by intentional injection of saline solution). Or he may present a confabulated history of serious illness, such as cancer, to specialists. Patients sometimes feign symptoms of rare neurodegenerative diseases, such as amyotrophic lateral sclerosis (ALS) or Parkinson's, and even generate fake medical records. Diagnostic criteria for the two factitious disorders appear in Boxes 5.3. and 5.4.

Persons suffering from these disorders reap emotional gains from their dysfunctional behaviors, as shown in Box 5.5. The behaviors, often attention-seeking, stem from unmet psychological needs, such as poor nurturing or attachment in infancy.

Box 5.3: Signs, symptoms, and treatment of factitious disorder imposed on another (formerly known as Munchausen syndrome by proxy)

Note: The perpetrator receives the diagnosis, not the victim.

DSM-5-TR criteria:

- Falsification of physical or psychological signs or symptoms or inducing injury or disease in another person, associated with identified deception
- Presenting another person (the victim) to others as ill, impaired, or injured
- Deceptive behavior is evident, even in the absence of obvious external rewards
- The behavior is not better explained by another mental disorder (e.g., delusional disorder) or other psychotic disorder

Specify:

- Single episode or recurrent episodes (two or more events of illness/injury falsification)

Treatments:

- Selective serotonin reuptake inhibitors (SSRIs) for depression or anxiety, though potential for overuse should be monitored
- Psychotherapy: CBT (individual therapy), family therapy, group therapy
- Monitor for manipulation and malingering

American Psychiatric Association, 2022, pp. 367-370

Box 5.4: Signs, symptoms, and treatment of factitious disorder imposed on self

DSM-5-TR criteria:

- Falsification of physical or psychological signs or symptoms or inducing injury or disease, associated with identified deception
- Individual presents as ill, impaired, or injured
- Deceptive behavior is evident, even in the absence of obvious external rewards
- The behavior is not better explained by another mental disorder (e.g., delusional disorder) or other psychotic disorder

Specify:

- Single episode or recurrent episodes (two or more events of illness/injury falsification)

Treatments:

- Selective serotonin reuptake inhibitors (SSRIs) for depression or anxiety, though potential for overuse should be monitored
- Psychotherapy: Cognitive behavioral therapy (individual), family therapy, group therapy
- Monitor for manipulation and malingering

American Psychiatric Association, 2022, pp. 367-370

Box 5.5: Common patient primary and secondary gains that drive factitious disorder

- Attention-seeking behaviors related to:
  - Pleasure derived from being in ill role, especially for individuals who sensed a lack of affection during childhood
  - Seeking and maintaining relationships
  - Enjoying being cared for by others
- A way to cope with stressful life events or a lack of identity
- Feeling a sense of accomplishment by duping physicians and other providers

Carnahan, 2023

FUNCTIONAL NEUROLOGICAL SYMPTOM DISORDER (FORMERLY CONVERSION DISORDER)

Consider this scenario: Mara is brought to the ED by her spouse, Jaye, for sudden onset of bilateral paralysis in her arms. "Mara was fine this morning. Then she called from work and said she had lost feeling in her arms," says Jaye. Upon exam, no overt medical etiology is identified. Mara is discharged to follow-up with her primary care provider. She is prescribed follow-up labs and diagnostic tests to rule out a stroke or other neurological or orthopedic etiology. Mara's condition worsens, however, and her disorder remains a mystery when neurodegenerative and neurocognitive conditions are ruled out. During a conversation with the MCO case manager, Jaye mentions that Mara recently attended a staff training on sexual assault prevention. He remarks, "She was fine at dinner, though seemed off. My wife is a good sleeper, but she tossed and turned all night. I heard her yell out a name but couldn't make it out." The case manager asks, "Do you know if your wife has ever been a victim of intimate partner violence or sexual assault?"

The case manager was correct to question Jaye about Mara's history, and she is eventually diagnosed with *functional neurological symptom disorder* (FNSD), previously known as conversion disorder. The condition is frightening, for it manifests as a sudden disruption to one of more of the five senses: numbness or loss of sensation, slurred speech or inability to express oneself, loss of vision or hearing, or cognitive disruption. Pain can result from any of the disorder's symptoms, often appearing as muscle cramps and spasms, migraine headaches, or esophageal discomfort.

Though not always, FSND can be triggered by a reaction to stress or an event that was perceived as traumatic, even when memories of the event have long stayed buried in the person's unconscious mind. (More on this topic in Chapter 10.) Fear of losing control or one's power may trigger symptoms. In Mara's case, it is likely she was the victim of a traumatic event. Her memories and associated emotions were internalized, stored within her unconscious, until being triggered by the sexual assault training. With FNSD, there is not usually damage to the brain's structure as in stroke, multiple sclerosis, infection, or other illness or injury, but rather is caused by what the brain perceives as a threat. FNSD can take months or years to diagnose.

The integration of physical and psychological symptoms in FNSD (and other disorders discussed in this chapter) provide a critical reminder for case managers to obtain a thorough biopsychosocial history for each patient and to gain knowledge of contributing pathophysiology, psychopathology, and psychosocial factors. Box 5.6 shows the range of symptoms for FNSD and treatment considerations.

Box 5.6: Signs, symptoms, and treatment of functional neurological symptom disorder

DSM-5-TR criteria:

- Diagnosis is only considered after a comprehensive medical examination and testing has ruled out neurologic or general medical disorders because they can't fully account for the symptoms and their effects
- Symptoms must be severe enough to cause significant distress or impair social, occupational, or other important areas of functioning
- Symptoms include:
    - Weakness or paralysis
    - Abnormal movement, tremors, difficulty ambulating
    - Loss of balance
    - Difficulty swallowing, or sensation of a lump in the throat
    - Seizures, loss of consciousness
    - Episodes of unresponsiveness
    - Numbness or loss of touch
    - Speech problems
    - Loss of or blurry vision
    - Deafness or loss of hearing
    - Memory loss, forgetfulness, or another cognitive dysfunction
- Symptoms and signs are not consistent with neurologic disease
    - A patient may have marked weakness of plantar flexion when tested in bed but can walk normally on tiptoes
    - In a supine patient, the examiner's hand under the heel of a "paralyzed" leg detects downward pressure when the patient lifts the unaffected leg against resistance (Hoover sign)
    - Tremors change or disappear when the patient is distracted (e.g., by having the patient copy a rhythmic movement with the unaffected hand)
    - Resistance to eye opening is detected during an apparent seizure
    - A visual field deficit is tubular (tunnel vision)

Treatments:

- Physical therapy
- Hypnosis
- Psychotherapy: Cognitive behavioral therapy
- Coexisting psychiatric disorders (e.g., depression) should be treated

American Psychiatric Association, 2022, pp. 360-364

ILLNESS ANXIETY DISORDER

Imagine you evaluate a patient who is appearing in the ED for the fifth time this month. The person complains of a freckle on his wrist, insisting, "It could bother me while I'm sleeping. I've heard that can happen. Or maybe it's melanoma; I could be dead in a few months." But the freckle has been present for several years and has not changed shape, color, or form. It's not painful, nor does it itch. The patient has visited a local dermatologist and his primary care physician repeatedly, and neither noted concern. This patient presents with *illness anxiety disorder* (IAD), formerly known as hypochondriasis, a mental health condition characterized by excessive worry or fear about having a serious illness, despite indicating no symptoms for the condition.

Many case managers have engaged with people who complain frequently about miscellaneous symptoms. The patients spend hours in providers' offices or urgent care centers. They may scour the internet for an explanation, but they are dissatisfied with lab and diagnostic test results, thinking there must be an alternative answer for the discomfort they feel. People with IAD can interpret normal bodily sensations (e.g., passing gas, heartburn) or minor health issues (e.g., common cold, constipation) as signs of severe medical conditions, even after a medical evaluation shows no etiology and yields a clean bill of health. Box 5.7 provides signs, symptoms, and treatment considerations for IAD.

Box 5.7: Signs, symptoms, and treatment of illness anxiety disorder

DSM-5-TR criteria:

The patient:

- Is preoccupied with having or acquiring a serious illness
- Has no or minimal somatic symptoms
- Is highly anxious about health and easily alarmed about personal health issues
- Repeatedly checks health status or maladaptively avoids doctor appointments and hospitals
- Has been preoccupied with illness ≥ 6 months, though a specific illness feared may change during that time
- Displays symptoms that are not better accounted for by depression or another psychiatric disorder

Treatments:

- Selective serotonin reuptake inhibitors (SSRIs) for depression or anxiety, though potential for overuse should be monitored
- Psychotherapy: Cognitive behavioral therapy

American Psychiatric Association, 2022, pp. 357-360

SOMATIC SYMPTOM DISORDER

People who chronically experience physical symptoms that intersect with excessive and maladaptive thoughts, emotions, and behaviors are diagnosed with *somatic symptom disorder.* These patients are emotionally dependent on their healthcare providers, craving response to their queries.

People prone to this attention-seeking behavior tend to reside alone, are isolated, or have limited interpersonal support, and they feel consoled and validated by support from physician's office or ED staff. Patients with somatic symptom disorder "provider-hop" from one practitioner to another seeking a diagnosis they feel explains their perceptions, or they may seek treatment from multiple practitioners simultaneously. These patients may become irate or desperate, even suicidal, if they feel their needs aren't met or their complaints aren't heard. Symptoms and treatment considerations for somatic symptom disorder are in Box 5.8.

Box 5.8: Signs, symptoms, and treatment of somatic symptom disorder

DSM-5-TR criteria:

Symptoms must be distressing or disruptive to daily life for greater than 6 months and be associated with at least one of the following:

- Disproportionate and persistent thoughts about the seriousness of the symptoms
- Persistently high anxiety about health or the symptoms
- Excessive time and energy spent on the symptoms or health concerns

Treatment:

- Psychotherapy: Cognitive behavioral therapy

American Psychiatric Association, 2022, pp. 351-356

PSYCHOLOGICAL FACTORS AFFECTING OTHER MEDICAL CONDITIONS

The body is an intricate system, and when people with chronic illnesses experience major life stressors like unemployment and loss of health insurance, the sudden angst can exacerbate the illness, even if it had been well-managed. A patient may require acute treatment to restabilize their symptoms, or they may need major adjustment to their pain medication dosage, prompting concern in the clinical team.

For example, a sudden, unexpected loss of a dwelling can put a person with an autoimmune disorder into autoimmune crisis, leading to tachycardia or uncontrolled inflammation. Both the physical condition and behavioral health must be stabilized. These individuals are often diagnosed with *psychological factors affecting other medical conditions,* the signs and symptoms of which appear in Box 5.9.

Box 5.9: Signs, symptoms, and treatment of psychological factors affecting other medical conditions

DSM-5-TR criteria:

- Patients have one or more clinically significant psychological or behavioral factors that adversely affect an existing general medical disorder (e.g., diabetes mellitus, heart disease) or symptom (e.g., pain).
- These factors may increase the risk of suffering, death, or disability; aggravate an underlying medical condition; or result in hospitalization or emergency department visit

Psychological or behavioral factors that can adversely affect a general medical disorder include:

- Denial of the significance or severity of symptoms
- Poor adherence to prescribed testing and treatment

Treatments:

- Psychotherapy: Cognitive behavioral therapy
- Selective serotonin reuptake inhibitors (SSRIs)

Financial impacts

Even though the behavioral health disorders discussed in this section are not widespread, their fiscal impact is massive. Factitious disorders affect less than three percent of the population but incur $40 million in medical expenses annually (Carnahan & Jha, 2023). This outsized impact makes the disorders a major priority in healthcare.

American Psychiatric Association, 2022, pp. 364-367

DIAGNOSTIC CONSIDERATIONS: MALINGERING AND MANIPULATION

Patients in any practice setting and age group may *malinger*—report physical symptoms they don't have, motivated by external incentives like missing work (Merriam-Webster, n.d.). Case managers and their teams struggle to distinguish between these fake symptoms and the patient's real ones. The patient isn't uncooperative but is manipulative. Malingering causes challenges for accurately diagnosing and treating patients.

Malingering presents in all populations, but 50 percent of cases occur in people with chronic illness and chronic pain (Punko et al. 2023). Reasons for malingering include avoiding employment, seeking financial compensation, or evading criminal prosecution. Medication- or drug-seeking behaviors are also common. Patients may malinger for other self-serving reasons, too, such as to defend against a provider dismissing their symptoms. Keep in mind, however, that a patient's attempts to derail evaluation or treatment through poor participation or nonadherence is not, in itself, malingering.

Case managers may become frustrated by deciphering malingering and manipulative behaviors; some professionals even avoid these patients altogether. But behavioral protocols exist to help healthcare workers manage malingering situations. To set these protocols in motion, the patient should be referred for a consultation with a behavioral health professional. Box 5.10 provides guidance for clinicians to consider.

Box 5.10: Patient presentation that may reflect malingering, manipulation, or factitious disorders

- Inconsistent information provided by the patient
- Symptoms that are especially dramatic or out of proportion with the suspected diagnosis
- Inconsistencies among symptoms and exam findings
- Inconsistencies in patient-provided information and past medical records
- Symptoms inconsistent with anatomy or physiology
- The patient resists the release of medical records
- The patient has an extensive past medical history and may have numerous ailments
- Extensive workup and no definite diagnosis
- Exam findings that contradict patient-provided information (e.g., patient denies history of surgeries but has surgical scars visible on a physical exam)

Carnahan, 2023

DATA AND DEMOGRAPHICS

When patients don't receive the care they need to manage chronic pain and chronic illness, many self-medicate, which leaves them susceptible to addiction, suicidal ideation, and suicide. Other general risk factors for these conditions appear below.

GENERAL RISK FACTORS

Lack of interdisciplinary care impedes thorough treatment of chronic illness and chronic pain. The U.S. Pain Foundation (2020) explored treatment realities for 1,500 adults. Over 74 percent of respondents had lived with some level of pain for 10 years or more, and 30 percent for over 20 years. Roughly 50 percent of respondents received Social Security Disability payments for their chronic pain (U.S. Pain Foundation, 2020). Some 50 percent of respondents were also diagnosed with a chronic illness.

Patients with access to pain management specialists reported that their healthcare team emphasized medicating the pain by prescription medication, epidural nerve blocks, and targeted injections, rather than offering restorative therapies or treatment by behavioral health specialists, nutritionists, and physical therapists. Alternative treatments (e.g., healing touch, neurofeedback, reiki) were not offered or covered by insurance (U.S. Pain Foundation, 2020).

DEVELOPMENTAL LIFE STAGES

Chronic illness and chronic pain manifest differently in each person and across age groups. This section provides an overview of the incidence, prevalence, and fiscal burden of these disorders across the lifespan.

Youth

The annual cost of pediatric pain management in the U.S. is almost $20 billion annually (Groenewald et al., 2019). Prevalence of chronic pain in youth vary by symptom presentation. For example, primary headache disorders span 19.4 to over 66 percent of children and adolescents, and gastrointestinal disorders affect 4.6 to 31.2 percent (Rikard et al., 2023). The lack of appropriate assessment by providers and limited access to specialists are among the causes for these disparate numbers.

Youth who present with chronic pain are at increased risk for co-occurring behavioral health conditions, especially depression and anxiety. They also have higher rates of school absenteeism. Unpredictable symptom presentation decreases a child's engagement with school and social activities, hinders development of peer relationships, and leads to a poorer quality of life, so behavioral health is a vital aspect of care. Parents of children with chronic illnesses and/or chronic pain can be overprotective, keeping a child home from school for worry about any symptom presentation. This behavior impedes the child's socialization and can cause dependence, rather than empowering the child's self-efficacy. Managing these patients is a delicate balance: Youth diagnosed with chronic pain and chronic illness are at higher risk of opioid dependence than the general population (Groenewald et al., 2019).

Adults

More than 50 million U.S. adults—24 percent—deal with chronic pain (Rikard et al., 2023). Globally, chronic pain reaches more than 30 percent of the population (Cohen et al., 2021). Lucas and Sohl (2024) reported that 8.5 percent of the population have lived with *high impact chronic pain,* defined as pain that frequently limits life or work activities, during the past 3 months. Chronic pain is also the most common reason adults seek medical care. Pain treatment has contributed to opioid and other substance misuse, increased incidence of anxiety and depression, and other mental health needs (Lucas & Sohl, 2024).

When chronic illness and chronic pain intersect, case managers' expertise on whole-person assessment, care coordination, resource management, and treatment planning can bring some relief. Viderman et al. (2023) reviewed pain prevalence in a set of chronic diseases: cancers, neurodegenerative disorders, congestive heart failure, COPD, kidney disease, traumatic brain injury, and other cerebrovascular diseases. Prevalence of pain occurred in all disease states, despite variations in diagnosis (e.g., type of cancer), acuity of disease, and demographics (e.g., age, race, ethnicity). A high-level view of this data is found in Figure 5.3.

Population demographics reveal additional drivers of chronic pain. For example, pain prevalence for recently divorced or recently separated adults (29.6 percent and 10.1 percent, respectively) is higher than for their married counterparts (5.2 percent). Recently divorced or separated patients also had higher intensity of pain and increased depression (Rikard et al., 2023).

Race and ethnicity also correlate with chronic pain. The data suggest opportunities to pay more attention to pain management for certain cultural groups. American Indian and Alaska Native non-Hispanic adults are more likely to experience chronic pain (30.7 percent), when compared with Asian non-Hispanic (11.8 percent) and Hispanic (17.1 percent) adults (Lucas & Sohl, 2024). White and Hispanic patients had lower prevalence of high-impact pain than Black patients (6.3 percent for White and Hispanic, 7.9 percent for Black), and multiracial patients had the highest prevalence of high-impact pain, at 12.0 percent (Zajacova et al., 2023). Adults in rural communities experience more chronic pain than adults in urban and suburban regions, with challenges often related to lack of access to specialists and delays in treatment (Zajacova et al., 2023). Provider bias is a constant theme in these communities, with concerns about drug-seeking behaviors (Zajacova et al., 2023).

Figure 5.3: *Prevalence of chronic pain with chronic disease*

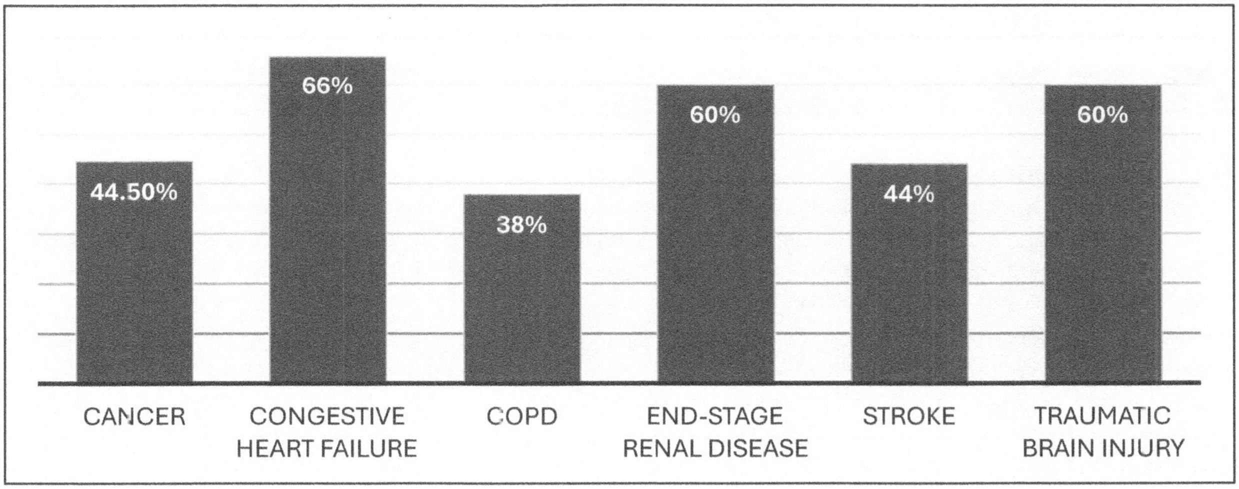

Data from Viderman et al., 2023

Older adults

The high incidence of pain associated with chronic illness is a concern for U.S. adults over age 65; 85 percent are diagnosed with at least one chronic condition, and 60 percent are diagnosed with two or more (Fong, 2019). Even still, they face challenges to identifying, managing, and treating chronic illness and chronic pain.

For example, older adults' symptoms may be wrongly associated with normal aging, rather than a serious condition, or they can be perceived as attention-seeking in response to loneliness or depression. They are also more susceptible to *medical gaslighting,* which refers to a misuse of power to disregard, dismiss, degrade, or otherwise devalue a patient's assertions (Ng et al., 2024). Note that the gaslighting dynamic is more than a simple difference of opinion or a negative interaction with a practitioner. Box 5.11 offers a medical gaslighting case scenario.

Levy et al. (2023) identified that older adults also frequently encounter *ageism,* or negative age stereotypes and discrimination, which impedes chronic pain management and other diagnostic considerations. For example, somatic symptom disorder may be inadvertently or incorrectly ruled out for older patients, since fatigue or pain are associated with aging. Such flawed assessments lead to poor clinical and fiscal outcomes. To reduce the likelihood of older adults becoming addicted to pain medication, providers often suggest non-pharmacological interventions, such as exercise, physical therapy, rehabilitation, and topical treatments of ice or heat.

Box 5.11: Medical gaslighting case scenario

An 85-year-old woman named Sam visits her long-standing primary care physician (PCP) for an annual visit. Sam has been in relatively good health, though complains of lower back pain, chronic nausea, and discomfort. Her pain level is an 8/10 and has intensified in recent weeks. Sam shares her symptoms, but the PCP interrupts: "You ARE 85 years old! Your labs were fine last year. These symptoms are arthritis." Sam tries to inform the PCP she doesn't have arthritis but is again interrupted.

Sam next tries to tell her PCP of ongoing nausea and 10-pound weight loss. The PCP responds, "This is related to pain and nothing more. How long have I known you? Call me if the meds don't help." Sam leaves the physician's office with a prescription for 800 mg of ibuprofen t.i.d. for pain. The medication provides little relief, which exacerbates underlying depression. Sam starts having bouts of constipation that worsen her nausea, decrease her appetite further, and add to the weight loss.

Some three months later, Sam's wife, Carol, emails the PCP through the patient portal: "Sam won't stop throwing up. The pain seems intolerable." The PCP replies, "Don't be so dramatic. A stomach flu is making the rounds. We know what a hypochondriac Sam is. Rest and fluids will do the trick."

One week later Carol brings Sam to the ED. The hospitalist orders a CT scan. He is alarmed by the radiologist's findings and immediately shares the results with Sam and Carol: the presence of a 7 cm renal mass on Sam's left kidney. Sam is admitted for an emergent workup and is diagnosed with stage 4 renal cancer that has metastasized to her liver and pancreas. The prognosis is less than a month to live, or a little longer with removal of the kidney and targeted chemotherapy and radiation. Sam denies treatment and asks to be discharged home with hospice care. She dies three weeks later.

POPULATION-FOCUSED MONITORING

When patients don't receive the care they need to manage chronic pain and chronic illness, many self-medicate, which leaves them susceptible to addiction, suicidal ideation, and suicide. Other general risk factors for these conditions appear below.

LGBTQIA+

The CDC's Behavioral Risk Factor Surveillance System (BRFSS) compiled research on 64,696 adults identifying as gay, lesbian, bisexual, other, and/or transgender and 1,369,681 persons identifying as cisgender/straight (Pinnamaneni et al., 2022). Patients in the LGBTQIA+ community had significantly higher rates of chronic illness across all diagnostic categories. Likewise, Zajacova et al. (2023) identified that LGBTQIA+ patients had higher prevalence of chronic pain at age 40 and again at age 64 than their straight or cisgender counterparts. See figures 5.4 and 5.5.

LGBTQIA+ people seeking healthcare encounter pronounced obstacles, such as invalidation of symptoms, provider rejection, and general inequity in access to care. They may experience delays in finding specialists, for example, because healthcare professionals can struggle to provide concordant care to the community. Healthcare workers may be unfamiliar with evolving LGBTQIA+ terminology and population norms, or they may be biased against the population (Lampe et al., 2023). Furthermore, older LGBTQIA+ adults may have difficulty accessing care due to economic insecurities. Poverty rates for the community are higher than for their cisgender/straight counterparts, at 21.6 percent versus 15.6 percent; poverty rates exceed 30 percent for trans persons (Badgett et al., 2019). Box 5.12 summarizes these issues.

Figure 5.4: *Prevalence of general chronic pain at age 40, by sexuality*

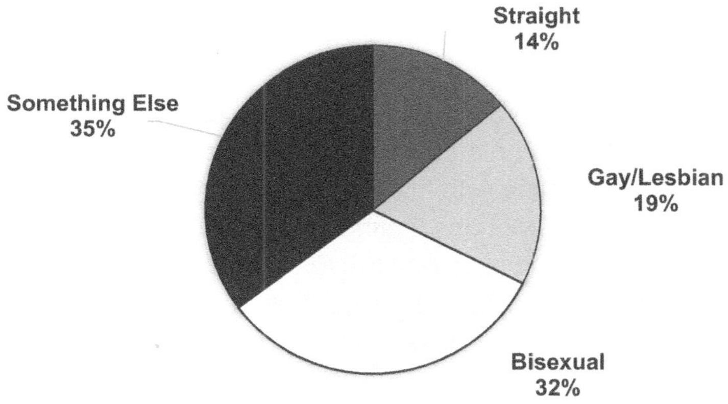

Figure 5.5: *Prevalence of general chronic pain at age 64, by sexuality*

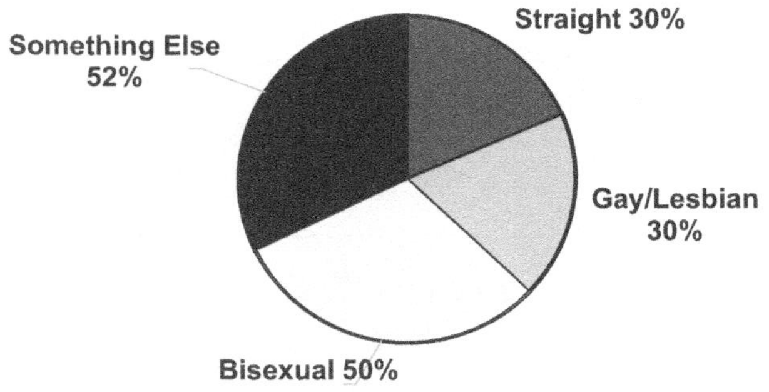

Data from Zajacova et al., 2023

Box 5.12: Chronic illness and chronic pain in LGBTQIA+

High incidence for:

- Chronic illness (all diagnoses) compared with cisgender and straight counterparts, and significantly higher rates of illness morbidity and mortality
- Chronic pain during every life stage
- Presence of high impact pain across all demographics
- Worsening symptoms as one ages

Distinct considerations:

- High incidence of medical gaslighting/invalidation by providers
- Rejection by providers
- Presence of health disparities related to SDoH (e.g., poverty, lack of stable employment or health insurance) that impact access to specialty care and medication management

Military members and veterans

Military members and veterans' chronic illness and chronic pain are frequently driven by trauma. Exposure to trauma exacerbates chronic conditions and worsens mental health. The number of military personnel and veterans dealing with this fierce triad is high. Some 44 percent of active-duty military live with chronic pain, with symptoms lasting, on average, 34 to 38 months (Ee et al., 2023). Over 35 percent of veterans with chronic pain are also diagnosed with PTSD, and 20 percent have an adjustment disorder (Hadlandsmyth et al., 2024; National Center for PTSD, 2025; Saluhuddin & Conti, 2022). Trauma, post-traumatic stress disorder (PTSD), and adjustment disorder will be addressed in Chapter 10.

Chronic pain's unrelenting discomfort and effect on a person's activities of daily life (ADLs) can be amplified by helplessness to manage the symptoms; that vulnerability runs counter to the military identity and its culture of control. Low self-esteem can result and lead to suicidal ideation. For military veterans who died by suicide, arthritis and back pain were the most common conditions: 38.5 percent and 33.3 percent, respectively (Boska et al., 2021).

Other diagnoses to note in military veterans include *psychogenic pain*—psychological pain caused primarily by a medical condition—as well as fibromyalgia (2.7 percent), neuropathy (4.4 percent), migraines (6.6 percent), and other headaches (7.2 percent) (Boska et el., 2021). Sleep disruption and deprivation due to pain is another critical consideration. As pain intensity decreases, sleep quality increases (Wilson et al., 2023). Mindfulness meditation and hypnosis have yielded better sleep for veterans. Veterans also have higher rates of obesity, diabetes, heart disease, stroke, cancers, COPD, and kidney disease compared with non-military (Betancort et al., 2023). For treatment, opioids and psychopharmacological agents can benefit veterans, but concerns about addiction complicate their use. Box 5.13 provides a snapshot of issues for military personnel and veterans.

Box 5.13: Chronic illness and chronic pain in military members and veterans

High incidence for:

- o Comorbid diagnoses of substance use and addiction, trauma, and stressor-related disorders
- o Chronic illness (across all diagnoses)
- o Chronic pain
- o Sleep disruption
- o Disability

Distinct considerations:

- o Medication mismanagement
- o Medication-seeking behaviors
- o High incidence of suicidal ideation and action
- o Inability to manage pain counter to the sense of control associated with military identityS

Persons with disabilities

Under the Americans with Disabilities Act, chronic pain is considered a disability when it limits one or more major life activities, mobility and ambulation, employment, or concentration (ADA, n.d.). The level of disability is defined by the intensity of pain and its disruption to functioning rather than any specific diagnoses. Over 82 percent of individuals with chronic pain view themselves as disabled (U.S. Pain Foundation, 2020).

Over 70 percent of adults who live with a disability and report poor quality of health also experience persistent chronic pain (Rikard et al., 2023). Due to bias about disabilities, their pain may be minimized by providers and by caregivers. Somatic concerns are often perceived as malingering, even when related to autoimmune disorders, traumatic accidents like motor vehicle crashes, or psychological trauma.

Since faulty assessment of a patient's pain, or invalidation of pain, impedes treatment, a screening tool exists to assess a patient's perception of his own pain and the possible faulty perceptions of the chronic pain by others (Nicola et al., 2022). The Pain-Invalidation Scale (P-IS) measures aspects of invalidation perceived by people with chronic pain. It appears in Table 5.2 with other screening tools. Considerations for working with persons with disabilities appear in Box 5.14.

Box 5.14: Chronic illness and chronic pain in persons with disabilities

High incidence for:

- Disability due to chronic pain
- Chronic pain, chronic illness, and poor quality of health
- Depression and anxiety

Distinct considerations:

- Medical gaslighting and pain/symptom invalidation
- Concerns of malingering and manipulating
- Use of the Pain-IS and other screening tools enhance symptom management
- Monitor for self-medication through substance use
- Advocacy for insurance approval of alternative/complementary treatment

Women's health

Pain varies greatly by sex. Gender-related pain mechanisms influence pain intensity, severity, and management, and tolerance to psychopharmacological dosing and medication half-life vary greatly (Casale et al., 2021).

Women and girls are more likely than men to admit to chronic pain—25.4 percent verses 23.2 percent. Women are also more likely to express their pain management needs to their providers. They also have higher prevalence of high impact chronic pain, at 10 percent compared to 7 percent of men (Lucas & Sohl, 2024). These issues impact a woman's socialization in platonic and intimate relationships. They can also exacerbate isolation and depression (Boggero et al., 2024).

Women also have higher rates of chronic illness than men. Over 51 percent of U.S. adults experience a chronic condition, and 6 of the 21 conditions defined by CMS as chronic occur more often in women than in men. These six conditions are hypertension, arthritis, depression, dementia, asthma, and osteoporosis (Temkin et al., 2023). Menstrual phases and reproductive status also affect pain ratings in women, particularly when the pain comes from migraines, arthritis, fibromyalgia, and bladder pain syndrome. Considerations for chronic illness and chronic pain for women appear in Box 5.15.

Box 5.15: Chronic illness and chronic pain in women's health

High incidence for:

- o Chronic pain in persons born as women compared to men (more than double the rate)
- o High impact pain
- o Complaints to providers about discomfort from pain

Distinct considerations:

- o Medical gaslighting and invalidation of symptoms
- o Dismissal of pain and providers perceiving drug-seeking behaviors
- o Attention to perimenopausal pain
- o Provider/case manager advocacy for insurance approval of alternative/complementary treatment
- o Concern for patient isolation
- o Embarrassment around symptoms that decrease socialization
- o Engagement in platonic and intimate relationships

SCREENING AND ASSESSMENT TOOLS FOR CHRONIC PAIN

Evidence-based tools assess pain and emotional discomfort caused by chronic illness. Table 5.2 provides screening tools for various aspects of pain, spanning intensity, quality, and impact on functioning in adults. Table 5.3 displays options for screening pediatric patients.

Table 5.2: *Screening tools for chronic pain (adults)*

Instrument	Focus	Source
Adult Non-Verbal Pain Scale (NVPS)	Quantifies patient pain in critical care using 5 measures scored from 0-2: facial expression activity level guarding behavior vital signs vocalizations	Odhner, M., Wegman, D., Freeland, N., Steinmetz, A., & Ingersoll, G.L. (2003). Assessing pain control in nonverbal critically ill adults. *Dimensions of Critical Care Nursing, 22*(6), 260-267. https://doi.org/10.1097/00003465-200311000-00010
Behavioral Pain Scale (BPS)	Quantifies patient pain in critical care settings across three categories scored from 1-4: facial expression upper limb movement ventilation compliance	Payen, J.F., Bru, O., Bosson, J.L., Lagrasta, A., Novel, E., Deschaux, I., Lavagne, P., & Jacquot, C. 2001). *Behavioral Pain Scale (BPS)* [Database record]. APA PsycTests. https://doi.org/10.1037/t65547-000
Brief Pain Inventory (BPI)	11-item self-report questionnaire (or 9-item short version) to assess the severity of pain (1-4) and how much it interferes with seven daily activities.	Cleeland, C.S., & Ryan, K.M. (1994). Pain assessment: Global use of the Brief Pain Inventory. *Annals of the Academy of Medicine Singapore, 23*(2), 129-138.

Instrument	Focus	Source
Defense and Veterans Pain Rating Scale (DVPRS)	A 5-item pain assessment tool using a numerical rating scale (0-10) enhanced by functional word descriptors, color coding, and pictorial facial expressions matched to pain levels. Four supplemental questions measure how much pain interferes with usual activity and sleep, affects mood, and contributes to stress.	Buckenmaier, C.C. III, Galloway, K.T., Polomano, R.C., McDuffie, M., Kwon, N., & Gallagher, R.M. (2013). Preliminary validation of the Defense and Veterans Pain Rating Scale (DVPRS) in a military population. *Pain Medicine 14*(1), 110-123. https://doi.org/10.1111/j.1526-4637.2012.01516.x
McGill Pain Questionnaire (MPQ)	Questionnaire with long (78 pain descriptors) and short versions (15 descriptors), used to assess three major measures of pain (sensory intensity, cognitive evaluation, and emotional impact). Pain intensity rated on a 1-5 scale.	Melzack R. (1975). The McGill Pain Questionnaire: Major properties and scoring methods. *Pain*, *1*(3), 277-299. https://doi.org/10.1016/0304-3959(75)90044-5
Numerical Rating Scale (NRS)	An 11-point numeric rating scale for mild, moderate, and severe pain. Patients receive a number noting average pain for the last week.	Downie, W.W., Leatham, P.A., Rhind, V.M., Wright, V., Branco, J.A., & Anderson, J.A. (1978). Studies with pain rating scales. *Annals of the Rheumatic Diseases*, *37*(4), 378-381. https://doi.org/10.1136/ard.37.4.378
Pain Assessment in Advanced Dementia Scale (PAINAD)	5-item scale for clinicians to observe and score the pain experience (0-2 points) in five domains: Breathing Negative vocalizations Facial expression Body language Consolability	Warden, V., Hurley, A.C., & Volicer, L. (2003). Development and psychometric evaluation of the Pain Assessment in Advanced Dementia (PAINAD) scale. *Journal of the American Medical Directors Association*, *4*(1), 9-15. https://doi.org/10.1097/01.JAM.0000043422.31640.F7
PainDETECT (for neuropathic pain)	A 9-item questionnaire to assess neuropathic pain with seven sensory descriptor items, plus two for spatial and temporal characteristics of pain.	Freynhagen, R., Baron, R., Gockel, U., & Tölle, T.R. (2006). painDETECT: a new screening questionnaire to identify neuropathic components in patients with back pain. *Current Medical Research and Opinion*, *22*(10), 1911-1920. https://doi.org/10.1185/030079906X132488
Pain Invalidation Scale (P-IS)	A 24-item patient self-report questionnaire with four subscales: Invalidation by the self Invalidation by immediate others Invalidation by healthcare professionals Invalidation by over-attentive others Each statement is rated on a Lickert scale spanning 1 (strongly disagree) to 7 (strongly agree). Patients respond to each statement in all four subscales.	Nicola, M., Correia, H., Ditchburn, G., & Drummond, P.D. (2022). The Pain-Invalidation Scale: Measuring patient perceptions of invalidation toward chronic pain. *The Journal of Pain*, *23*(11), 1912-1922. https://doi.org/10.1016/j.jpain.2022.06.008

Instrument	Focus	Source
Visual Analog Scale (VAS)	Measurement tool to assess the intensity of a subjective experience, like pain, by asking a person to mark a point on a continuous line, where the ends represent the extremes of that experience.	Langley, G.B., & Sheppeard, H. (1985). The visual analogue scale: Its use in pain measurement. *Rheumatology International*, *5*(4), 145-148. https://doi.org/10.1007/BF00541514

Table 5.3: *Screening tools for chronic pain (youth)*

Instrument	Focus	Source
CRIES	Tool assesses pain in infants, particularly newborns, by evaluating five indicators: Crying Requires increased oxygen Increased vital signs Facial expression Sleeplessness	Krechel, S.W., & Bildner, J. (1995). CRIES: A new neonatal postoperative pain measurement score. Initial testing of validity and reliability. *Paediatric Anaesthesia*, *5*(1), 53-61. https://doi.org/10.1111/j.1460-9592.1995.tb00242.x
Neonatal/Infant Pain Scale (NIPS)	Used to assess pain in infants less than 1 year old. The behavioral scale evaluates six indicators of pain: facial expression crying breathing patterns arms legs state of arousal	Lawrence, J., Alcock, D., McGrath, P., Kay, J., MacMurray, S.B., & Dulberg, C. (1993). The development of a tool to assess neonatal pain. *Neonatal Network*, *12*(6), 59-66.
Non-Communicating Children's Pain Checklist (NCCPC-R)	Measures chronic pain for children with cognitive impairments. Originally 30-items across seven subscales, with modified versions (e.g., 15 items) developed.	Breau, L.M., McGrath, P.J., Camfield, C.S., & Finley, G.A. (2002). *Non-communicating Children's Pain Checklist—Revised (NCCPC-R)* [Database record]. APA PsycTests. https://doi.org/10.1037/t69554-000
Revised—Faces, Legs, Activity, Cry, Consolability (r-FLACC)	Uses a scale of 0-10 to assess pain in children who are too young to speak, don't understand questions, or may not know how to report their pain. Also used for children with developmental differences or cognitive impairments.	Merkel, S.I., Voepel-Lewis, T., Shayevitz, J.R., & Malviya, S. (1997). The FLACC: A behavioral scale for scoring postoperative pain in young children. *Pediatric Nursing*, *23*(3), 293-297.

CONCLUSION

The intersection of chronic illness, chronic pain, and mental health is a challenging space to navigate. However, an influx of research on the realities of life for these patients has led to better treatments. As ICD-11 shifts some chronic pain diagnoses, we'll likely see greater industry awareness and identification of these intersecting conditions, while reducing prevailing stigmas.

Now we transition to another challenging diagnosis to navigate, depression. Like anxiety disorders, depression has assorted presentations and manifestations, which may provide pause for any case manager.

CONTEMPLATION QUESTIONS

1. Consider a situation where you worked with a patient who experienced chronic pain. Answer the following prompts:
   a) Using Figure 5.2 as a guide, which type of pain was the patient experiencing?
   b) How did culture factor into how the patient expressed his or her pain?
2. Review the screening tools for adults and pediatric patients in Tables 5.2 and 5.3.
   a) Which of the tools are you familiar with?
   b) Pick one tool you are not familiar with for each age group, and work through the tool.
   c) Reflect on how using a standardized tool for symptoms of chronic pain will inform your future efforts.
3. Review the diagnoses listed in Table 5.1.
   a) Which diagnoses are you most familiar with, personally or professionally?
   b) Reflect on professional experiences you have had with patients diagnosed with chronic pain disorders.
   c) Consider how bias might impact your assessment of a patient's symptoms and treatment plan.

Consider the following case scenario for questions 4-5.

Markia presents to the ED with self-reported pain "that is off the charts." The patient has a history of rheumatoid arthritis and fibromyalgia. Markia's electronic health record shows she has had repeated visits over the past year for uncontrolled joint and back pain.

1. Review the content in Box 5.10 on patient malingering or manipulation. Consider what recommendations you might make to the treatment team to assess and determine next steps for Markia.
2. Using Case Management's Behavioral Health Conversation Map in Table 1.4, reflect on how the phases would support your work with Markia.

RESOURCES

- **American Chronic Pain Association**
  https://www.acpanow.com
- **Centers for Disease Control and Prevention (CDC)**
  https://www.cdc.gov/chronic-disease/index.html
- **International Association for the Study of Pain (IASP)**
  https://www.iasp-pain.org/resources/terminology/
- **U.S. Pain Foundation**
  https://uspainfoundation.org

REFERENCES

- ADA.gov. (n.d.) Introduction to the Americans with Disabilities Act. Retrieved October 26, 2025, from https://www.ada.gov/topics/intro-to-ada/
- Armstrong, S.A. & Herr, M.J. (2023). Physiology, Nociception. [Updated 2023 May 1]. StatPearls Publishing: Treasure Island, FL. Available from https://www.ncbi.nlm.nih.gov/books/NBK551562/
- American Psychiatric Association. (2022). *Diagnostic and Statistical Manual of Mental Disorders* (5th ed., text rev.).
- Badgett, M.V.L., Choi, S.K., & Wilson, B.D.M. (2019). LGBT poverty in the United States: A study of differences between sexual orientation and gender identity groups. The Williams Institute.
- Betancourt, J.A., Dolezel, D.M., Shanmugam, R., Pacheco, G.J., Stigler Granados, P., & Fulton, L.V. (2023). The health status of the US veterans: A longitudinal analysis of surveillance data prior to and during the COVID-19 pandemic. *Healthcare*, *11*(14), 2049. https://doi.org/10.3390/healthcare11142049
- Boggero, I.A., Sangalli, L., Brasch, L., & King, C.D. (2024). Social health in young women with chronic pain. *Pain Reports*, *9*(2), e1146. https://doi.org/10.1097/PR9.0000000000001146
- Boska, R.L., Bishop, T.M., & Ashrafioun, L. (2021). Pain conditions and suicide attempts in military veterans: A case-control design. *Pain Medicine*, *22*(12), 2846-2850. https://doi.org/10.1093/pm/pnab287
- Carnahan, K.T., & Jha A. (2023). Factitious Disorder. StatPearls Publishing: Treasure Island, FL. Available from https://www.ncbi.nlm.nih.gov/books/NBK557547/
- Casale, R., Atzeni, F., Bazzichi, L., Beretta, G., Costantini, E., Sacerdote, P., & Tassorelli, C. (2021). Pain in women: A perspective review on a relevant clinical issue that deserves prioritization. *Pain and Therapy*, *10*(1), 287-314. https://doi.org/10.1007/s40122-021-00244-1
- Centers for Disease Control and Prevention. (2024a). About Chronic Diseases. Retrieved October 9, 2025, from https://www.cdc.gov/chronic-disease/about/index.html

- Centers for Disease Control and Prevention. (2024b). ICD-10-CM Official Guidelines for Coding and Reporting FY 2025 -- Updated October 1, 2024 (October 1, 2024 - September 30, 2025). Retrieved from https://www.cdc.gov/nchs/icd/icd-10-cm/files.html.
- Coady, A., Godard, R., & Holtzman, S. (2024). Understanding the link between pain invalidation and depressive symptoms: The role of shame and social support in people with chronic pain. *Journal of Health Psychology*, *29*(1), 52-64. https://doi.org/10.1177/13591053231191919
- Cohen, S.P., Vase, L., & Hooten, W.M. (2021). Chronic pain: An update on burden, best practices, and new advances. *The Lancet*, *397*(10289), 2082-2097. https://doi.org/10.1016/S0140-6736(21)00393-7
- Dohenny, K. (2022). Chronic pain gets its own condition under ICD-11, *MedCentral*. Retrieved December 27, 2024, from https://www.medcentral.com/guidelines/chronic-pain-gets-its-own-condition-under-icd-11
- Dydyk, A.M., & Conermann, T. (2024). Chronic Pain. [Updated 2024 May 6]. StatPearls Publishing: Treasure Island, FL. Available from https://www.ncbi.nlm.nih.gov/books/NBK553030/
- Ee, J.S., Dogbey, G.Y., Fitzpatrick, J.K., Agnello, R.N., Skelly, S.K., Chang, M.H., & Frost, L.S. (2023). Factors associated with chronic pain intensity in U.S. Army soldiers. *Military Medicine*, *188*(Suppl 6), 340-345. https://doi.org/10.1093/milmed/usad137
- Fong, J.H. (2019). Disability incidence and functional decline among older adults with major chronic diseases. *BMC Geriatrics*, *19*(1), 323. https://doi.org/10.1186/s12877-019-1348-z
- Groenewald, C.B., Essner, B.S., Wright, D., Fesinmeyer, M.D., & Palermo, T.M. (2014). The economic costs of chronic pain among a cohort of treatment-seeking adolescents in the United States. *The Journal of Pain*, *15*(9), 925-933. https://doi.org/10.1016/j.jpain.2014.06.002
- Hadlandsmyth, K., Zhuang, C., Driscoll, M.A., & Lund, B.C. (2024). Comorbid chronic pain and post-traumatic stress disorder: Current rates and psychiatric comorbidities among U.S. military veterans. *Military Medicine*, *189*(11-12), 2303-2306. https://doi.org/10.1093/milmed/usae313
- Hoffman, K.M., Trawalter, S., Axt, J.R., & Oliver, M.N. (2016). Racial bias in pain assessment and treatment recommendations, and false beliefs about biological differences between blacks and whites. *Proceedings of the National Academy of Sciences of the United States of America*, *113*(16), 4296-4301. https://doi.org/10.1073/pnas.1516047113
- Hollingshead, N.A., Ashburn-Nardo, L., Stewart, J.C., & Hirsh, A.T. (2016). The pain experience of Hispanic Americans: A critical literature review and conceptual model. *The Journal of Pain*, *17*(5), 513-528. https://doi.org/10.1016/j.jpain.2015.10.022
- International Association for the Study of Pain. (2020). Terminology revised. Retrieved from https://www.iasp-pain.org/resources/terminology/
- Levy, B.R., Pietrzak, R.H., & Slade, M.D. (2023). Societal impact on older persons' chronic pain: Roles of age stereotypes, age attribution, and age discrimination. *Social Science & Medicine (1982)*, *323*, 115772. https://doi.org/10.1016/j.socscimed.2023.115772
- Lucas, J.W., & Sohi, I. (2024). Chronic pain and high-impact chronic pain in U.S. adults, 2023. *NCHS Data Brief*, (518), CS355235. https://doi.org/10.15620/cdc/169630

- Merriam-Webster. (n.d.). Malingering, definition. Retrieved December 28, 2024, from https://www.merriam-webster.com/dictionary/malingering
- National Center for PTSD. (2025). Chronic Pain and PTSD; VA/U.S. Department of Veterans Affairs. Retrieved February 10, 2025, from https://www.ptsd.va.gov/index.asp
- Ng, I.K., Tham, S.Z., Singh, G.D., Thong, C., & Teo, D.B. (2024). Medical gaslighting: A new colloquialism. *The American Journal of Medicine*, *137*(10), 920-922. https://doi.org/10.1016/j.amjmed.2024.06.022
- Osborne, N.R., & Davis, K.D. (2022). Sex and gender differences in pain. *International Review of Neurobiology*, *164*, 277-307. https://doi.org/10.1016/bs.irn.2022.06.013
- Pinnamaneni, M., Payne, L., Jackson, J., Cheng, C.I., & Cascio, M.A. (2022). Disparities in chronic physical health conditions in sexual and gender minority people using the United States Behavioral Risk Factor Surveillance System. *Preventive Medicine Reports*, *28*, 101881. https://doi.org/10.1016/j.pmedr.2022.101881
- Rikard, S.M., Strahan, A.E., Schmit, K.M., & Guy, G.P. Jr. (2023). Chronic pain among adults — United States, 2019-2021. *Morbidity Mortality Weekly Report*, *72*, 379-385. http://dx.doi.org/10.15585/mmwr.mm7215a1
- Rogger, R., Bello, C., Romero, C.S., Urman, R.D., Luedi, M.M., & Filipovic, M.G. (2023). Cultural framing and the impact on acute pain and pain services. *Current Pain and Headache Reports*, *27*(9), 429-436. https://doi.org/10.1007/s11916-023-01125-2
- Salahuddin, D., & Conti, T. (2022). Trauma and behavioral health care for patients with chronic pain. *Primary Care*, *49*(3), 415-423. https://doi.org/10.1016/j.pop.2022.04.001
- Treede, R.D., Rief, W., Barke, A., Aziz, Q., Bennett, M.I., Benoliel, R., Cohen, M., Evers, S., Finnerup, N.B., & First, M.B. et al. (2019). Chronic pain as a symptom or a disease: The IASP classification of chronic pain for the International Classification of Diseases (ICD-11). *Pain*, *160*(1), 19-27. https://doi.org/10.1097/j.pain.0000000000001384
- U.S. Pain Foundation. (2020). Understanding Barriers to Multidisciplinary Pain Care. Retrieved February 17, 2025, from https://uspainfoundation.org/surveyreports/accesstocare/
- Wade, D.T., & Halligan, P.W. (2004). Do biomedical models of illness make for good healthcare systems? *BMJ (Clinical Research Ed.)*, *329*(7479), 1398-1401. https://doi.org/10.1136/bmj.329.7479.1398
- Wan, J., Chua, E.Y.C., Soon, W.S.W., Xie, Y., & Tang, W.E. (2021). The impact of a mental health service on chronic disease management in primary care. *Singapore Medical Journal*, *62*(5), 235-239. https://doi.org/10.11622/smedj.2021063
- Wilson, M., Skeiky, L., Muck, R.A., Miller, M.A., Hansen, D.A., Williams, R.M., Jensen, M.P., & Van Dongen, H.P.A. (2023). Sleep and pain in veterans with chronic pain: Effects of psychological pain treatment and temporal associations. *Nature and Science of Sleep*, *15*, 1061-1077. https://doi.org/10.2147/NSS.S418532
- Zajacova, A., Grol-Prokopczyk, H., & Fillingim, R. (2022). Beyond Black vs White: Racial/ethnic disparities in chronic pain including Hispanic, Asian, Native American, and multiracial US adults. *Pain*, *163*(9), 1688-1699. https://doi.org/10.1097/j.pain.0000000000002574

- Zinboonyahgoon, N., Luansritisakul, C., Eiamtanasate, S., Duangburong, S., Sanansilp, V., Korwisi, B., Barke, A., Rief, W., & Treede, R.D. (2021). Comparing the ICD-11 chronic pain classification with ICD-10: How can the new coding system make chronic pain visible? A study in a tertiary care pain clinic setting. *Pain*, *162*(7), 1995-2001. https://doi.org/10.1097/j.pain.0000000000002196

CHAPTER 6

DEPRESSION

INTRODUCTION

Depression is a long and winding road of terms and diagnoses. DSM-5-TR includes over 40 diagnoses that include a symptom of depression, from periodic sulking to chronic despair, withdrawal, and isolation. This chapter will explore the most common conditions case managers see. (Note: Bipolar disorder, as an SMI, appears in Chapter 7.)

Case managers will interact with people displaying such manifestations of depression. Depression evokes concern in a patient, his or her family, and certainly members of the care team. Let's dig into the intricacies of this common behavioral health condition.

BEHAVIORAL LEARNING OBJECTIVES

1. Identify the depression continuum
2. Distinguish between presentations of depression
3. Relate symptoms and treatment recommendations for common DSM diagnoses
4. Understand how depression appears across developmental life stages
5. Analyze the incidence of depression across life stages and populations
6. Identify screening tools used to assess for depression
7. Apply Case Management's Behavioral Health Conversation Map to patients and their families living with depression

ESSENTIAL TERMS

- Ableism
- Anhedonia
- Biogenic depression
- Bipolar disorder
- Endogenous depression
- Depression
- Depressive disorder due to another medical condition
- Despair
- Disruptive mood dysregulation disorder (DMDD)

- Dysphoria
- Dysthymic disorder
- Major depressive disorder (MDD)
- Melancholy
- Other specified or unspecified depressive disorder
- Persistent depressive disorder
- Premenstrual dysphoric disorder (PMDD)
- Premenstrual syndrome (PMS)
- Prodromal
- Sadness
- Seasonal patterns
- Social isolation
- Substance/medication-induced depressive disorder

TERMS AND FEATURES OF DEPRESSION

Sad, moody, irritable, hopeless, and morose: terms of *depression.* With these emotions go depressive behaviors, spanning isolation to loss of appetite—or, sometimes, increased food intake. Patients present with decreased endurance and motivation, as well as treatment non-adherence. They may express passive suicidal ideation through language like "I'm just done with it" or "Everyone would be better off without me." The condition may be a direct cause of substance or medication use.

THE DEPRESSION CONTINUUM

> **Author's Note**
> *Case managers mention that current resources lack common diagnoses for children and adolescents, so I made it a point to include some this book. The topic is especially important to me because I trained clinically with youth and their families.*

The symptoms and conditions associated with depression cover quite a range. They spread across a continuum, like anxiety in Figure 4.1. The continuum begins with sadness on the mild end. Sadness is a natural, prevalent human emotion, experienced regularly by over 30 percent of the population (Tebeka et al., 2021). For some people, sadness can follow seasonal patterns, such as the wintertime blues caused by fewer hours of sunshine each day, or the change between daylight saving's time and standard time, which wreaks havoc on many a person's mood.

When, then, does normal sadness or sulking become a diagnoseable mental illness? The degree of sadness intensifies along the depression continuum, as seen in Figure 6.1, with sustained unhappiness characterizing most types of depression.

Sadness can be a *prodromal* sign of depression disorders—that is, an initial symptom before diagnosable onset (Tebeka et al., 2021). A person who experiences occasional feelings of hopelessness may transition to chronic frustration, profound sorrow, or *anhedonia,* a decreased interest in activities that previously provided pleasure. The individual no longer enjoys socializing and finds excuses to stay home, eventually becoming withdrawn. The withdrawal becomes debilitating, wherein he is unable to attend school or work or participate in life activities. He may conceive suicidal ideation, either passively or intrusively. These symptoms may be more severe and indicative of an intense *biogenic* or *endogenous* depression, stemming from internal or genetic causes rather than related to external stress or other life events.

It's common that case managers' patients present with *melancholy* or hopelessness and intermittent sadness. After all, frequent visits with PCPs and specialists can be overwhelming, and uncertainty about illness disrupts work schedules and the sense of employment security. Repeated hospital admissions can leave the family unit feeling *despair* or loss of hope that health and quality of life will improve. Feelings get internalized over time, as the illness status passes from months to years. What's more, case management patients frequently experience events, like new and unexpected diagnoses, that further upend regular life and exacerbate sadness and other manifestations of depression.

Figure 6.1: *The depression continuum*

Mild

- Minor distress, low mood, and feelings of sadness
- May spend periods of time alone or lose interest in engaging with others
- Increasing fatigue, decreased ability to concentrate, increased sleep
- Increasing frustration, irritability, or preoccupation

Moderate

- Increased hopelessness, malaise and/or sadness
- Decreased enjoyment or participation in activities of interest
- Increased challenges at school, work, and/or socialization
- Somatic complaints (e.g., stomach pains, body aches) or rapid speech

Severe

- Marked feelings of hopelessness and sadness; feeling life is not worth living
- Full lost of interest in any activity of interest or pleasure
- Suicidal ideation
- Intense physical symptoms of vomiting, chest pain, or diarrhea

COMMON DEPRESSION DISORDERS

A case manager's practice setting will dictate the incidence of various depressive disorders in their patients. Table 6.1 displays the most common diagnoses in the DSM-5-TR depressive disorders category and a lengthy list of specifiers. As covered in Chapter 1 (Box 1.2), specifiers are extensions to a diagnosis. They clarify the course, severity, and special features of mental disorders.

Table 6.1: *DSM-5-TR depressive disorders*

DSM-5-TR Diagnosis	Code		
Disruptive mood dysregulation disorder	F34.81		
Major depressive disorder			
Specifiers:	Single episode		Recurrent episode
Mild	F32.0		F33.0
Moderate	F32.1		F33.1
Severe	F32.2		F33.2
With psychotic features	F32.3		F33.3
In partial remission	F32.4		F33.41
In full remission	F32.5		F33.42
Unspecified	F32.9		F33.9
With: Anxious distress Mixed features Melancholic features Atypical features Mood-congruent psychotic features Mood-incongruent psychotic features Peripartum onset Seasonal pattern			
Persistent depressive disorder	F34.10		
Specify if: Mild, Moderate, Severe: With anxious distress With atypical features Specify if: In partial or full remission Specify if: Early onset (under 21 years of age) Late onset (21 year of age or older) Within the 2 most recent years: Pure dysthymic syndrome Persistent major depressive episodes Intermittent major depressive episodes with current episode Intermittent major depressive episodes without current episode			
Premenstrual dysphoric disorder	F32.81		
Substance/medication-induced depressive disorder	Mild use	Moderate-severe use	Without use disorder

DSM-5-TR Diagnosis	Code		
Alcohol	F10.14	F10.24	F10.94
Phencyclidine	F16.14	F16.24	F16.94
Other hallucinogen	F16.14	F16.24	F16.94
Inhalant	F18.14	F18.24	F18.94
Opioid	F11.14	F11.24	F11.94
Sedative, hypnotic, or anxiolytic	F13.14	F13.24	F13.94
Amphetamine-type substance (or another stimulant)	F15.14	F15.24	F15.94
Cocaine	F14.14	F14.24	F14.94
Other (or unknown substance)	F.19.14	F19.24	F19.94
Depressive disorder due to another medical condition			
Specify: With depressive features With major depressive-like episode With mixed features			
Other specified depressive disorder	F32.89		
Unspecified depressive disorder	F32.A		
Unspecified mood disorder	F39		

Adapted from American Psychiatric Association, 2022, pp. 163-214

DISRUPTIVE MOOD DYSREGULATION DISORDER

Disruptive mood dysregulation disorder (DMDD) primarily affects the pediatric population. Imagine a parent bringing his child to the ED for hand injuries. The child sustained the wounds when she punched a wall following a routine discussion about her day. This scenario demonstrates more than a bad mood or a tantrum. The parent describes other violent, aggressive outbursts during which the child throws household objects or punches walls. The eruptions are disproportional to the triggers and occur several days a week. The child always apologizes for the behavior after. Box 6.1 summarizes the symptoms and treatments for DMDD.

Box 6.1: Signs, symptoms, and treatment of disruptive mood dysregulation disorder (DMDD)

DSM-5-TR criteria:

Age at onset: 6 to 10 years; diagnosis excluded after 18 years of age

The presence of the following for 12 months or more, with no symptom-free periods for longer than 3 months

- Severe recurrent temper outbursts (e.g., verbal rage and/or physical aggression toward people or property) that are grossly out of proportion to the situation and that occur 3 times or more per week on average
- Temper outbursts are inconsistent with developmental level

- An irritable, angry mood presents every day for most of the day and is observed by others (e.g., parents, teachers, peers)

  The outbursts and angry mood must occur in 2 of 3 settings (e.g., home or school, with peers).

Treatments:

- For preadolescents:
  - Psychotherapy, followed by antidepressants if needed
  - Expressive therapies (e.g., art or play) and dialectical behavior therapy (individual and group) may be recommended
- For adolescents:
  - Evaluation for antidepressants such as selective serotonin reuptake inhibitors (SSRIs), stimulants, or antipsychotics may be recommended, combined with
  - Psychotherapy such as cognitive behavioral therapy, dialectical behavior therapy, or traditional talk therapy
  - Behavioral management and parent training
- Homeopathic and medicinal herb use is increasingly common (e.g., ashwagandha, chamomile, kava kava, lavender, passionflower, omega-3 fatty acids, St. John's wort), though should be openly reviewed with prescribing practitioners to ensure safety. Careful monitoring and mitigation with other current prescriptions, over-the-counter medications, and other substances should be discussed prior to initiating use to avoid interactions, complications, etc.
- Monitoring of diet, exercise, and activity

Author's Note

Case managers mention that current resources lack common diagnoses for children and adolescents, so I made it a point to include some this book. The topic is especially important to me because I trained clinically with youth and their families.

Adapted from American Psychiatric Association, 2022, pp. 177-179; Cui et al., 2024; Noori et al., 2022

MAJOR DEPRESSIVE DISORDER

A patient presents to the ED complaining of abdominal discomfort and periodic headaches. The patient's partner complains, "My husband is so distractable. He spends more time scrolling social media than on work tasks. We used to cook meals together, but now I can't get him off the couch. He's too exhausted to do anything and isn't sleeping, which only makes things worse. He claims to be bored and unmotivated, but it feels like more is up. Last week he blurted out, 'We're all going to die sometime.' He's become the oldest 24-year-old I know! We went to our PCP last month and his lab work was negative, but this has been going on for the past few months. Enough is enough!"

One explanation for the above behaviors is *major depressive disorder* (MDD). It's among the most common diagnoses in this category. Symptoms and treatments appear in Box 6.2.

The integrated care connection: mental illness, physical illness, or both?

As an integrated care professional, I must call attention to the puzzle of distinguishing a mental illness from a physical one. I hope you'll read one or more of the many books on this topic, and on the models of care for clinical assessment and intervention. Several of these are listed in the chapter resources. But for the purposes of this topic, here is what case managers should know: Your patients' symptoms will most likely exist at the complex intersection of pathophysiology, neuropathophysiology, and psychopathology.

For this reason, case managers should engage with practitioners and specialists who diagnose a patient's overall health condition. In lieu of such access, this book provides foundational knowledge to conduct behavioral health assessments. Yet a higher level of clinical expertise may be required to understand a patient's presentation, such as consideration of other mental health disorders or medical disorders that mimic depression. Case managers should ensure patients undergo a thorough biopsychosocial assessment by trained clinicians, as presented in Chapter 1.

For example, physical disease states that mimic depression include endocrine disorders; neurological disorders like Parkinson's, multiple sclerosis, or strokes; and vitamin deficiencies. Respiratory disorders that cause decreased breathing capacity and low oxygenation can cause patients to present as lethargic, weary, and lackluster; in these cases, a diagnosis of depression may be wrongly presumed. Chronic pain conditions (Chapter 5), such as fatigue, decreased endurance, or mood lability, can resemble depression symptoms. Substance use notoriously contributes to depressive episodes, as well as anxiety, agitation, and mania. Side effects of prescription drugs and over-the-counter medications yield mental health symptoms, too.

In women's health, a seemingly endless list of reproductive health conditions yield co-occurring physical and mental health symptoms, including endometriosis, peri- and postpartum, perimenopause, and menopause. The list may also include premenstrual dysphoric disorder, discussed below. Hormonal imbalances alone can be confused for mental health conditions, due to agitation, despair, frustration, or potential psychotic thinking.

Box 6.2: Signs, symptoms, and treatment of major depressive disorder

DSM-5-TR criteria:

Age at onset: May occur at any age, though more common after puberty

≥ 1 of the following must be present for most of the day nearly every day during a single 2-week period:

- Feeling sad or being observed by others to be sad or irritable
- Loss of interest or pleasure in almost all activities (often expressed as profound boredom)

In addition, ≥ 4 of the following must be present:

- Decrease in weight (in children, failure to make expected weight) or decrease or increase in appetite
- Insomnia or hypersomnia
- Psychomotor agitation or retardation observed by others (not self-reported)
- Fatigue or loss of energy
- Decreased ability to think, concentrate, and make choices
- Recurrent thoughts of death (not just fear of dying) and/or suicidal ideation or plans

- Feelings of worthlessness (e.g., feeling rejected and unloved) or excessive or inappropriate guilt

Treatments:

- Antidepressants: Selective serotonin reuptake inhibitors (SSRIs); for severe symptoms may be used in tandem with antipsychotics
  - MAO inhibitors may be considered, though need careful reconciliation with SSRIs and other psychopharmacological and prescription drugs
- Homeopathic and medicinal herb use is increasingly common (e.g., ashwagandha, chamomile, kava kava, lavender, passionflower, omega-3 fatty acids, St. John's wort), though should be openly reviewed with prescribing practitioners to ensure safety. Careful monitoring and mitigation with other current prescriptions, over-the-counter medications, and other substances should be discussed prior to initiating use to avoid interactions, complications, etc.
- Monitoring of diet, exercise, and activity
- Psychotherapy: Cognitive behavioral therapy, expressive therapies (e.g., art or sand)
  - Electroconvulsive therapies (ECT) for extreme symptoms are increasingly considered

Adapted from American Psychiatric Association, 2022, pp. 183-185; Cui et al., 2024; Noori et al., 2022

PERSISTENT DEPRESSIVE DISORDER

Most people know at least one person they might call a "Debbie Downer." They suck the life out of gatherings by their gloomy, pessimistic, or humorless presentation. They may be passive, lethargic, and introverted. A prominent Debbie Downer feature is frequent, wide-ranging criticism, of others and themselves. The person seems incapable of seeing positivity anywhere.

This type of prolonged, unceasing, low-level depression is diagnosed as *persistent depressive disorder.* Prior versions of the DSM called this group of symptoms *dysthymic disorder*; the diagnostic classification was changed in DSM-5. Common signs, symptoms, and treatments for persistent depressive disorder appear in Box 6.3.

Box 6.3: Signs, symptoms, and treatment for persistent depressive disorder

DMS-5-TR criteria:

Patients must have had a depressed mood for most of the day, for more days than not, for ≥ 2 years

In addition, ≥ 2 of the following must be present:

- Poor appetite or overeating
- Insomnia or hypersomnia
- Low energy or fatigue
- Low self-esteem
- Poor concentration or difficulty making decisions
- Feelings of hopelessness

Treatments:

- Antidepressants: Selective serotonin reuptake inhibitors (SSRIs); for severe symptoms may be used in tandem with antipsychotics
    - MAO inhibitors may be considered, though need careful reconciliation with SSRIs and other psychopharmacological and prescription drugs
- Homeopathic and medicinal herb use is increasingly common (e.g., ashwagandha, chamomile, kava kava, lavender, passionflower, omega-3 fatty acids, St. John's wort), though should be openly reviewed with prescribing practitioners to ensure safety. Careful monitoring and mitigation with other current prescriptions, over-the-counter medications, and other substances should be discussed prior to initiating use to avoid interactions, complications, etc.
- Monitoring of diet, exercise, and activity
- Psychotherapy: Cognitive behavioral therapy, expressive therapies (e.g., art or sand)
    - Electroconvulsive therapies (ECT) for extreme symptoms are increasingly considered

Adapted from American Psychiatric Association, 2022, pp. 193-197; Cui et al., 2024; Noori et al., 2022

PREMENSTRUAL DYSPHORIC DISORDER

Imagine you are reviewing the EMR of an adult female patient who has recurrent visits to her PCP for the following symptoms: physical bloating and joint pain, intense mood swings, inability to control her emotions, distractibility, and periodic brain fog. The EMR documents her recent college graduation, moving back into her parents' home, and starting a "high-pressure" job. The PCP documented that the stress of the transitions has exacerbated the patient's symptoms, with a final recommendation to start an anti-depressant.

Stress from life transitions wreaks havoc on the body. But you are correct if you considered other etiology. The patient had tracked her symptoms over the past six months and noticed they appeared up to a week before starting her monthly menses and stopped when her period ended. The patient preferred to meet with her gynecologist before starting medication.

For decades, the symptoms described for this patient had been considered *premenstrual syndrome,* or PMS. In 2013, however, *premenstrual dysphoric disorder* (PMDD) was added to DSM-5. Box 6.4 provides PMDD details case managers should know.

Many patients and psychiatrists supported the inclusion of PMDD in DSM-5, but there were critics, too. Schroll and Lauritson (2022) described many of the concerns: They noted that behavioral health clinicians and PCPs worried about overuse of the diagnosis and pathologizing of normal hormonal changes. There was concern that the pharmaceutical industry would benefit more than patients, due to prescribing of medication. They also highlighted that misdiagnosis could cause harm by unnecessary use of antidepressants, many with adverse effects such as sexual dysfunction. And feminist leaders felt PMDD devalued women by categorizing aspects of ordinary life as mental illness.

Box 6.4: Signs, symptoms, and treatment of premenstrual dysphoric disorder

DSM-5-TR criteria:

A. At least five of the symptoms below must be present in the final week before the onset of menses, start to improve within a few days after the onset of menses, and become minimal or absent in the week following menses.

B. At least one of the following symptoms must be present:
   - Marked mood swings (e.g., suddenly feeling sad or tearful)
   - Marked irritability or anger or increased interpersonal conflicts
   - Marked depressed mood, feelings of hopelessness, or self-deprecating thoughts
   - Marked anxiety, tension, or an on-edge feeling

C. And one or more of the following symptoms must also be present to reach the total of five symptoms when combined with those in group B.
   - Decreased interest in usual activities (e.g., school, work, friends, interests)
   - Difficulty concentrating
   - Lethargy, easy fatigue, or marked lack of energy
   - Noticeable change in appetite; overeating or specific food cravings
   - Hypersomnia or insomnia
   - Feeling overwhelmed or out of control
   - Physical symptoms (e.g., breast tenderness, swelling, joint or muscle pain, bloating)

Note: Symptom criteria must have been met for most menstrual cycles occurring in the preceding year

Treatments:

- Antidepressants: Selective serotonin reuptake inhibitors (SSRIs); for severe symptoms may be used in tandem with antipsychotics
  - MAO inhibitors may be considered, though need reconciliation with SSRIs and other psychopharmacological and prescription drugs
- Homeopathic and medicinal herb use is increasingly common (e.g., ashwagandha, chamomile, kava kava, lavender, passionflower, omega-3 fatty acids, St. John's wort), though should be openly reviewed with prescribing practitioners to ensure safety. Careful monitoring and mitigation with other current prescriptions, over-the-counter medications, and other substances should be discussed prior to initiating use to avoid interactions, complications, etc.
- Monitoring of diet, exercise, and activity
- Psychotherapy: Cognitive behavioral therapy, dialectical behavior therapy, mindfulness, relaxation strategies, sleep hygiene

Adapted from American Psychiatric Association, 2022, pp. 197-198; Cui et al., 2024; Noori et al., 2022

OTHER SPECIFIED AND UNSPECIFIED DEPRESSIVE DISORDERS

As with other mental illnesses, patients can present with a cluster of depressive symptoms but don't meet the criteria for any single disorder. Imagine a patient admitted to the hospital amid a medical crisis. She lacks full knowledge of her history of symptoms and is unable to provide accurate information. There may be pressure within the practice setting to render a diagnosis, whether for utilization management or other reasons. Like other similar (though limited) and incomplete presentations of psychopathology, the patient may be diagnosed with "other depressive disorders (specified or unspecified)." A brief description of this disorder appears in Box 6.5.

Box 6.5: Signs, symptoms, and treatment of other depressive disorders (specified or unspecified)

DSM-5-TR criteria:

Patient has recurrent periods of dysphoria with ≥ 4 other depressive symptoms that last < 2 weeks in people who have:

- never met criteria for another mood disorder (e.g., recurrent brief depression), and
- depressive periods that last longer but include insufficient symptoms for diagnosis of another depressive disorder

Symptoms cause clinically significant distress.

Treatments:

- Homeopathic and medicinal herb use is increasingly common (e.g., ashwagandha, chamomile, kava kava, lavender, passionflower, omega-3 fatty acids, St. John's wort), though should be openly reviewed with prescribing practitioners to ensure safety. Careful monitoring and mitigation with other current prescriptions, over-the-counter medications, and other substances should be discussed prior to initiating use to avoid interactions, complications, etc.
- Monitoring of diet, exercise, and activity
- Psychotherapy: Cognitive behavioral therapy, dialectical behavior therapy, mindfulness, relaxation strategies, sleep hygiene

Adapted from American Psychiatric Association, 2022, pp. 209-210; Cui et al., 2024

DEPRESSIVE DISORDER DUE TO ANOTHER MEDICAL CONDITION

Another common diagnosis is depressive disorder due to another medical condition. A cause-and-effect relationship can be identified between a patient's presenting medical condition and his or her mood, meaning the depressive disorder is the direct result of another other health condition.

Think of patients who have been admitted to the hospital, their lives turned upside down by sudden onset of a health condition. Questions like How will this condition impact my life? blaze through their minds, but they can't verbalize those concerns in the moment. Coping can be difficult, and some individuals act dismissive, while others worry incessantly.

The upset over unfamiliar health conditions is understandable. After all, neurological and neurocognitive conditions such as Alzheimer's, Huntington's, multiple sclerosis, Parkinson's, or stroke can grossly limit a person's thinking and independence of mobility and activities of daily living.

Endocrine disorders may cause weight gain or acne and negatively impact self-esteem and mood. Infections can limit one's functioning and quality of life, prompting emotional lability and despair.

A snapshot of the symptoms and treatment considerations for depressive disorder due to another medical condition appear in Box 6.6.

Box 6.6: Signs, symptoms, and treatment for depressive disorder due to another medical condition

DSM-5-TR criteria:

The patient presents with:

- Prominent and persistent disturbance in mood that predominates the clinical picture and is characterized by depressed mood or markedly diminished interest or pleasure in all or most of one's activities
- Evidence exists from a patient's history, physical exam, labs, or other diagnostic findings that the presentation is the direct pathophysiological consequence of another defined medical condition
- The presentation is not better explained by another mental disorder (e.g., adjustment disorder with depressed mood)
- The presentation does not occur only during a course of delirium
- The presentation causes clinically significant distress or impairment in the patient's social, educational, occupational, or social domains of functioning

The diagnosis should note the specifiers as presented in Table 6.1.

Treatments:

- Antidepressants: Selective serotonin reuptake inhibitors (SSRIs); for severe symptoms may be used in tandem with antipsychotics
  - MAO inhibitors may be considered, though need careful reconciliation with SSRIs and other psychopharmacological and prescription drugs
- Homeopathic and medicinal herb use is increasingly common (e.g., ashwagandha, chamomile, kava kava, lavender, passionflower, omega-3 fatty acids, St. John's wort), though should be openly reviewed with prescribing practitioners to ensure safety. Careful monitoring and mitigation with other current prescriptions, over-the-counter medications, and other substances should be discussed prior to initiating use to avoid interactions, complications, etc.
- Monitoring of diet, exercise, and activity
- Psychotherapy: Cognitive behavioral therapy, expressive therapies (e.g., art and sand)

Adapted from American Psychiatric Association, 2022, pp. 206-207; Cui et al., 2024

DATA AND DEMOGRAPHICS

Depression is among the most common mental health conditions worldwide, impacting more than 280 million people, or some 4 percent of the global population (World Health Organization, 2023). Barely 30 percent of people diagnosed receive treatment, however, due to disparities in population health measures for identification, treatment, and intervention. Most people (75 percent) diagnosed with depression in low- and middle-income countries receive little to no treatment whatsoever (Mekonen et al., 2021).

GENERAL RISK FACTORS

General risk factors for depression encompass several domains. From a population health perspective, biology and genetic predisposition are certainly contributing factors. But as with anxiety in Chapter 4, case managers should consider Engel's (1977) biopsychosocial lens when they consider the drivers of depressive disorders.

For example, environmental stress takes its own psychological toll. Multiple environmental factors influence depression, such as the quality of social and intimate relationships, employment status, income level, and housing sufficiency and stability. Furthermore, developmental factors associated with attachment, adversity, aging, bereavement, or trauma either promote or detract from mood stability and the intensity of symptoms. Suffice to say, persons struggling with psychosocial life stressors are more vulnerable to mood lability. The behavioral manifestations of these risk factors play out differently among populations and will be discussed in the following sections.

Of note for this discussion is how unstable mood, poor medication adherence, or inaccessible treatment heighten a patient's risk for self- or public harm. Suicide is a major worry for providers, especially when assessing for imminent or foreseeable risk of doing harm. This topic requires a dedicated chapter; assessment, presentation, screening, and management of suicide is covered in Chapter 9.

DEVELOPMENTAL LIFE STAGE

Depression presents differently during the developmental life stages. This section provides a brief review of incidence, prevalence, and manifestation of depression across the lifespan.

Youth

Youth depression is among the most pressing population health priorities. Over 3 percent of U.S. children experience depression, with onset occurring as young as 2 years old. More than 75 percent of adult mental health conditions, particularly depression, are diagnosed during childhood (Mulraney et al., 2021).

Proactive and early identification of depression is critical for effective symptom management. Even still, when depression is first identified in a child, the child's likelihood for depressive disorders in adulthood quadruples. Looked at another way, upwards of 70 percent of adolescents with diagnosed depressive disorder experience a recurrence of symptoms within 5 years (Xiang et al., 2024).

The most pressing challenge for adolescent depression involves the variety of symptoms that can present with it, as well as their intensity across the population. This makes it more difficult for practitioners to distinguish typical or age-appropriate moodiness from depression. Adolescents often present with intense dysphoria, or general dissatisfaction with life. This presentation can be viewed as “adolescent angst” and dismissed. Adolescents can also have a mixed presentation of depression and anxiety, which makes accuracy of the diagnosis more difficult. However, case managers and other clinicians should be on the lookout for symptoms that impede the academic performance, social relationships, or overall functioning of adolescent patients.

Poor self-esteem can often be at the core of depression in youth. Newer approaches to assessment are emerging that account for factors that impact patient vulnerability to poor self-esteem. These factors include bullying, attachment, and early family stability (Rikard-Bell et al., 2022).

Adults

Depression can be a lifelong struggle, even with consistent medication and psychotherapy. The disorder is a major cause of disability worldwide, impacting 5 percent of the adult population (World Health Organization, 2023). The CDC’s Behavioral Risk Factor Surveillance System data (Lee et al., 2023) show 18.5 percent of U.S. adults have depression, and the prevalence ranges from 12.7 to 27.5 percent in various states. The prevalence of depressive disorders by age appears in Figure 6.2, with differences by gender shown in Figure 6.3.

Chronic illness co-occurs with depressive disorders at high rates. Case managers should be aware that patients with depressive disorders have a 40 percent greater chance of premature death than their counterparts who are not depressed (Alotaibi et al., 2024; Zenebe et al., 2021). For the following conditions, depressive disorders co-occur in 9 to 25 percent of patients: hypertension, cardiovascular diseases, diabetes, and chronic kidney diseases.

Chronic pain also exacerbates depression, with 85 percent of patients diagnosed with chronic pain also diagnosed with moderate to severe depression (Ma et al., 2021). As presented in Chapter 5, chronic illness and chronic pain wear on patients’ resilience and quality of life and shrink their self-worth. The depression can be quite severe and become a major obstacle to wellness.

Figure 6.2: *Age-specific prevalence of depression for adults*

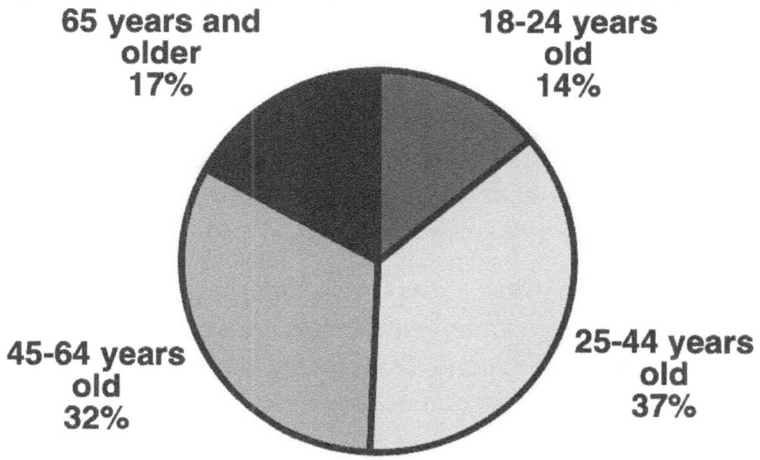

Figure 6.3: *Gender variations in depression*

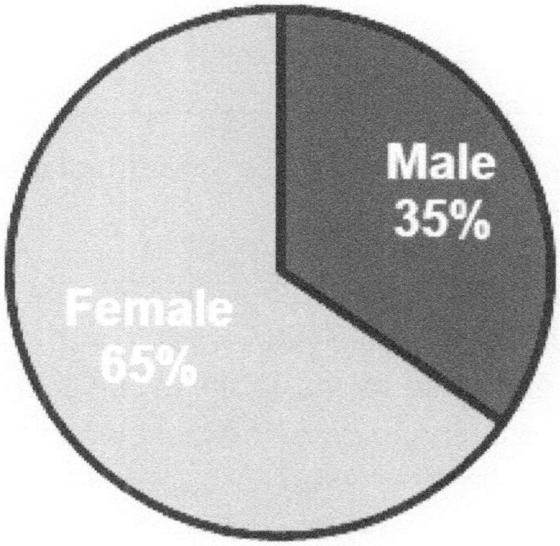

Lee et al., 2023

Older adults

Depression is a priority for older adults, too, though many are not formally diagnosed. Despite being a common behavioral health condition, depression is diagnosed only inconsistently, in about 50 percent of geriatric cases (Zenebe et al., 2021). Part of this rationale is explained by the focus of providers, patients, and their families on physical health symptoms. What's more, depression symptoms like hyposomnia, self-isolation, or limited endurance can be mistaken for other chronic health conditions common in older adults.

The intersection of depression with injurious falls yields damaging consequences in older adults. Over 30 percent of older adults suffer falls each year, with 50 percent of those falling 80 years or older (Feng et al., 2023). Depression is particularly prevalent in individuals who have fallen and require hospitalization, surgery, and rehabilitation, as their recovery can be slowed by despair over their quality of life, independence, and self-sufficiency.

Worry about the aging process can be enough to exacerbate a prior mental illness or prompt depressive episodes for patients. Treatment-resistant depression is common in older adults, and can be related to chronic medical conditions, cerebrovascular disease, co-existing anxiety, history of MDD, onset of or increase in substance abuse, or bereavement (Steffens, 2024).

POPULATION-FOCUSED MONITORING

Depression manifests in unique ways in distinct populations. We now explore what case managers should keep in mind to address the needs of their patients, especially those who are traditionally marginalized and minoritized.

LGBTQIA+

Discrimination, victimization, and family rejection are drivers of depressive disorders for the LGBTQIA+ community.

Youth. Depression is common in LGBTQIA+ youth—a full 58 percent of the population experiences the disorder (The Trevor Project, 2024). LGBTQIA+ youth are easy targets at school or in their communities for presenting their authentic selves. Bullying can be intense and unrelenting, occurring in person and on social media, resulting in psychological insecurity during the school years. The child is deprived of the sense of belonging, which results in limited social relationships (Garcia et al., 2020). The student is subjected to *social isolation* due to others' damaging actions.

They also face criticism, disbelief, and challenges from trusted allies and kin, including parents. Less than 30 percent of LGBTQ youth attain parental acceptance when they come out; many deal with ultimatums and other forced decisions (Katz-Wise, 2016). Parental expectations of heterosexuality or gender norms clash with a child's autonomy, and the difference of opinion leads to dissension in the family. The Family Acceptance Project, PFLAG, and The Trevor Project provide resources and guidance for families during the coming-out process.

Adults. Roughly 10 percent of adults who identify as sexual minorities experience moderately severe to severe depression; of those adults, 64 percent identify as women and 36 percent as men (Sarharkar & Friday, 2022). Some 32 percent of the population have been formally diagnosed with MDD (Cai et al., 2024).

The transgender and non-binary community, especially, is at greater risk for mental health issues, due to barriers to employment, rejection by family, societal discrimination, and rejection by healthcare providers. Repeated negative life experiences may devalue their self-worth. Social interactions with the general public also cause stress due to unknown intent; that is, interactions may be driven by uncharitable curiosity or stigma about their gender identity. Increased vigilance demanded by social interactions contributes to depression prevalence as high as 59 percent (Liles et al., 2024).

Orlov and Calixte (2024) researched the co-occurrence of depression with other chronic illnesses in LGBTQIA+ adults. Multimorbidity LGBTQIA+ patients are four times more likely to be depressed than patients with a single chronic illness or no chronic illness, with decreased quality of life and increased isolation (Orlove & Calixte, 2024).

Upstream factors (e.g., HRSNs, SDoH) greatly influence overall functioning and behavioral health for sexual minorities. LGBTQIA+ people are challenged in the workplace by internalized stigma, job stress, and low income, according to Tomic et al. (2025). Secure employment, and thus health insurance, can become a casualty. Box 6.7 provides a snapshot of depression-related concerns for the LGBTQIA+ community.

Box 6.7: Depression and LGBTQIA+

High incidence for:

- Depressive symptoms in youth due to bullying, family rejection, social isolation
- Major depressive disorder
- Increased risk of suicidal ideation and action

Distinct considerations:

- Concealment of sexual identity, especially for youth and young adults
- Worry about rejection by family members and friends
- Worries by trans and non-binary individuals about access to gender-affirming care
- Worries about ability to live an authentic life
- Worry about the policy and legal climate and its impact on autonomy
- Access to concordant care providers who respect their autonomy
- Contribution of HRSNs to high incidence of depression (e.g., employment and financial stability, housing sufficiency and access)

Military members and veterans

The military environment has long been viewed as "a catalyst for the development and progression of depression, and the exacerbation of pre-existing mental health conditions" (Moore et al., 2023). This reality is due to a range of factors, such as:

- Witnessing high-risk situations
- Discord among command or leadership
- Frequent relocations and change of station
- Combat stressors
- Separation from family and support systems
- Physical fitness requirements

(Moore et al., 2023)

More than 9 percent of ambulatory military health appointments are for incident-specific depression. Following deployments, diagnosed depressive disorders increase, jumping to 15 percent from 11.4 percent pre-deployment (Moore et al., 2023). During times of active conflict or war, prevalence of depression rises to almost 30 percent for active-duty military (Finnegan & Randles, 2022).

Despite the military's increased attention to mental health, accuracy of diagnosis remains low. Barely 50 percent of military members are correctly diagnosed by their providers due to missed symptoms or inconsistent use of screening tools (Moore et al., 2023).

Co-occurring substance use is addressed in Chapter 8. Case managers should be vigilant in assessing veterans and military personnel for substance use in cases of depression. Self-medication by alcohol, opioids, or other substances can intensify depression, including increased mood lability. Some 30 percent of active military personnel meet criteria for substance use disorder, and 32 percent of veterans are officially diagnosed (Boden et al., 2018; Judkins et al., 2022). These numbers speak to clear opportunities for additional mental health screening and assessment protocols, as well as access to treatment.

Military spouses and families. Military spouses and family members face considerable psychological hardship; 5 percent of military spouses are diagnosed with MDD (Donoho et al., 2018). Children feel chronic worry about their parent's safety and suffer insomnia, sadness, and reactivity, prompting DMDD diagnoses. Family members encounter isolation and loneliness due to frequent moves (Wooten et al., 2019). It can feel easier to just not make friends when arriving in a new location, knowing they'll be left later. Box 6.8 offers insight on depression in military and veteran populations.

Box 6.8: Depression and military members and veterans

High incidence for:

- Disruptive mood dysregulation disorder (in youth)
- Major depressive disorder
- Co-occurring substance use for military members, veterans, and family members

Distinct considerations:

- Stress related to being put high risk situations* or witnessing others in these situations

- Command or leadership discord
- Frequent relocations and change of station*
- Combat stressors
- Separations from family and support systems*
- Pressure to maintain physical fitness*

* Denotes risks for family members

Persons with disabilities

Persons with developmental, intellectual, physical, and other disabilities are more prone to depressive symptoms than the general population. Global research validates the correlation between a disability (learning, sensory, or neurodegenerative) and amplified depression (Asdaq et al., 2024). Persons with physical disabilities are almost twice as likely to express depression symptoms than the general population—41 percent compared to 22 percent (Shen et al., 2017).

Driving this prevalence are lack of access to stable employment, limitations on education and career trajectory, and societal prejudice and stigma (Karki et al., 2023). Disability-related prejudice is common and is known as *ableism.* It occurs in all employment sectors. Teachers, healthcare practitioners, and employers may stereotype persons with disabilities and dismiss their symptoms and voice.

Depression is the most common behavioral health disorder in children with a developmental disability (Ugwu et al., 2022). Common symptoms are depressed mood and affect, anhedonia, poor appetite, crying, and fatigue (Eaton et al., 2021).

Depression screening tools, such as the Beck Depression Inventory and PHQ-9, are helpful to assess severity of symptoms. See severity prevalence for persons with intellectual disabilities in Figure 6.4.

Case managers, particularly those specializing in workers' compensation, may work with patients who have suffered injuries that led to disability. The incidence of depressive disorders rises when patients have endured work-related accidents, traumatic injuries, and musculoskeletal disorders. Patients frequently require outpatient intervention to manage depression, as well as anxiety (López Gómez et al., 2020).

Hospitalization or unanticipated treatments can prompt strong behavior responses in patients with disabilities, and in their families. Since this population is at great risk for such circumstances, case managers should pay attention to their physical, behavioral, and psychosocial health. Worries about physical regression, reduced independence, and threats to quality of life can worsen a patient's mood and derail his or her progress and prognosis.

Case management departments may need to advocate for patients' accommodations or expanded services by collaborating with MCO and community-based case managers. This could include, but is not limited to:

- Accessible housing or other residential requirements
- Increased homecare, durable medical equipment, or other home supports
- Individualized education plans or homebound education
- Referral to vocational rehabilitation for employment allowances

Box 6.9 provides the issues case managers should keep on their radar for persons with disabilities.

Figure 6.4: *Degrees of depression in persons with intellectual disabilities*

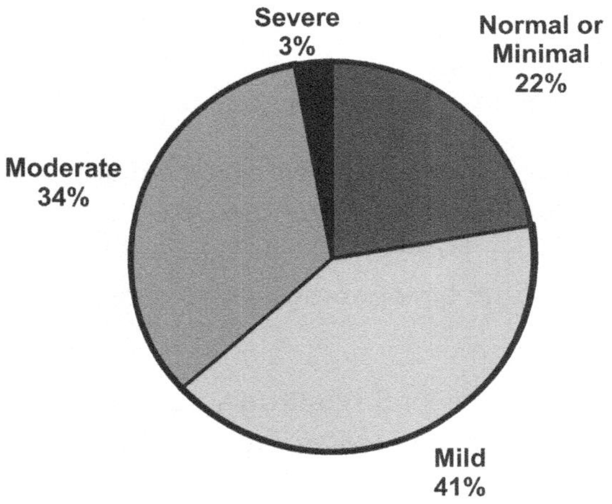

Karki et al., 2023

Box 6.9: Depression and persons with disabilities

High incidence for:

- Disruptive mood dysregulation disorder (in youth)
- Major depressive disorder
- Depressive disorder due to another medical condition

Distinct considerations:

- Presentation of depressive symptoms upon hospitalization or provider visits due to regression in physical or cognitive abilities or reduced independence
- Worry about access to education, stable employment, or accessible housing
- Reconciling ableism and stigma by educators, providers, practitioners, or employers
- Advocacy and coordination with MCO and community-based CMs and providers

Women's health

This topic fills plenty of large books. For our purposes, here's a 35,000-foot view of the topic. People born as women are twice as likely as those born as men to develop depression. Biological causes, hormonal variations, and psychosocial stressors have been cited as contributing factors (DiBennedetto, 2024; Gao et al., 2024; Keuhner, 2017). To be sure, people born as males are less likely to report their depressive feelings or to seek help.

Higher occurrence of female depression starts in adolescence (Gao et al., 2024). Alongside biochemical and hormonal factors, psychosocial stressors add fuel to the fire and continue into adulthood. Stressors include gaps in pay and employment equity and pressure related to career and parenting choices (Gao et al., 2024). Bracke et al. (2020) note that gender inequality has a cumulative effect on women, leading to greater prevalence of depression later in life. Trauma-related depression caused by physical and sexual abuse, assault, and family and intimate partner violence is also higher in women. Trauma is covered in Chapter 10.

PMDD. Recent research has yielded new perspectives on PMDD, with the diagnosis being more readily viewed as a gender-specific depressive disorder. Despite menstruation being a normal biological process, cultural beliefs can stigmatize the diagnosis as one that is a taboo or shameful presentation.

PMDD diagnosis occurs as early as mid- or late adolescence (Akyuk-Cim & Cim, 2023), but on average, women are diagnosed with PMDD when they're 33-35 years old. Many women have endured years of mood lability and physical and emotional discomfort before diagnosis.

Economic burden of PMDD is sizeable with direct and indirect costs. Patients with this diagnosis often need multiple and repeated practitioner visits annually with many diagnostic studies and lab tests to ascertain symptom etiology. Absenteeism rates for patients with PMDD are over 8 hours per menstrual cycle and may impair productivity, with indirect costs estimated at $4,000 per person annually (Islas-Preciado et al., 2025).

Medical gaslighting can happen to PMDD sufferers, as providers dismiss symptoms. This dismissal intensifies feelings of discomfort, demoralization, and despair, with suicidal ideation common (Chan et al., 2023). Getting a PMDD diagnosis and treatment typically requires prolific self-advocacy to navigate the healthcare maze and the stigma. It is difficult for patients, especially patients experiencing the debilitating indicators of PMDD, to amass the emotional fortitude to persevere to diagnosis. A high-level summary of issues regarding depression and women's health appears in Box 6.10.

Box 6.10: Depression and women's health

High incidence for:

- Major depressive disorder
- Premenstrual dysphoric disorder

Distinct considerations:

- Hormonal imbalances and shifts
- Effective management of the menopause continuum (e.g., perimenopause, menopause, and post menopause)
- Medical gaslighting
- Misdiagnosis of PMDD
- Societal stigma prompts stress related to career-or-homemaker choices, gender pay inequities, and related pressures
- Trauma (e.g., bullying, intimate partner violence, physical and sexual abuse and assault)

SCREENING AND ASSESSMENT TOOLS FOR DEPRESSION

Most case managers are familiar with one or more screening tools for depression, primarily the PHQ-9. An array of options is provided. The screening tools in Table 6.2 are for adults or general use across the lifespan. The tools in Table 6.3 are for youth.

Table 6.2: *Screening tools for depression (youth and adults)*

Instrument	Focus	Source
Beck Depression Inventory (BDI)	Self-report questionnaire of 21 items that screens for the presence and severity of depression For ages 13 to 80 years old	Beck, A.T., Ward, C.H., Mendelson, M., Mock, J., & Erbaugh, J. (1961). An inventory for measuring depression. *Archives of General Psychiatry, 4*(6), 561-571. http://dx.doi.org/10.1001/archpsyc.1961.01710120031004
Beck Hopelessness Scale	Self-report questionnaire of 20 items to assess a person's negative expectations about the future; true or false responses For adults	Beck, A.T., Weissman, A., Lester, D., & Trexler, L. (1974). The measurement of pessimism: The Hopelessness Scale. Journal of Consulting and Clinical Psychology, 42(6), 861-865. http://dx.doi.org/10.1037/h0037562
Center for Epidemiologic Studies Depression Scale (CES-D)	20-item self-report questionnaire to measure major dimensions of depression in the past week, scored on a 4-point scale For ages 6 to older adults	Radloff, L.S. (1977). The CES-D Scale: A self-report report depression scale for research in the general population. *Applied Psychological Measurement, 1*(3), 385-401. http://dx.doi.org/10.1177/014662167700100306

Instrument	Focus	Source
EQ-5D	Standardized, non-disease specific instrument to describe and evaluate health-related quality of life The instrument measures quality of life in 5 dimensions: mobility self-care usual activities pain/discomfort anxiety/depression Versions for youth (ages 8-15) and adults (age 16 and up)	The EuroQol Group (1990) EuroQol — A new facility for the measurement of health-related quality of life. *Health Policy, 16*(3), 199-208. https://doi.org/10.1016/0168-8510(90)90421-9
Geriatric Depression Scale (GDS)	4-, 10-, 15-, and 30-item questionnaires (yes/no responses) to screen and measure depression in older adults	Yesavage, J.A., Brink, T.L., Rose, T.L., Lum, O., Huang, V., Adey, M., & Leirer, V.O. (1982-1983). Development and validation of a Geriatric Depression Screening Scale: A preliminary report. *Journal of Psychiatric Research, 17*(1), 37-49. http://dx.doi.org/10.1016/0022-3956(82)90033-4
Hamilton Depression Rating Scale (HDRS, HRSD, or HAM-D)	21-item questionnaire used by healthcare professionals to measure depression in individuals before, during, and after treatment; scored on a 5-point or 3-point scale Ages: not specified	Hamilton, M. (1960). A rating scale for depression. *Journal of Neurology, Neurosurgery & Psychiatry, 23*, 56-61. http://dx.doi.org/10.1136/jnnp.23.1.56
Montgomery-Asberg Depression Rating Scale (MADRS)	10-item questionnaire that uses a 7-point rating scale to measure the severity of depression For ages 18 and up	Montgomery, S.A., & Åsberg, M. (1979). A new depression scale designed to be sensitive to change. *The British Journal of Psychiatry, 134*, 382-389. http://dx.doi.org/10.1192/bjp.134.4.382
Patient Health Questionnaire (PHQ)	Self-report measuring system used in primary/specialty care to screen for the presence and severity of depression: Part 1 PHQ-2: Preliminary brief 2-item screen Part 2 PHQ-9: 9-item screen to assess symptom severity over the past two weeks	Spitzer, R.L., Kroenke, K., Williams, J.B.W., & Patient Health Questionnaire Primary Care Study Group. (1999). Validation and utility of a self-report version of PRIME-MD: The PHQ primary care study. *JAMA 282*(18), 1737-1744. http://dx.doi.org/10.1001/jama.282.18.173

Table 6.3: *Screening tools for depression (youth)*

Instrument	Focus	Source
Behavioral Assessment System for Children (BASC)	Assesses emotional disorders, personality constructs, and behavioral problems in individuals from ages 2 to 21, and from 3 perspectives: teacher, parent, and self (starting at age 8)	Merenda, P.F. (1996). BASC: Behavior Assessment System for Children. *Measurement and Evaluation in Counseling and Development, 28*(4), 229-232.
Child Behavior Checklist (CBCL)	Standardized questionnaire administered to parents to obtain reports of their children's social competence and behavioral problems	Achenbach, T.M. (1978). The child behavior profile: An empirically based system for assessing children's behavioral problems and competencies. *International Journal of Mental Health, 7*(3-4), 24-42. https://doi.org/10.1080/00207411.1978.11448806
Childhood Depression Inventory (CDI)	A modification of the Beck Depression Inventory for adults, this version assesses depression severity in children and adolescents, ages 7-17 2 scales measure emotional and functional problems with a rater form for teachers, parents, and patient self-report	Kovacs, M. (1981). Rating scales to assess depression in school-aged children. *Acta Paedopsychiatrica: International Journal of Child & Adolescent Psychiatry, 46*(5-6), 305-315. http://dx.doi.org/10.1037/t00788-000
Patient Health Questionnaire Adolescent Version (PHQ-A)	A distinct version of the PHQ-9 used to screen for depression and other mental health conditions in adolescents in primary care settings Focus is on whether the adolescent is experiencing symptoms related to anxiety, mood, eating, or substance use disorders	Johnson, J.G., Harris, E.S., Spitzer, R.L., & Williams, J.B. (2002). The patient health questionnaire for adolescents: Validation of an instrument for the assessment of mental disorders among adolescent primary care patients. *Journal of Adolescent Health, 30*(3), 196-204. doi:10.1016/s1054-139x(01)00333-0

CONCLUSION

Depression is a complex and expansive topic. This chapter has provided the basic information for case managers to better understand and screen for depression and facilitate quality-driven and inclusive care. Our next stop on the behavioral health highway is SMI and a population of heavy users of healthcare and case management intervention.

CONTEMPLATION QUESTIONS

1. 1. Consider a time when you experienced feelings of depression. Answer the following prompts:
   a) Where did your symptoms fall on the depression continuum?
   b) How did the symptoms impact your social, occupational, or academic functioning?
   c) What did you do to resolve the depression?
   d) What did you learn about yourself as you moved through the process?
2. Access one of the screening tools for depression from the MD+CALC website (found in the resources list at the end of the chapter).
   a) Review the screening tool.
   b) Complete it for yourself, then total your score.
   c) How will a standardized depression screening tool inform your future efforts?
3. Review the depressive disorders in Table 6.1.
   a) Which diagnoses are you most familiar with, personally or professionally?
   b) Reflect on professional experiences you have had with patients diagnosed with depressive disorders.

Use the following case scenario and the Behavioral Health Conversation Map in Table 1.4 to respond to questions 4 and 5.

Napoleon is an MCO case manager who has just been assigned Maya, an adult female who resides alone and has a 3-year history of multiple sclerosis. Maya was recently hospitalized for left wrist and ankle fractures, sustained when she slipped in the bathroom. She spent 3 weeks in acute rehab and was emphatic about a discharge home. She currently lives independently, with ambulation using a quad cane within her apartment and supervision when in the community.

Napoleon's colleague, Michael, worked with Maya and the rehab case manager to complete a home safety evaluation prior to Maya's discharge. The safety evaluation resulted in installation of DME for the bathroom, including a shower seat, grab bars, and 3-in-1 commode placed by Maya's bed for use as needed.

Napoleon held a virtual meeting with Maya immediately after her discharge. While still expressing sadness over her ongoing physical limits and potential future deterioration, Maya vocalized her determination to return to her baseline functioning before the fall: "I hate this but am starting to cope with this new norm. My online therapist has been a big help. I was simply moving too fast and knew better. I get impatient and still think that I can move at the speed of sound."

Then Napoleon reviewed the documentation completed by the home health nurse following her recent intake visit: "Patient is alert and oriented, though defensive to suggestions for long-term placement. The topic was broached, but the interview could not be completed. The patient escorted this nurse to the door and requested she leave immediately. She became rude and slammed the door."

Napoleon is left wondering, "What happened?"

1. Reflect on how ableism is relevant in this situation.
2. Use the Behavioral Health Conversation Map to guide Napoleon's interactions with Maya moving forward.

RESOURCES

- **Family Acceptance Project**
  https://familyproject.sfsu.edu/
- **MD+CALC**
  https://www.mdcalc.com
- **National Institute of Mental Health - Depression**
  https://www.nimh.nih.gov/health/topics/depression
- **PFLAG**
  https://pflag.org
- **The Trevor Project**
  https://www.thetrevorproject.org
- **World Health Organization**
  https://www.who.int/news-room/fact-sheets/detail/depression

Integrated Care further reading

- Amelung, V.E., Stein, V., Suter, E., Goodwin, N., Balicer, R. & Beese, A. (Eds). (2025). *Handbook of Integrated Care*, 3rd ed. Springer: New York, New York.
- English, C., Baldwin, U.G., Fink-Samnick, E. (Eds). (2026). *Integrated Behavioral Health: Applying the Biodyne Model in Healthcare.* Routledge/Taylor & Francis, United Kingdom.
- Hunter, C.L., Goodie, J.L., Oordt, M.S., & Dobmeyer, A.C. (2024). *Integrated Behavioral Health in Primary Care: Step-by-step Guidance for Assessment and Intervention*, 3rd ed. American Psychological Association, Washington, D.C.
- Mancini, M.A. (2021). *Integrated Behavioral Health Practice.* Springer Nature Publishing: New York, New York.

REFERENCES

- Akyuz Cim, E.F., & Cim, N. (2023). The effect of premenstrual dysphoric disorder diagnosis and severity on depression sensitivity. *The Journal of Nervous and Mental Disease*, *211*(11), 862-865. https://doi.org/10.1097/NMD.0000000000001736
- Alotaibi, R., Halbesma, N., Wild, S.H., & Jackson, C.A. (2024). Severe depression and all-cause and cause-specific mortality in Scotland: 20-year national cohort study. *BJPsych Open*, *10*(1), e28. https://doi.org/10.1192/bjo.2023.633
- American Psychiatric Association. (2022). *Diagnostic and Statistical Manual of Mental Disorders* (5th ed., text rev.).
- Asdaq, S.M.B., Alshehri, S., Alajlan, S.A., Almutiri, A.A., & Alanazi, A.K.R. (2024). Depression in persons with disabilities: A scoping review. *Frontiers in Public Health*, *12*, 1383078. https://doi.org/10.3389/fpubh.2024.1383078
- Boden, M.T., & Hoggatt, K.J. (2018). Substance use disorders among veterans in a nationally representative sample: Prevalence and associated functioning and treatment utilization. *Journal of Studies on Alcohol and Drugs*, *79*(6), 853-861. https://doi.org/10.15288/jsad.2018.79.853
- Boland, R., Verduin, M.L., & Ruiz, P. (2022). *Kaplan and Sadock's Synopsis of Psychiatry* (12th ed.). Lippincott Williams & Wilkins, Wolters Kluwer.
- Bracke, P., Delaruelle, K., Dereuddre, R., & Van de Velde, S. (2020). Depression in women and men, cumulative disadvantage and gender inequality in 29 European countries. *Social Science & Medicine (1982)*, *267*, 113354. https://doi.org/10.1016/j.socscimed.2020.113354
- Cai, H., Xie, X.M., Zhang, Q., Cui, X., Lin, J.X., Sim, K., Ungvari, G.S., Zhang, L., & Xiang, Y.T. (2021). Prevalence of suicidality in major depressive disorder: A systematic review and meta-analysis of comparative studies. *Frontiers in Psychiatry*, *12*, 690130. https://doi.org/10.3389/fpsyt.2021.690130
- Cai, H., Chen, P., Zhang, Q., Lam, M.I., Si, T.L., Liu, Y.F., Zheng, W.Y., Su, Z., Cheung, T., & Jackson, T. et al. (2024). Global prevalence of major depressive disorder in LGBTQ+ samples: A systematic review and meta-analysis of epidemiological studies. *Journal of Affective Disorders*, *360*, 249-258. https://doi.org/10.1016/j.jad.2024.05.115
- Chan, K., Rubtsova, A.A., & Clark, C.J. (2023). Exploring diagnosis and treatment of premenstrual dysphoric disorder in the U.S. healthcare system: A qualitative investigation. *BMC Women's Health*, *23*(1), 272. https://doi.org/10.1186/s12905-023-02334-y
- Cui, L., Li, S., Wang, S., Wu, X., Liu, Y., Yu, W., Wang, Y., Tang, Y., Xia, M., & Li, B. (2024). Major depressive disorder: Hypothesis, mechanism, prevention and treatment. *Signal Transduction and Targeted Therapy*, *9*(1), 30. https://doi.org/10.1038/s41392-024-01738-y
- Di Benedetto, M.G., Landi, P., Mencacci, C., & Cattaneo, A. (2024). Depression in women: Potential biological and sociocultural factors driving the sex effect. *Neuropsychobiology*, *83*(1), 2-16. https://doi.org/10.1159/000531588
- Donoho, C.J., LeardMann, C., O'Malley, C.A., Walter, K.H., Riviere, L.A., Curry, J.F., & Adler, A. B. (2018). Depression among military spouses: Demographic, military, and service member

psychological health risk factors. *Depression and Anxiety, 35*(12), 1137-1144. https://doi.org/10.1002/da.22820

- Eaton, C., Tarver, J., Shirazi, A., Pearson, E., Walker, L., Bird, M., Oliver, C., & Waite, J. (2021). A systematic review of the behaviours associated with depression in people with severe-profound intellectual disability. *Journal of Intellectual Disability Research, 65*(3), 211-229. https://doi.org/10.1111/jir.12807
- Engel, G.L. (1977). The need for a new medical model: A challenge for biomedicine. *Science, 196*(4286), 129-136. https://doi.org/10.1126/science.847460
- Feng, Z., Chen, Q., Li, Y., Xue, Z., & Hao, X. (2023). The association between falls and depressive symptoms among older adults: Evidence from the China Health and Retirement Longitudinal Study. *Frontiers in Public Health, 11*, 1248551. https://doi.org/10.3389/fpubh.2023.1248551
- Finnegan, A., & Randles, R. (2023). Prevalence of common mental health disorders in military veterans: Using primary healthcare data. *BMJ Military Health, 169*(6), 523-528. https://doi.org/10.1136/bmjmilitary-2021-002045
- Garcia, J., Vargas, N., Clark, J.L., Magaña Álvarez, M., Nelons, D.A., & Parker, R.G. (2020). Social isolation and connectedness as determinants of well-being: Global evidence mapping focused on LGBTQ youth. *Global Public Health, 15*(4), 497-519. https://doi.org/10.1080/17441692.2019.1682028
- Glette, M., Stiles, T.C., Jensen, M.P., Nilsen, T.I.L., Borchgrevink, P.C., & Landmark, T. (2021). Impact of pain and catastrophizing on the long-term course of depression in the general population: The HUNT pain study. *Pain, 162*(6), 1650-1658. https://doi.org/10.1097/j.pain.0000000000002168
- Islas-Preciado, D., Ramos-Lira, L., & Estrada-Camarena, E. (2025). Unveiling the burden of premenstrual dysphoric disorder: A narrative review to call for gender perspective and intersectional approaches. *Frontiers in Psychiatry, 15*, 1458114. https://doi.org/10.3389/fpsyt.2024.1458114
- Judkins, J.L., Smith, K., Moore, B.A., & Morissette, S.B. (2022). Alcohol use disorder in active duty service members: Incidence rates over a 19-year period. *Substance Abuse, 43*(1), 294-300. https://doi.org/10.1080/08897077.2021.1941512
- Karki, P., Shahi, P.V., Sapkota, K.P., Bhandari, R., Adhikari, N., & Shrestha, B. (2023). Depressive symptoms and associated factors among persons with physical disabilities in disability care homes of Kathmandu district, Nepal: A mixed method study. *PLOS Global Public Health, 3*(1), e0001461. https://doi.org/10.1371/journal.pgph.0001461
- Kuehner C. (2017). Why is depression more common among women than among men? *The Lancet Psychiatry, 4*(2), 146-158. https://doi.org/10.1016/S2215-0366(16)30263-2
- Lee, C.S., & Wong, Y.J. (2020). Racial/ethnic and gender differences in the antecedents of youth suicide. *Cultural Diversity & Ethnic Minority Psychology, 26*(4), 532-543. https://doi.org/10.1037/cdp0000326
- Lee, B., Wang, Y., Carlson, S.A., Greenlund, K.J., Lu, H., Liu, Y., Croft, J. B., Eke, P. I., Town, M., & Thomas, C.W. (2023). National, state-level, and county-level prevalence estimates of adults

aged ≥18 years self-reporting a lifetime diagnosis of depression - United States, 2020. *Morbidity and Mortality Weekly Report, 72*(24), 644-650. https://doi.org/10.15585/mmwr.mm7224a1

- Liles, S.M., Olsavsky, A.L., Chen, D., Grannis, C., Hoskinson, K.R., Leibowitz, S.F., Nelson, E. E., Stanek, C.J., Strang, J.F., & Nahata, L. (2024). Depression and anxiety in transgender and non-binary adolescents: Prevalence and associations between adolescent and caregiver reports. *European Journal of Pediatrics, 183*(11), 4711-4719. https://doi.org/10.1007/s00431-024-05723-z
- Lim, I.C.Z.Y., Tam, W.W.S., Chudzicka-Czupała, A., McIntyre, R.S., Teopiz, K.M., Ho, R.C., & Ho, C.S.H. (2022). Prevalence of depression, anxiety and post-traumatic stress in war- and conflict-afflicted areas: A meta-analysis. *Frontiers in Psychiatry, 13*, 978703. https://doi.org/10.3389/fpsyt.2022.978703
- López Gómez, M.A., Williams, J.A.R., Boden, L., Sorensen, G., Hopcia, K., Hashimoto, D., & Sabbath, E. (2020). The relationship of occupational injury and use of mental health care. *Journal of Safety Research, 74,* 227-232. https://doi.org/10.1016/j.jsr.2020.06.004
- Ma, Y., Xiang, Q., Yan, C., Liao, H., & Wang, J. (2021). Relationship between chronic diseases and depression: The mediating effect of pain. *BMC Psychiatry, 21*(1), 436. https://doi.org/10.1186/s12888-021-03428-3
- Mekonen, T., Chan, G.C.K., Connor, J.P., Hides, L., & Leung, J. (2021). Estimating the global treatment rates for depression: A systematic review and meta-analysis. *Journal of Affective Disorders, 295*, 1234-1242. https://doi.org/10.1016/j.jad.2021.09.038
- Moore, M.J., Shawler, E., Jordan, C.H., & Jackson, C.A. (2023). Veteran and Military Mental Health Issues. StatPearls Publishing: Treasure Island, FL. Available from https://pubmed.ncbi.nlm.nih.gov/34283458/
- Mulraney, M., Coghill, D., Bishop, C., Mehmed, Y., Sciberras, E., Sawyer, M., Efron, D., & Hiscock, H. (2021). A systematic review of the persistence of childhood mental health problems into adulthood. *Neuroscience and biobehavioral reviews, 129*, 182–205. https://doi.org/10.1016/j.neubiorev.2021.07.030
- Noori, T., Sureda, A., Sobarzo-Sánchez, E., & Shirooie, S. (2022). The role of natural products in treatment of depressive disorder. *Current Neuropharmacology, 20*(5), 929-949. https://doi.org/10.2174/1570159X20666220103140834
- Pederson A.B. (2023). Management of depression in Black people: Effects of cultural issues. *Psychiatric Annals, 53*(3), 122-125. https://doi.org/10.3928/00485713-20230215-01
- Ong, M.S., Lakoma, M., Gees Bhosrekar, S., Hickok, J., McLean, L., Murphy, M., Poland, R.E., Purtell, N., & Ross-Degnan, D. (2021). Risk factors for suicide attempt in children, adolescents, and young adults hospitalized for mental health disorders. *Child and Adolescent Mental Health, 26*(2), 134-142. https://doi.org/10.1111/camh.12400
- Orlov, D. & Calixte, R. (2024). The association of sexual minority status with the prevalence, diagnosis, and treatment of depression among NYC adults. *Journal of Community Health, 49,* 954-958. https://doi.org/10.1007/s10900-024-01336-7

- Rikard-Bell, C., Hunt, C., McAulay, C., Hay, P., Morad, A., Cunich, M., & Touyz, S. (2022). Adolescent depression from a developmental perspective: The importance of recognizing developmental distress in depressed adolescents. *International Journal of Environmental Research and Public Health*, *19*(23), 16029. https://doi.org/10.3390/ijerph192316029
- Sakharkar, P., & Friday, K. (2022). Examining health disparities and severity of depression among sexual minorities in a national population sample. *Diseases*, *10*(4), 86. https://doi.org/10.3390/diseases10040086
- Schroll, J.B., & Lauritsen, M.P. (2022). Premenstrual dysphoric disorder: A controversial new diagnosis. *Acta Obstetricia et Gynecologica Scandinavica*, *101*(5), 482-483. https://doi.org/10.1111/aogs.14360
- Shen, S.C., Huang, K.H., Kung, P.T., Chiu, L.T., & Tsai, W.C. (2017). Incidence, risk, and associated factors of depression in adults with physical and sensory disabilities: A nationwide population-based study. *PloS One*, *12*(3), e0175141. https://doi.org/10.1371/journal.pone.0175141
- Steffens, D.C. (2024). Treatment-resistant depression in older adults. *The New England Journal of Medicine*, *390*(7), 630-639. https://doi.org/10.1056/NEJMcp2305428
- Tebeka, S., Geoffroy, P.A., Dubertret, C., & Le Strat, Y. (2021). Sadness and the continuum from well-being to depressive disorder: Findings from a representative US population sample. *Journal of Psychiatric Research*, *132*, 50–54. https://doi.org/10.1016/j.jpsychires.2020.10.004
- The Trevor Project. (2024). U.S. national survey on the mental health of LGBTQ+ young people. Retrieved May 26, 2025, from https://www.thetrevorproject.org/survey-2024/
- Tomic, D., O'Dwyer, M., Keegel, T., & Walker-Bone, K. (2025). Mental health of LGBTQ+ workers: A systematic review. *BMC Psychiatry*, *25*(1), 114. https://doi.org/10.1186/s12888-025-06556-2
- Ugwu, G.C., Ugwuanyi, C.S., Okeke, C.I.O., Uzodinma, U.E., & Aneke, A.O. (2022). Efficacy of rational emotive behavior therapy on depression among children with learning disabilities: Implications for evaluation in science teaching. *Journal of Rational-Emotive & Cognitive-Behavior Therapy, 40,* 313-333. https://doi.org/10.1007/s10942-021-00417-z
- U.S. Centers for Disease Control and Prevention. (2024). Anxiety and Depression in Children: Children's Mental Health. Retrieved December 17, 2024, from https://www.cdc.gov/children-mental-health/about/about-anxiety-and-depression-in-children.html
- Wooten, N.R., Brittingham, J.A., Sumi, N.S., Pitner, R.O., & Moore, K.D. (2019). Behavioral health service use by military children during Afghanistan and Iraq Wars. *The Journal of Behavioral Health Services & Research*, *46*(4), 549-569. https://doi.org/10.1007/s11414-018-09646-0
- World Health Organization. (2023). Depressive Disorder: Key Facts. Retrieved May 20, 2025, from https://www.who.int/news-room/fact-sheets/detail/depression
- Zenebe, Y., Akele, B., W/Selassie, M., & Necho, M. (2021). Prevalence and determinants of depression among old age: A systematic review and meta-analysis. *Annals of General Psychiatry*, *20*(1), 55. https://doi.org/10.1186/s12991-021-00375-x

CHAPTER 7

SEVERE MENTAL ILLNESS

INTRODUCTION

Patients with SMI are among largest and most difficult patient populations case managers work with, and the population is prioritized for case management. The financial, personal, and emotional costs of these illnesses are massive. Patients with SMI may appear as "frequent flyers" in hospital EDs or community-based clinics. After hospitalization, they may require post-acute placement for short-term skilled nursing needs. Safe discharge plans often must be provided, and questions about clinical capacity, autonomy, and treatment non-adherence can involve ethics committees. Patients who live with SMI are more likely to face chronic co-occurring conditions, but primary and specialty care access can be hampered by insurance limits, coverage gaps, and other factors. When youth are diagnosed with an SMI, families must manage staggering clinical, fiscal, emotional, and human burdens. This chapter addresses the moving parts of SMI.

A note: The topic of SMI covers enormous range, which required a shift in this chapter's organization. To provide the most comprehensive information to guide case management practice, I replaced population-based material specific to the LGBTQIA+, military, disability, and women's communities with more information on general risks and developmental life stages.

BEHAVIORAL LEARNING OBJECTIVES

1. Know which disorders are considered severe mental illnesses (SMI)
2. Identify the SMI continuum
3. Relate symptoms and treatment recommendations for common DSM diagnoses
4. Understand how SMI appears across developmental life stages
5. Analyze the incidence of SMI across life stages and populations
6. Identify screening tools to assess for SMI
7. Apply Case Management's Behavioral Health Conversation Map to patients and their families living with SMI

ESSENTIAL TERMS

- Anosognosia
- Attenuated
- Avolition
- Bipolar disorder I
- Bipolar disorder II
- Compulsions
- Delusional disorder
- Delusions
- Disability
- Disorganized thinking
- Hallucinations
- Hypersomnia
- Mania
- Multimorbidity
- Obsessions
- Obsessive compulsive disorder
- Psychosis
- Psychotic disorders
- Relapse
- Remission
- Schizoaffective disorder
- Schizophrenia
- Schizophrenia spectrum
- Schizophreniform disorder
- SMI spectrum
- Social Security Disability Income (SSDI)
- Social Security Insurance (SSI)
- Subthreshold

TERMS AND FEATURES OF SMI

SMIs are not restricted to a single category of the DSM. They appear across several categories, spanning the schizophrenia spectrum, other psychotic disorders, and depressive, anxiety, personality, trauma, and stressor-related disorders. They form a distinct subset of mental disorders that share a common thread: serious functional impairment that substantially interferes with or limits one or more major life activities (National Institute of Mental Health, 2024a).

THE SMI SPECTRUM

Unlike the other mental illness categories discussed so far in this book, disorders categorized as SMI do not progress linearly along a continuum. Instead, the conditions present as a spectrum of symptoms with varying frequency and severity. Patients may have periods of stability, then experience relapse or regression of degrees of impairment, as shown in Figure 7.1.

Discerning normal behaviors from SMI symptoms is a challenge; SMI behaviors appear very different from person to person. What may present as mania in one person may be a steady personality trait for another. Imagine an exuberant, outgoing individual, always in overdrive, whose energies are channeled entirely into work. She's viewed as an ambitious and determined professional—not someone on the verge of a manic episode. When does exuberance become mania? It turns manic when that ambitious professional stays up all night working and continues the behavior over days. Her mood becomes erratic, and she begins to struggle with motivation. She socializes less and withdraws more often. Colleagues may rationalize the change as exhaustion, but the behaviors have crossed a diagnostic line.

This woman's symptoms represent a critical marker, the prodromal phase of bipolar I, with mixed features or rapid cycling. With SMIs, any symptoms are a critical assessment opportunity.

Remember, the prodromal period precedes a patient's first episode of psychosis. Prodromal periods are especially characteristic of schizophrenia and bipolar disorder, and the periods can last from months to years (Conroy et al., 2018).

During psychosis, patients may report hearing voices or seeing images that they believe are real. These events can be frightening to witnesses. Patient can experience *delusions*, or false beliefs, despite evidence to the contrary. *Hallucinations* are also common, where a person believes he sees, hears, smells, tastes, or senses an external reality that nobody else does. These symptoms disrupt socialization and relationships by impeding the ability to attend work or classes or engage in discussions. Thus, they impact employment stability as well. SMIs escalate in severity when symptoms become more frequent or intense.

Another common symptom of SMI is *anosognosia,* or profound lack of awareness of their condition or situation. A person may present with impaired judgment, labile or uncontrolled emotions, lapses in or absence of memory, or lack of executive functioning. They may show disrupted language or poor balance, motor ability, or coordination. Anosognosia is among the most common reasons patients diagnosed with an SMI don't seek treatment or adhere to it (Acharya & Sánchez-Manso, 2023).

Case managers often meet patients who have reported various, disconnected symptoms of SMI over repeated ED visits and encounters with healthcare. This varied presentation can confuse the diagnostic process and sometimes leads to misdiagnosis. When people's symptoms are less intense or occur less often than those typically seen in a full-blown psychotic state, such as schizophrenia, they are referred to as *subthreshold* or *attenuated* symptoms. The symptoms still warrant clinical evaluation and attention, however. Consider a patient who discloses she stayed up all night reading a new book or binging on a TV show. Who hasn't gotten engaged in an activity and lost track of time? The short-term occurrence of these behaviors is less concerning than if they span long periods or happen frequently.

Figure 7.1: *The SMI spectrum*

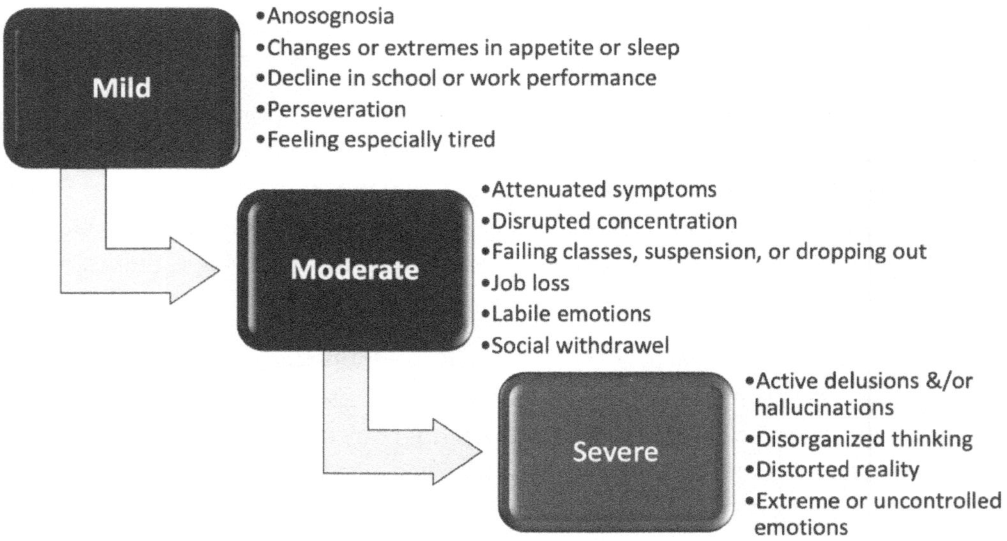

COMMON SMI DISORDERS

The most common SMIs are bipolar disorder (bipolar I and severe or recurrent bipolar II), severe or recurrent MDD, delusional disorders, disorders on the schizophrenia spectrum, and conditions in the 'other psychotic disorders' classification. Case managers may interact with patients who have other diagnosed mental illnesses that also meet the criteria for SMI, such as post-traumatic stress disorder, panic disorder (severe), obsessive-compulsive disorder, certain neurocognitive disorders, or intellectual disorders. Table 7.1 shows DSM-5-TR diagnoses commonly considered SMI. Bookmark this page, as you will refer to the table throughout the chapter.

Note how bipolar II uses a single code. The specifiers of patient severity, presence of psychotic features, and course are not identified by unique diagnostic codes, but rather in written form. For example, case managers might read, "F31.81, hypomanic, severe, with mood-congruent features."

This section includes information on those diagnoses not addressed elsewhere in this text. MDD and panic disorder appear with their primary DSM categories of depressive disorders (Chapter 6) and anxiety disorders (Chapter 4), respectively. Post-traumatic stress disorder (PTSD) is addressed in Chapter 10.

Table 7.1: *DSM-5-TR diagnoses for severe mental illness*

DSM-5-TR Diagnosis	Code			
Bipolar I disorder	Current/most recent episode manic	Current/most recent episode hypomanic	Current/most recent episode depressed	Current/most recent episode unspecified
Specifiers:				
• Mild	F31.11	N/A	F31.31	N/A
• Moderate	F31.12	N/A	F31.32	N/A
• Severe	F31.13	N/A	F31.4	N/A
• With psychotic features	F31.2	N/A	F31.5	N/A
• In partial remission	F31.73	F31.71	F31.75	N/A
• In full remission	F31.74	F31.72	F31.76	N/A
• Unspecified	F31.9	F31.9	F31.9	N/A
With:				
• Anxious distress				
• Mixed features				
• Rapid cycling				
• Melancholic features				
• Atypical features				
• Mood-congruent psychotic features				
• Mood-incongruent psychotic features				
• With catatonia				
• Peripartum onset				
• Seasonal pattern				
Bipolar II disorder	F31.81			
Specifiers				
• Mild, moderate, or severe				
• Hypomanic or depressed				
• In partial remission or full remission				
With				
• Anxious distress				
• Mixed features				
• Rapid cycling				
• Melancholic features				
• Atypical features				
• Mood-congruent psychotic features				
• Mood-incongruent psychotic features				
• With catatonia				
• Peripartum onset				
Seasonal pattern				
Delusional disorder	F22			

Table 7.1: *DSM-5-TR diagnoses for severe mental illness*

DSM-5-TR Diagnosis	Code	
Specifiers:	Major themes of each delusion specifier:	
• Erotomanic	Another person is in love with the patient	
• Grandiose	Belief one has a great talent or insight that is unrecognized by others	
• Jealous	View that a spouse, lover, or partner is unfaithful	
• Persecutory	Belief one is conspired against, spied on, followed, poisoned or drugged, maligned, harassed, or obstructed in pursuit of long-term goals	
• Somatic	Belief involves bodily functions or sensations (e.g. body odor, deformity)	
• Mixed type	Multiple beliefs with no single dominant theme	
• Unspecified type	Dominant theme cannot be determined	
Specify if bizarre or implausible content		
Specify episode, whether: • First episode: currently in acute episode, partial remission or full remission • Multiple episodes, currently in acute episode, partial remission, or full remission		
Major depressive disorder (severe or recurrent)		
Specifiers:	Single episode	Recurrent episode
Severe	F32.2	F33.2
With psychotic features	F32.3	F33.3
Panic disorder (severe)	F41.0	
Obsessive compulsive disorder (OCD)	F42.2	
Specify if: • With good or fair insight • With poor insight • With absent insight/delusional beliefs Specify if tic-related		
Post-traumatic stress disorder	F43.10	
Specify with: • Dissociative symptoms • Depersonalization • Derealization		

Table 7.1: *DSM-5-TR diagnoses for severe mental illness*

DSM-5-TR Diagnosis	Code
Schizoaffective disorder	Bipolar type F25.0; Depressive type F25.1
Specify episode, whether: • First episode, currently in acute episode, partial remission, or full remission • Multiple episodes, currently in acute episode, partial remission, or full remission • Continuous • Unspecified Specify with catatonia (note: add F06.1)	
Schizophreniform disorder	F20.81
Specify • With or without good prognostic features • With catatonia (Note: add F06.1) Severity using Clinician-Rated Dimensions of Psychosis Symptom Severity for DSM-5-TR	
Schizophrenia	F20.9
Specify episode, whether: • First episode, currently in acute episode, partial remission, or full remission • Multiple episodes, currently in acute episode, partial remission, or full remission • Continuous • Unspecified Specify with catatonia (Note: add F06.1) Severity using Clinician-Rated Dimensions of Psychosis Symptom Severity for DSM-5-TR	

BIPOLAR I DISORDER

Imagine you are riding a roller coaster. You anticipate the ascents and drops along the track, but they feel sudden and terrifying anyway. You move at a steady speed then feel the gears shift; the cars are now at the highest point of the track. Time feels infinite before the drop to the lowest point begins. Just as your nerves settle and you anticipate getting off the ride, the cycle begins all over again. Your lack of control evokes anxiety and fear. Patients with *bipolar I* disorder face similar rapid and inexplicable cycling.

The population hit hardest by bipolar I disorder is young adults, up to their 30s. They may experience an acute phase of either depressive symptoms or mania, with repeated courses of *remission*—or being symptom-free. There may also be periods of total *relapse,* when symptoms recur and functioning further deteriorates. Persons with bipolar I disorder may attain total remission, but even then can experience residual symptoms that impede their functioning and quality of life. Treatment of bipolar disorders traditionally follows a phased response, as shown in Figure 7.2. Symptoms and treatment for bipolar I are found in Box 7.1.

Challenges between manic, hypomanic, and depressive episodes. Patients with bipolar I may have manic, hypomanic, or depressive episodes. Patients with severe mania or depression often warrant inpatient treatment for safety and stabilization. The extreme behavioral manifestations leave patients vulnerable to physical or emotional harm, as in:

- Impulsive, high-risk, or unsafe behaviors (e.g., gambling, binge-spending, hypersexual desires or impulsive sexual encounters, reckless driving), which
- Potentially lead to financial, legal, and relationship consequences
- Substance use that exacerbates euphoria
- Sleep deprivation that reduces a person's insight or awareness of danger or risk

Feeling elated and omnipotent impacts a person's judgement, which negatively affects treatment adherence, particularly medication management (Lintunen et al., 2023).

By comparison, individuals undergoing hypomanic episodes are often treated as outpatients. Their symptoms may appear closer to the norm, and thus not as evident to others. Individuals in hypomania may express heightened confidence in their abilities or demonstrate enhanced social functioning. Some patients function optimally during hypomanic states and do not notice impairment in functioning, while others feel distractible and irritable. It is common for a person to not notice anything wrong with him- or herself. But mood lability can make it difficult to focus on schoolwork, a job, or social relationships.

Figure 7.2: *Treatment phases of bipolar disorders*

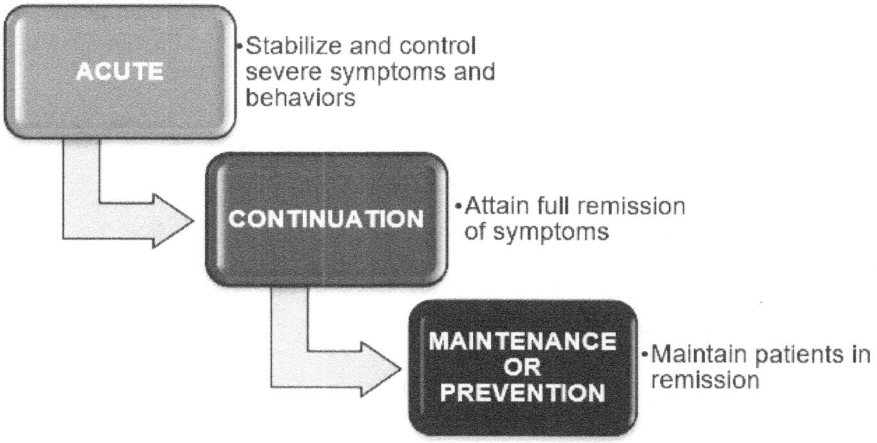

Box 7.1: Signs, symptoms, and treatment of bipolar I disorder

7.1 Signs, symptoms, and treatment of bipolar I disorder

DSM-5-TR criteria:

- Occurrence of a manic episode; may also be preceded and followed by a hypomanic or major depressive episode

Manic episode:

Marked by ≥ 1 week of:

- Persistently elevated, expansive, or irritable mood, and
- Persistently increased goal-directed activity, or
- Noticeable increase of energy, as well as ≥ 3 additional symptoms (or ≥ 4 if the mood is only irritable)
- Inflated self-esteem or grandiosity
- Decreased need for sleep
- Greater talkativeness than usual
- Flight of ideas or racing of thoughts
- Distractibility
- Increased goal-directed activity or psychomotor agitation
- Excessive involvement in activities with high potential for risky consequences (e.g., buying sprees, impulsive business investments, binge purchases or spending, reckless driving, unsafe sex)

Hypomanic episode:

Lesser type of mania involving a distinct episode that lasts ≥ 4 days with behavior that is:

- Distinctly different from the patient's usual nondepressed self, and
- Encompasses ≥ 3 symptoms from the list of manic episode symptoms or any of the following:
  - Brightening mood

- Decreased need for sleep with increased energy
- Acceleration of psychomotor activity

Major depressive episode:

This episode must have ≥ 5 of the following symptoms over a single 2-week period; one symptom must be depressed mood or loss of interest or pleasure, and all symptoms, except suicidal thoughts or attempts, must occur almost daily:

- Depressed mood most of the day
- Markedly diminished interest or pleasure in all or almost all activities for most of the day
- Significant (> 5 percent) weight gain or loss or decreased or increased appetite
- Insomnia (often sleep-maintenance insomnia) or hypersomnia
- Psychomotor agitation or retardation observed by others (not self-reported)
- Fatigue or loss of energy
- Feelings of worthlessness or excessive or inappropriate guilt
- Diminished ability to think or concentrate, or indecisiveness
- Recurrent thoughts of death or suicide, a suicide attempt, or a specific plan for suicide

Age at onset:

- Most commonly appears in young adulthood

Treatments:

- Mood stabilizers (e.g. lithium, certain antiseizure medications, second-generation antipsychotics)
- Antidepressants for severe depression (e.g., SSRIs)
    - Homeopathic and medicinal herb use is increasingly common (e.g., ashwagandha, chamomile, kava kava, lavender, passionflower, omega-3 fatty acids, St. John's wort), though should be openly reviewed with prescribing practitioners to ensure safety. Careful monitoring and mitigation with other current prescriptions, over-the-counter medications, and other substances should be discussed prior to initiating use to avoid interactions, complications, etc.
    - Monitoring of diet, exercise, activity, and sleep hygiene are recommended
    - Group, individual, and family psychotherapy: CBT, expressive therapies (e.g., art therapy, sand therapy)
        - Electroconvulsive therapies (ECT) for extreme symptoms is an option increasingly used
        - Phototherapy
        - Transcranial magnetic stimulation

American Psychiatric Association, 2022, pp.140-141

BIPOLAR II DISORDER

Patients with *bipolar II* disorder have major depressive episodes and at least one hypomanic episode. Yet unlike bipolar I, they do not experience full manic episodes. In fact, confirming the occurrence of a hypomanic episode is a challenge of diagnosing a patient with bipolar II. These episodes may be misevaluated as a time of wellness. For example, a patient diagnosed with MDD may experience a time of increased socialization and work productivity. Friends may be so relieved the person has re-engaged that they dismiss the hypomanic symptoms as nothing out of the ordinary. Misdiagnosis occurs roughly 25 percent of the time, with symptoms attributed to other conditions or factors, such as anxiety, stress, or substance use (Jiang et al., 2024). Box 7.2. provides further information on bipolar II disorder.

Box 7.2: Signs, symptoms, and treatment of bipolar II disorder

DSM-5-TR criteria:

- The presence of major depressive episodes, as noted for bipolar I, and
- At least one current or past hypomanic episode but no full-fledged manic episodes
- Symptoms must be severe enough to markedly impair social or occupational functioning or require hospitalization to prevent harm to oneself or others

Age at onset:

- Adolescence through young adulthood, most commonly

Treatments:

- Mood stabilizers to regulate mood (e.g., lithium, lamotrigine)
- Careful attention to the severity of depression
- Closely monitor for suicidality
- See Box 7.1 for other treatment guidance

American Psychiatric Association, 2022, pp. 150-152

OBSESSIVE-COMPULSIVE DISORDER (OCD)

Imagine feeling intense stress each time you leave your apartment; you are certain something bad will happen to your personal belongings left behind. The worry is overwhelming, so you conduct a series of actions to feel it's safe to leave. You check that every electric switch is off and every pet accounted for, several times each. After you leave, you stop, think, and recall locking the door, but feel an impulse to turn back and recheck the lock—often repeatedly—before feeling comfortable to depart again. You may already be in the car or on public transportation yet feel compelled to go home and check *again*. You know logically your belongings are safe, but your anxiety drives the illogical actions. Patients with OCD are unable to banish these *obsessions,* or profound concerns, from their minds. Imagine the disruption to their lives, and the lives of family members and friends.

The intrusive and all-encompassing anxiety, thoughts, or worries associated with OCD drive individuals to engage in ritualistic behaviors, or *compulsions*. Patients may feel driven to repeat behaviors a set number of times before moving on. For example, a person apprehensive about the safety of his personal effects may recite a certain phrase as he departs home to ease his mind, neutralize negative thoughts, and instill confidence in his actions. For other people, anxiety about germs prompts hand-washing so often they suffer abrasions, burns, and scarring of the skin. The distinction between obsessions and compulsions appears in Figure 7.3. Further elaboration of the signs, symptoms, and treatment considerations for persons diagnosed with OCD appear in Box 7.3.

Figure 7.3: *Obsessions versus compulsions*

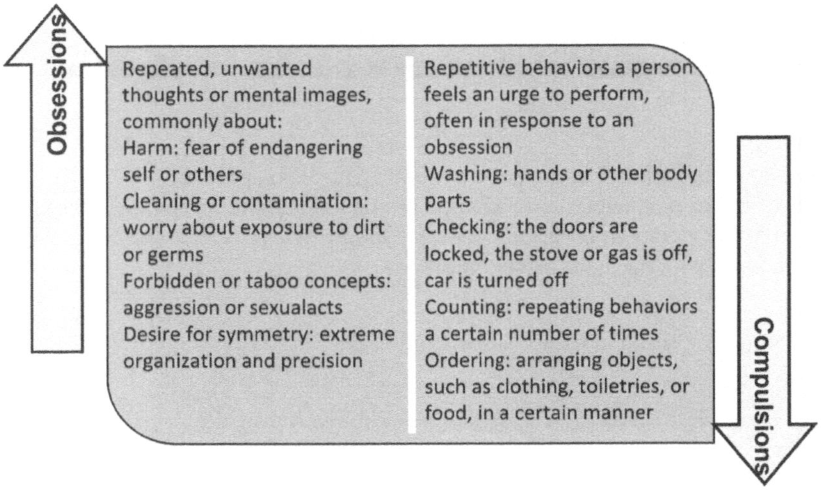

National Institute of Mental Health, 2024b

Box 7.3: Signs, symptoms, and treatment of obsessive-compulsive disorder (OCD)

DSM-5-TR criteria:

Clinical presentation is based on the presence of obsessions, compulsions, or both.

- The presenting obsessions or compulsions must be time-consuming; > 1 hour a day or causing clinically significant distress or impairment of functioning
- They cannot be attributed to the physiological effects of a substance (e.g., medications, illicit drugs) or other medical condition
- The disturbance is not better explained by the symptoms of another mental disorder (e.g., GAD, body dysmorphic disorder, eating disorders, illness anxiety disorder, or ASD)

Age at onset:

- Evidence notes 2 peak periods:
- 9-10 years of age
- 18-21 years of age

Treatments:

- SSRIs or tricyclic (e.g., clomipramine). Patients may require higher doses than typically used for depression and anxiety.
- Neuroleptics can manage severe symptoms, particularly for patients with tic disorders
- Psychotherapy:
  - CBT and other behavioral therapies
  - Exposure and response prevention (ERP)
  - Individual and collateral sessions with support systems

American Psychiatric Association, 2022, pp. 265-266; Carolan et al., 2019; Geller et al., 2021; Roh et al., 2023

DELUSIONAL DISORDER

Imagine a patient who presents with limited insight into their health condition. The person is employed and has a supportive long-term intimate partner. Yet there's a hitch. She challenges all information presented by the case manager or interprofessional care team members. She claims the PCP and team members are part of a conspiracy to misdiagnose her illness—a falsehood. The patient believes her private health information is being shared with researchers and funders, even though team members repeatedly repudiate the notion. In reality, lab results and diagnostic studies confirm the patient has pneumonia and should be treated with IV antibiotics. But the patient's irrational thoughts, or *delusions,* continue to impact communication, assessment, intervention, and treatment.

Delusional disorder is an SMI on the front-end of the DSM-5-TR *schizophrenia spectrum*, a series of *psychotic disorders* that share some essential symptoms of schizophrenia, including *hallucinations,* or false sensations of reality involving any of the five senses. Hallucinations may be somatic, as when a person feels an animal or alien crawling inside his or her body. *Disorganized thinking* can also occur, including incoherent speech, non-linear thought processes, or disjointed or unclear communication. The schizophrenia spectrum of disorders appears in Figure 7.4.

Not all practitioners agree that delusional disorder should be included as an SMI. Yet the disorder does significantly impair a person's ability to distinguish what is real from what is not. The delusions are driven by themes, found in Table 7.1, and are usually more disruptive to others than they are to the patient. Of critical importance: The delusions rarely obstruct the person's quality of life. This is counter to other SMIs, such as bipolar I, MDD, or schizophrenia, which can wreak havoc on quality of life factors like relationships, employment, or housing.

Case managers may experience strained communications with patients with delusional disorder. They are unaware of their own delusions, so a case manager's good intent may be confused or misinterpreted by the patient. Their irrational thoughts are based on the theme of their delusion(s). For example, patients with erotomanic delusions may romanticize their involvement with members of the healthcare team. A case manager's interest in their care or an urgent communication, such as an insurance denial of care, may be mistaken for flirtation. Further information on delusional disorders appears in Box 7.4.

Figure 7.4: *The schizophrenia spectrum*

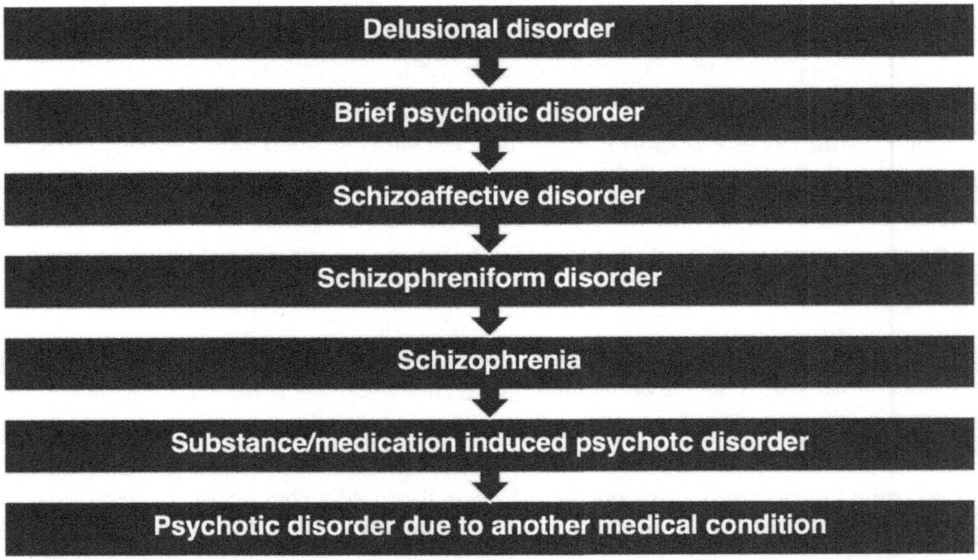

Box 7.4: Signs, symptoms, and treatment of delusional disorder

DSM-5-TR criteria:

- Presence of one or more delusions lasting ≥ 1 month, and
  - Patient has not met item A for schizophrenia (see Box 7.6)
  - If hallucinations are present, they are not prominent and are related to the delusion's theme
  - Distinct from the delusion's impact and ramifications, a person's functioning is not markedly impaired, and behavior is not bizarre or dysfunctional
  - If there have been manic or major depressive episodes, they are brief relative to the duration of the delusional periods
  - The disturbance is not related or attributed to the physiological effects of a substance or another medical condition, and not better explained by another mental disorder

Age at onset:

Any age, though common in late adolescence and early adulthood; mean age of onset is 49 years of age

Treatments:

- Medication evaluation: anti-psychotics
- Psychotherapy:
  - Prioritize therapeutic alliance to enhance insight and challenge cognitive distortions
  - CBT and other behavioral therapies: individual, family, group

American Psychiatric Association, 2022, pp. 104-108

SCHIZOAFFECTIVE DISORDER

We've discussed the disruption caused by mental illnesses that affect mood or prompt anxiety. Imagine then how overwhelming life is when a mood disorder co-occurs with a psychotic disorder. Practitioners commonly address the most distressing behavioral health symptoms first, such as psychotic thinking or suicidal ideation. But when a patient is thought to have *schizoaffective disorder,* assessment, intervention, and treatment become incredibly complex. Patients report that accurate diagnosis often takes upwards of 5-10 years. Bipolar disorders and schizophrenia are common differential diagnoses.

Consider a few examples of schizoaffective disorder presentations: A patient with profound sadness and depression simultaneously hears voices directing her to self-harm. Another patient with a history of child neglect and abandonment suffers from periods of profound agitation, as well as paranoid hallucinations, where he swears his treatment providers are plotting to kill him. An outgoing adolescent suddenly stops attending parties and social events because she claims to have "special friends" that nobody can see and who only speak to her, and she experiences severe anxiety with panic attacks when forced to socialize. Each scenario portrays a different facet of schizoaffective disorder, with further signs, symptoms, and treatment considerations in Box 7.5.

Box 7.5: Signs, symptoms, and treatment for schizoaffective disorder

DMS-5-TR criteria:

Coexistence of a major mood episode (major depressive or manic), and

2 or more of the following, each present for a significant time over 1 month (or less if successfully treated). At least one of the following must be delusions, hallucinations, or disorganized speech.

- Delusions
- Hallucinations
- Disorganized speech (e.g., consistent and frequent derailment or incoherence)
- Grossly disorganized or catatonic behavior
- Negative symptoms (e.g., diminished emotional expression, avolition or lack of motivation, initiative, or drive)

Age at onset:

- Late adolescence to early adulthood, primarily 16-30 years of age

Treatments:

- Combination of medication, psychotherapy, and community support
  - Manic type: Second generation antipsychotics often used, though may also need lithium, carbamazepine, or valproate
  - Depressive type: Second generation antipsychotics often used; upon stabilization add an anti-depressant
- Psychotherapy:
  - CBT: individual, family, and group
  - DBT: mindfulness, emotional regulation
  - Relaxation strategies
  - Lifestyle management and structured activities

Emerging research validates dietary management of symptoms using a ketogenic diet
American Psychiatric Association, 2022, pp. 121-125; Laurent et al., 2025

SCHIZOPHRENIA

Consider this scenario: A staff member looks out the healthcare clinic's window and notices a person sitting on the curb, speaking to someone. No one is physically present, so the staff member assumes the person is wearing ear buds and talking on the phone. Upon closer attention, she sees no ear buds. The person begins to gesture wildly and disrobe. Local law enforcement is called to the scene, and the individual is taken to an ED for evaluation. The patient's EMR reflects similar visits to other facilities and a diagnosis of an SMI.

If you have case managed in an acute care facility—especially the ED—this scenario likely sounds familiar. This is the classic presentation of *schizophrenia* that case managers often encounter. The reality represents one of the unfortunate consequences of a fragmented U.S. healthcare system and a faulty mental health continuum of care.

The diagnostic process for schizophrenia is often anything but straightforward and linear. As mentioned, symptoms and behaviors for SMI, especially schizophrenia, can be mistaken for other disorders. Two symptoms, flat affect and no expressed emotion, may be considered depression, rather than a psychotic disorder. Or perhaps the patient is in the prodromal phase, during which symptoms are unintentionally dismissed. Remember, the behaviors of patients with SMI fluctuate in their severity and presentation. The schizophrenic population can experience remission and relapse countless times within weeks, months, or years.

Diagnosis is also impeded by certain cultural or religious views by patients and families. Some people dismiss psychotic features like delusions, hallucinations, or disorganized thinking because they believe the person is acting or is making up stories to avoid accountability for their actions. Massive stigma often leads families to seek spiritual healers instead of assessment by mental health practitioners, to hide embarrassment or as a prioritization of faith.

Even after diagnosis, patients with schizophrenia face inordinate issues with treatment and medication non-adherence. Patients fortunate to be diagnosed in adolescence age out of academic and community-support services once they reach adulthood, and gaps in services ensue. People with schizophrenia also experience far greater incidence of comorbid conditions, including substance use disorders, anxiety disorders, and other chronic health conditions. These factors contribute to chronic difficulties with stabilization and consistent intervention for healthcare workers.

More will appear on this topic later in the chapter. For now, Box 7.6 summaries critical symptoms and treatment considerations for patients living with schizophrenia.

Box 7.6: Signs, symptoms, and treatment of schizophrenia disorder

DSM-5-TR criteria:

A. 2 or more of the following, each present for a significant portion of time over 1 month (or less if successfully treated). At least one of the following must be delusions, hallucinations, or disorganized speech.
   - Delusions
   - Hallucinations
   - Disorganized speech (e.g., consistent and frequent derailment or incoherence)
   - Grossly disorganized or catatonic behavior
   - Negative symptoms (e.g., diminished emotional expression, avolition or lack of motivation, initiative, or drive)

A. For a major portion of time since onset of the disturbance, level of functioning in one or more major life areas (e.g., school, work, socialization, self-care) is less than the level attained prior to onset.
B. Ongoing signs of the disturbance for a least 6 months, with at least 1 month of symptoms noted in item A. May include periods of prodromal or residual symptoms.
C. Schizoaffective disorder and depressive or bipolar disorder with psychotic features have been ruled out.
D. The disturbance is not attributed to the physiological effects of a substance (e.g., drug abuse, medication) or other medical condition.
E. If patient has a history of autism spectrum disorder or a communication disorder beginning during childhood, a diagnosis of schizophrenia is only made if prominent delusions or hallucination are present for at least one month.

Age at onset:

- Primarily late adolescence to adulthood, 18-35 years of age; late onset after 40 years of age

Treatments:

- Medication
  - Use of first and second generation antipsychotics to reduce severity of psychotic symptoms
- Structured community-based residential and day programs to preserve psychosocial function
- Psychotherapy
  - Group, individual, and family psychotherapy, CBT, expressive therapies (e.g., art therapy, sand therapy)
  - Electroconvulsive therapies (ECT) for extreme symptoms is a rising option

American Psychiatric Association, 2022, pp. 115-119; Zhan et al., 2024

SCHIZOPHRENIFORM DISORDER

Schizophreniform disorder is often viewed as a milder version or an early version of schizophrenia. Patients experience psychotic symptoms for a shorter duration of time—one to six months, rather than continuously for six months or more. Patients diagnosed with schizophreniform disorder often receive better prognoses for recovery than other SMI patients, but there are caveats. Practitioners often view schizophreniform disorder as a prodromal phase of schizophrenia, due to the high incidence (66 percent) of patients whose diagnosis advances to schizophrenia or schizoaffective disorder over time (Naz et al., 2003). Box 7.7 provides a snapshot of critical considerations for schizophreniform disorder.

Box 7.7: Signs, symptoms, and treatment of schizophreniform disorder

DSM-5-TR criteria:

2 or more of the following, each present for a significant portion of time over 1 month (or less if successfully treated). At least one of the following must be delusions, hallucinations, or disorganized speech.

- Delusions
- Hallucinations
- Disorganized speech (e.g., consistent and frequent derailment or incoherence)
- Grossly disorganized or catatonic behavior
- Negative symptoms (e.g., diminished emotional expression, avolition or lack of motivation, initiative, or drive)

An episode of the disorder lasts at least 1 month but less than 6 months

- Schizoaffective disorder and depressive or bipolar disorder with psychotic features have been ruled out
- The disturbance is not attributed to the physiological effects of a substance (e.g., drug abuse, medication) or other medical condition

Age at onset:

- Late adolescence to adulthood, 18-35 years of age

Treatments:

- Combination of antipsychotics and structured community support
  - Antipsychotics to manage psychotic symptoms until stabilization, then tapering of medications for at least 1 year

American Psychiatric Association, 2022, pp. 111-112; Bañón González et al., 2024

DATA AND DEMOGRAPHICS

SMIs pose inordinate challenges for every population, transcending every age group and demographic. Here is what case managers need to know about the vast impact of SMIs on society.

GENERAL RISK FACTORS

A series of biopsychosocial factors put patients with SMI at greater risk for illness than the general population, as shown in Figure 7.5. The intersection of biology and genetic predisposition to SMI are amplified by psychosocial factors that impede access to basic human needs and financial resources.

Other influences factor into this equation: nurturing and attachment with family, a history of traumatic and adverse experiences, and the quality of peer and family relationships. Severed family ties, common for patients with SMI, results in isolation and reduces access to dependable support systems. When these patients get older and require more frequent and invasive care, discharge can be difficult because they often lack family caregivers. This impediment increases hospital length of stay, prompts greater utilization of care, and adds to the economic and human burden of treatment.

Figure 7.5: *Biopsychosocial intersection with SMI*

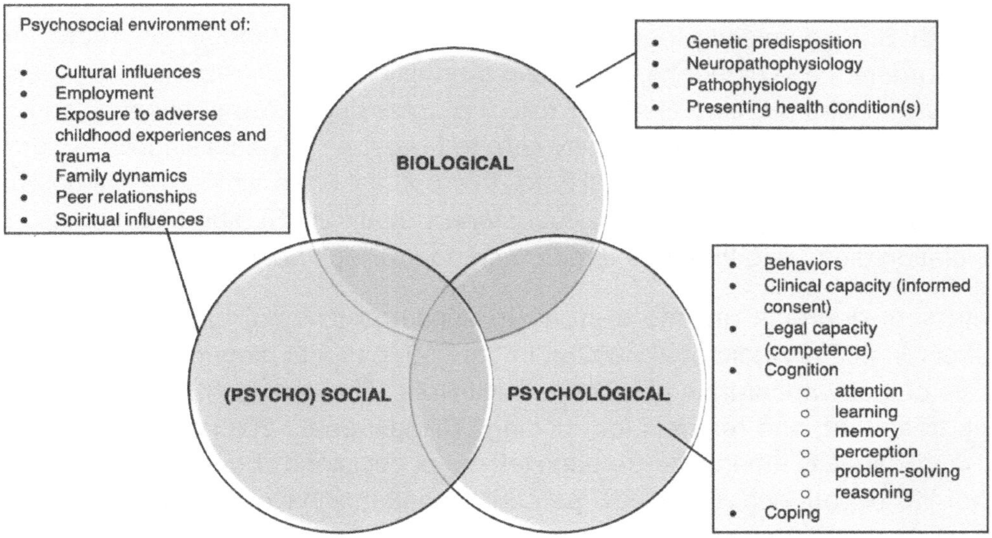

Treatment adherence

Upwards of 31 percent of patients with bipolar disorders are non-adherent with their mood stabilizers (Lintunen et al., 2023). Further, just over 50 percent of persons diagnosed with other SMIs do not consistently take their medications (Forma et al., 2020), leading to relapse, acute reevaluation and rehospitalization, and negative social outcomes, such as incarceration, unemployment, or self-harm.

SMI and disability

Some 20 percent of persons who receive *Social Security Disability Income (SSDI)* are eligible due to a mental illness. SSDI provides monthly income to individuals whose ability to work is limited due to a physical or mental disability and who have contributed Social Security tax through prior employment. By contrast, *Social Security Insurance (SSI)* is a need-based program that provides financial assistance to individuals with disabilities and low incomes. Eligibility requires the individual receive a determination of both disability and financial need determined by income and current assets. Currently, roughly 8 million individuals receive SSI benefits, including many people with an SMI (National Alliance of Mental Illness, 2025). Case managers can refer patients to state or local resources, non-profits, and other advocacy groups for further information about SSI/SSDI. The chapter resource list provides a variety of these options.

Interplay of chronic illness and SMI

Individuals with SMI, especially persons with schizophrenia, bipolar disorders, and severe depressive disorders, have higher morbidity and mortality due to physical illnesses (Grassi et al., 2023). Patients with SMI are also at higher risk of progressing to terminal conditions because of inconsistent or limited primary and specialty care to treat their physical illness—a data point that mandates attention. The all-cause mortality for this population is almost four times higher than other demographic groups (Shalev et al., 2020; Vinais et al., 2025). The data consistently shows that the population dies 10 to 25 years earlier than populations not impacted by SMI.

Persons with schizophrenia are more prone to succumb to lung, breast, and colon cancers (Nordentodt et al., 2021; Vinais et al., 2025). In general, patients diagnosed with SMIs are twice as likely to die of their cancer than persons without SMIs. They are less likely to receive standard assessment, treatment, and referrals for oncology (Grassi et al., 2023). Concerns about patient clinical and legal capacity means they're often left out of decisions about care or treatment options or the end-of-life experience. Barely 36 percent of patients have end-of-life care discussions documented in the medical record, compared to 63 percent of non-SMI patients (McFarland et al., 2021). Patients may not understand the scope and severity of their diagnosis or prognosis and can be denied advance care planning (advance directives, living wills). Referrals to palliative care programs can be delayed and appropriate pain management limited (Shalev et al., 2022).

Costs of care

Even amid decreased life expectancy, these populations yield high costs for care (Launders et al., 2022; Sporinova et. al., 2019). Hospitalization and physician billing claims were reviewed for adults with chronic diseases and mental illnesses, including SMIs, over a 3-year period. The data showed these patients are prone to multiple chronic illnesses, or *multimorbidity,* resulting in increased healthcare use and high expenditures. For patients with chronic diseases, the presence of an SMI was directly associated with higher rates of hospitalization and ED visits. Average expenditures across diagnostic groups were significantly higher for persons with SMIs: $38,250 versus $22,280 for acute care hospitalizations, prescription drugs, and physician visits (Sporinova, et al., 2019).

Figueroa et al. (2020) studied Medicare beneficiaries and dual eligibles. Over 12 percent of total spending was for mental health disorders alone, with 4.2 percent spent on mental health services and 8.5 percent related to mental illness.

Chronic ED admissions, discharge disposition, and poverty

Hospitalization and 30-day readmission rates—and, particularly, avoidable admissions—are more than double for patients with SMIs, compared to other populations (Launders et al., 2022). In general, patients with SMIs use EDs for their physical health more frequently than other patients.

The SMI population struggles financially. Over 38 percent of individuals with serious mental illness earned less than $10,000 annually, compared to 23 percent without an SMI (Luciano & Meara, 2014). Almost 40 percent live at or near the poverty level (Yu et al., 2020). In this reality, healthcare is altogether unaffordable. These persons also struggle with insufficient nutrition and unstable housing and rely on shelters, hotels, or tent cities.

Inconsistent treatment impedes consistent employment. Increased severity of mental illness and especially SMI translates to decreased rates of employment, as shown in Figure 7.6. As the population ages, employment rates plummet, particularly after 49 years of age (Luciano & Meara, 2014).

Figure 7.6: *Full-time employment rates of adults (18-64 years of age) with mental illness, by severity of mental health symptoms*

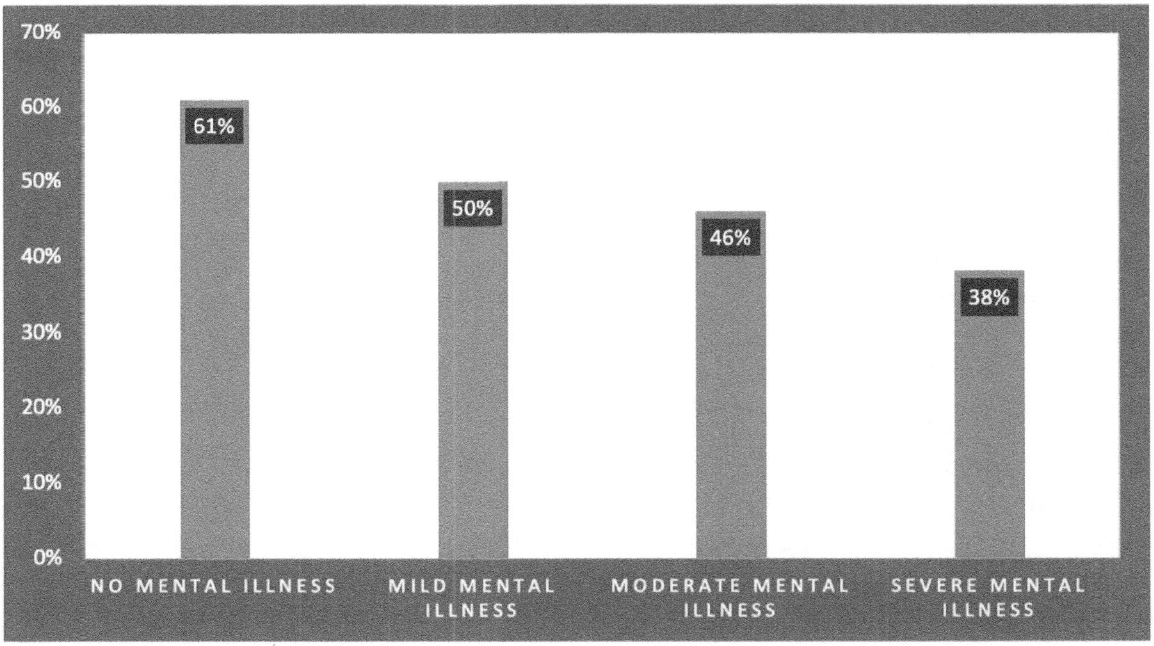

Luciano & Meara, 2014

DEVELOPMENTAL LIFE STAGE

The manifestations of SMIs transcend life stages. Case managers must understand a bundle of factors to achieve successful outcomes for patients and families.

Youth

SMIs are typically diagnosed after 18 years of age, so are youth excluded? They aren't—several disorders (e.g., bipolar, MDD, schizophrenia) can develop in childhood and adolescence, with the incidence ranging from 10-13 percent of children (Bitsko et al., 2022).

Family impact of SMI. Families experience massive upheaval when a child is diagnosed with MDD or bipolar disorder. They must manage the child's school attendance and academic performance while reconciling sudden absences from work for ED visits or other unscheduled appointments. They also struggle with the havoc of extreme mood lability, either highs or lows. They are highly attuned to comments reflecting patient self- or public harm.

It's also difficult for families to distinguish between normal adolescent behaviors and behaviors indicating SMI. Think of how often typical adolescents present as moody and prefer isolation to socialization. They may naturally experience *hypersomnia,* or excessive sleep, another common symptom of depression or depressive disorders.

Dickson et al. (2020) explored families' fiscal burden of managing SMIs, considering the average 14 episodes experienced by patients annually (e.g., emergent practitioner visits, ED admissions, hospitalizations). The mean total cost per episode for youth, using publicly funded outpatient mental health services, is $2,673, with the average cost per service type as follows:

- Psychotherapy: $1,079
- Assessment: $683
- Collateral services: $227
- Medication support: $186
- Community-based case management: $161

Note :the separation of collateral support and case management services in this research. Case managers should prioritize aligning these resources often. In this study, collateral support refers to parents, peer mentors with lived experience, school personnel, or individualized education plans (IEPs). Case management refers to community-based programs. Figure 7.7 shows the public cost breakdowns for youth with SMI.

Figure 7.7: *Percent of total cost for various publicly-funded, outpatient services for youth mental health treatment*

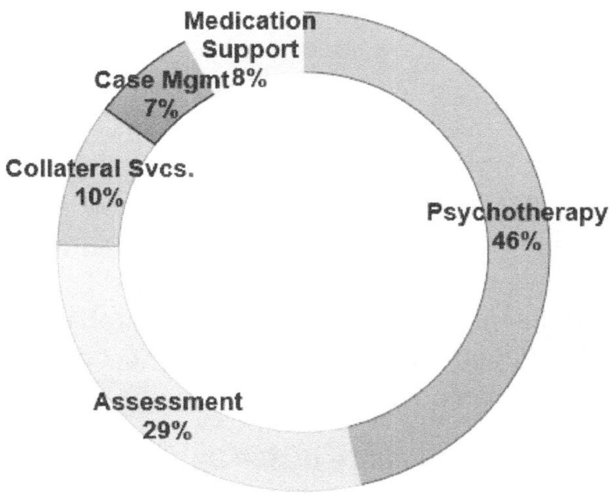

Bitsko et al., 2022

Diagnostic trends for youth. The number of children and adolescents presenting with moderate to severe levels of mental health impairment has risen over the past 15 years. Research shows some 9-10 percent of youth experience severe levels of depression and anxiety that are reflective of a potential SMI (Liu & Kuai, 2025; Lu et al., 2024; Olfson et al., 2024). Globally, this number is 1 in 5 of all youth (Lu et al., 2024). Approximately 3 percent of adolescents are diagnosed with bipolar I and II, with a higher prevalence identified for individuals born as females compared to males, 3.3 percent versus 2.6 percent (National Institute of Mental Health, n.d.).

The increase in youth with diagnoses on the schizophrenia spectrum is notable. Practitioners may be wary of diagnosing children with a psychotic disorder, even though criteria have been met. From 7.5 to 17 percent of children under 15 years old present with schizophrenia spectrum symptoms, but barely .05 percent are diagnosed with schizophrenia specifically (Kelleher et al., 2012; Sunshine & McClellan, 2023). Early onset of schizophrenia (under 16 years of age) has been diagnosed in only .2 percent of age-related population cohorts (Jerrell et al., 2016).

Schizoaffective disorder is typically diagnosed later in adolescence, though patients may endure years of mismanaged symptoms due to underdiagnosis and misdiagnosis. Mania can be mistaken for impulsivity, which may be attributed to ADHD. Agitation and perseveration may be associated with panic attacks or panic disorder. Episodes of psychosis are blamed on substance use and experimentation.

Medication trial and error is common with SMIs. Youth diagnosed with schizoaffective and bipolar disorders often endure a balancing act of symptom management until appropriate treatments for mood disturbance and psychosis are defined (Miller et al., 2020). Family members may present to EDs and practitioners with a lengthy history of antipsychotics, antidepressants, and other mood stabilizers. It may take several years of psychopharmacology adjustments before the right medications and dosages are defined for a specific patient.

Adults

Over 15.4 million adults with SMI live in the U.S.—6 percent of all adults (National Institute of Mental Health, 2024a). Prevalence by age range appears in Figure 7.8. Young adults 18-25 have the highest prevalence of SMI, compared with adults 26-49 and 50 years and older. Adult women have higher prevalence of SMI than males, 7.1 percent compared to 4.8. Prevalence across racial and ethnic groups appears in Figure 7.9. Prevalence is highest among adults who report two or more races and lowest among Asian adults.

Figure 7.8: *Prevalence of SMI by adult age groups*

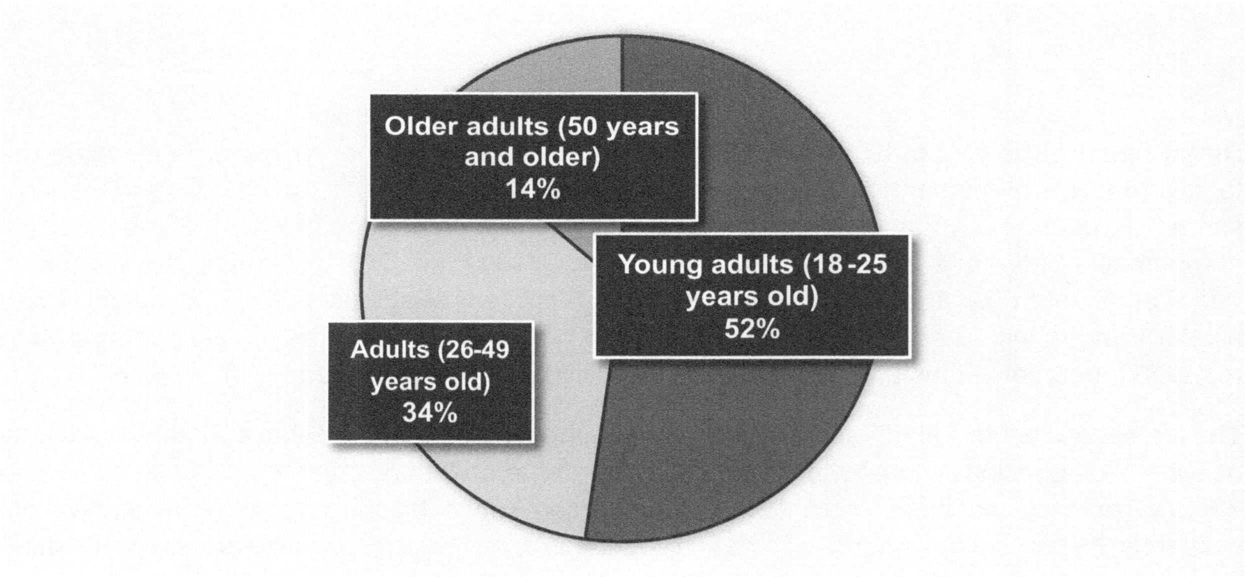

National Institute of Mental Health, 2024a

Figure 7.9: *Prevalence of SMI by race and ethnicity*

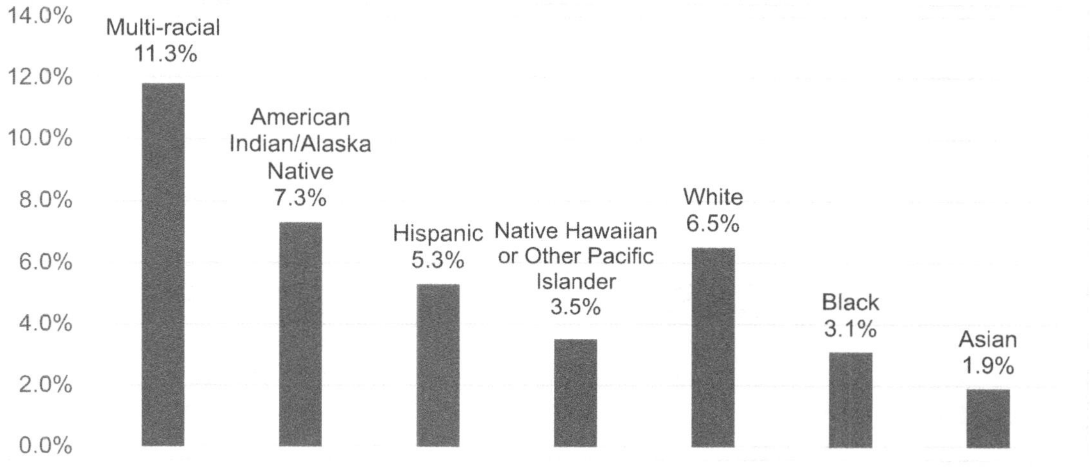

National Institute of Mental Health, 2024a

Older adults

Just under 5 percent of older adults are diagnosed with an SMI (Bartel et al., 2018) Chapter 2 addressed how deinstitutionalization in the 1970s led to SMI patients being placed in nursing homes, often due their inability to live independently with mental illness. Long-term care settings continue to house high numbers of individuals with SMIs, especially patients with chronic schizophrenia, recurrent and severe MDD, and severe bipolar disorder. Of the more than 800,000 individuals residing in assisted living communities, over 10 percent are diagnosed with an SMI; in nursing homes almost 19 percent of all residents have an SMI (Hua et al., 2021).

SCREENING TOOLS AND ASSESSMENT FOR SMI

Screening tools for SMI diagnoses appear in the following tables. Note that several tools are used by the family or caregiver to assess family functioning amid a crisis. This information allows care team members, case managers, and support systems to understand the acuity and severity of patient psychopathology. Table 7.2 provides tools primarily for adults, and Table 7.3 provides tools primarily for working with youth.

The DSM-5-TR also provides a tool called Clinician-Rated Dimensions of Psychosis Symptom Severity. This tool and others appear in Section III Assessment Measures. Screening tools for PTSD appear in Chapter 10.

CONCLUSION

We have reached the end of this lengthy and robust journey through SMIs. Your brain might need a recharge at this point, and you've earned it. These patients can try the skills and patience of even the most experienced, expert case manager. Know that your brain cells will recharge quickly, just in time for you to engage in critical thinking through the chapter contemplation questions. Chapter 8 is next up, on an equally complex topic: substance use and addiction.

Table 7.2: *Screening tools for SMI (adults)*

Instrument	Focus	Source
Brief Psychiatric Rating Scale (BPRS)	An 18-item, semi-structured interview rating scale for clinicians, noting the presence or absence of: • positive symptoms • general psychopathology • affective symptoms The three domains are measured for severity between 1 (absent) and 7 (extremely severe)	Overall, J.E., & Gorham, D.R. (1962). *Brief Psychiatric Rating Scale (BPRS)* [Database record]. APA PsycTests. https://doi.org/10.1037/t01554-000
Clinical Global Impression-Schizophrenia (CGI-SCH)	A 3-item, clinician-rated scale used to assess global illness severity in patients with schizophrenia, their overall improvement from the start of treatment, and therapeutic response	Haro, J.M., Kamath, S.A., Ochoa, S., Novick, D., Rele, K., Fargas, A., Rodríguez, M.J., Rele, R., Orta, J., & Kharbeng, A. et al. (2003). The Clinical Global Impression-Schizophrenia scale: A simple instrument to measure the diversity of symptoms present in schizophrenia. *Acta Psychiatrica Scandinavica, 107*, 16-23. https://doi.org/10.1034/j.1600-0447.107.s416.5.x
Family Attitude Scale* (FAS) * for youth to adults	A 30-item self-report to measure critical or hostile attitudes and behaviors toward a family member. Demonstrates ability to predict relapse in psychoses	Kavanagh, D.J., O'Halloran, P., Manicavasagar, V., Clark, D., Piatkowska, O., Tennant, C., & Rosen, A. (1997). *Family Attitude Scale (FAS)* [Database record]. APA PsycTests. https://doi.org/10.1037/t49946-000

Instrument	Focus	Source
Family Environment Scale* (FES) * for youth to adults	A 90-item inventory with 10 subscales measuring: • Interpersonal relationship dimension • Personal growth • System maintenance Used to understand how family members perceive the family and how each member's behavior affects the family unit during a time of crisis or transition	Moos, R.H. (1974). *Family Environment Scale (FES)* [Database record]. APA PsycTests. https://doi.org/10.1037/t27699-000
Level of Expressed Emotion (LEE) Scale	A 4-factor questionnaire to measure expressed emotion (EE) as perceived by the patient perceived lack of emotional support perceived intrusiveness perceived irritation perceive criticism	Cole, J.D., & Kazarian, S.S. (1988). The level of expressed emotion scale: A new measure of expressed emotion. *Journal of Clinical Psychology, 44*(3), 392-397. https://doi.org/10.1002/1097-4679(198805)44:3<392::AID-JCLP2270440313>3.0.CO;2-3
Mood Disorder Questionnaire	A brief, 3-part self-report tool to screen for lifetime history of manic or hypomanic symptoms. Includes: 1. Symptom checklist 2. Symptom clustering 3. Functional impairment and interference with daily functioning Differentiates bipolar disorder from unipolar depression Supports referral for further psychiatric evaluation	Hirschfeld, R.M.A. (2010). Mood Disorder Questionnaire: Its impact on the field. *Depression and Anxiety, 27*(7), 627-630. https://doi.org/10.1002/da.20697
Positive and Negative Syndrome Scale (PANSS)	A 30-item, standardized, clinician-administered interview tool to assess psychopathology of patients with schizophrenia and other psychotic disorders over the past week. Uses 3 subscales: • Positive scale: presence of hallucinations, delusions, or unusual thoughts • Negative scale: symptoms like blunted affect, social withdrawal, and lack of spontaneity • General psychopathology: evaluates for somatic concerns, anxiety, or depression	Kay, S.R., Opler, L.A., & Lindenmayer, J.-P. (1989). The Positive and Negative Syndrome Scale (PANSS): Rationale and standardisation. *The British Journal of Psychiatry, 155*(Suppl 7), 59-65.

Table 7.2: *Screening tools for SMI (adults) (continued)*

Instrument	Focus	Source
Schedule for Affective Disorders and Schizophrenia (SADS) • Regular SADS • Lifetime (SADS-L) • Changes in symptoms (SADS-C)	A semi-structured diagnostic clinician interview with questions that assess the presence, severity, and history of affective (mood) disorders and schizophrenia-spectrum disorders. Each screen focuses on identification of current and past episodes of psychiatric symptoms, such as depression, mania, anxiety, and psychosis, and is based on the standardized diagnostic criteria in the DSM.	Endicott, J., & Spitzer, R.L. (1978). A diagnostic interview: The schedule for affective disorders and schizophrenia. *Archives of General Psychiatry*, *35*(7), 837-844. https://doi.org/10.1001/archpsyc.1978.01770310043002
Structured Interview for Psychosis Risk Syndromes (SIPS) • **Mini-SIPS****	A semi-structured clinical interview to assess persons at high clinical risk for developing psychosis, with 2 main sections: 1. SOPS (Scale of Psychosis-Risk Symptoms): Assesses symptom severity across 4 domains: • Positive symptoms (e.g., unusual thought content, suspiciousness) • Negative symptoms (e.g., social withdrawal, decreased emotion) • Disorganized symptoms (e.g., odd behavior, disorganized communication) • General symptoms (e.g., mood disturbance, sleep issues) 2. Diagnostic criteria: Assesses if a person meets criteria for specific psychosis-risk syndromes: • Attenuated Positive Symptom Syndrome (APSS) • Brief Intermittent Psychotic Syndrome (BIPS) • Genetic Risk and Deterioration Syndrome (GRDS)	Miller, T.J., McGlashan, T.H., Rosen, J.L., Cadenhead, K., Cannon, T., Ventura, J., McFarlane, W., Perkins, D.O., Pearlson, G. D., & Woods, S.W. (2003). Prodromal assessment with the structured interview for prodromal syndromes and the scale of prodromal symptoms: Predictive validity, interrater reliability, and training to reliability. *Schizophrenia Bulletin*, *29*(4), 703-715. https://doi.org/10.1093/oxfordjournals.schbul.a007040 **Woods, S.W., Lympus, C., McGlashan, T.H., Walsh, B.C., & Cannon, T.D. (2022). The MiniSIPS: Development of a brief clinical structured interview guide to diagnosing DSM5 Attenuated Psychosis Syndrome and training outcomes. *BMC Psychiatry, 22,* Article 784. https://doi.org/10.1186/s12888-022-04406-z
The Prodromal Questionnaire-Brief (PQ-B)	A 21-item self-report questionnaire derived from the longer PQ (which contains 92 items), with screens for attenuated psychosis symptoms and risk for developing a psychotic disorder. Each endorsed symptom is followed by a distress rating; combined symptom and distress scores determine risk.	Loewy, R. L., Pearson, R., Vinogradov, S., Bearden, C. E., & Cannon, T. D. (2011). *Prodromal Questionnaire—Brief Version (PQ--B)* [Database record]. APA PsycTests. https://doi.org/10.1037/t11725-000

Table 7.3: *Screening tools for SMI (youth)*

Instrument	Focus	Source
Bech-Rafaelsen Mania Rating Scale (MAS)	An 11-item, clinician-administered questionnaire using a 5-point Likert-scale. Core symptoms or behaviors associated with mania are rated from 0 (absent) to 4 (severe): 1. Elevated mood 2. Increased motor activity 3. Increased speech 4. Increased social interaction 5. Increased sexual interest 6. Distractibility 7. Decreased sleep 8. Hostility or irritability 9. Grandiosity 10. Lack of insight 11. Appearance (e.g., dress, grooming)	Bech, P. (2002). The Bech-Rafaelsen Mania Scale in clinical trials of therapies for bipolar disorder: A 20-year review of its use as an outcome measure. *CNS Drugs, 16*(1), 47-63. https://doi.org/10.2165/00023210-200216010-00004
Comprehensive Assessment of At-Risk Mental States 23 (CAARMS 23)	A semi-structured assessment used by mental health professionals and researchers to identify youth at ultra-high risk of developing psychosis. 15 symptoms are assessed across: A. Primary symptom dimensions • Intensity of symptoms • Conviction (for symptoms 1-8) • Source (for symptoms 9 - 14) • Self-correction (for symptom 15) B. Secondary symptom dimensions • Distress due to the symptoms Interference due to the symptoms	Yung, A.R., Yuen, H.P., McGorry, P.D., Phillips, L.J., Kelly, D., Dell'Olio, M., Francey, S.M., Cosgrave, E.M., Killackey, E., Stanford, C., et al. (2005). *Comprehensive Assessment of At-Risk Mental States (CAARMS)* [Database record]. APA PsycTests. https://doi.org/10.1037/t52053-000
Early Psychotic Symptoms screening scale (EPSy)	A scale to assess the early prodromal psychotic symptoms in children aged 4-13 years, including levels of trust and disorganization	Babinet, M.-N., Demily, C., & Michael, G.A. (2023). A new scale for the screening of childhood early psychotic symptoms. *Psychiatry Research, 327,* 1-12. https://doi.org/10.1016/j.psychres.2023.115418

Instrument	Focus	Source
Kiddie-Schedule for Affective Disorders and Schizophrenia Present and Lifetime versions (K-SADS-PL)	A semi-structured interview for youth 6-18 years old aimed at early diagnosis of affective and psychotic disorders. The number of items depends on the version being administered. There are several sections per version: Unstructured interview Diagnostic-specific interview aligned with current DSM criteria Parent and child interviews	Kaufman, J., Birmaher, B., Brent, D., Rao, U., Flynn, C., Moreci, P., Williamson, D., & Ryan, N. (1997). Schedule for Affective Disorders and Schizophrenia for School-Age Children-Present and Lifetime Version (K-SADS-PL): Initial reliability and validity data. *Journal of the American Academy of Child and Adolescent Psychiatry, 36*(7), 980-988. https://doi.org/10.1097/00004583-199707000-00021
PRIME-5 Screener for Early Psychosis	A 5-item, clinician-administered, Likert-scale questionnaire to screen for early signs of psychosis, particularly for those in the prodromal phase and for 11 years of age and up	Miller, T.J., McGlashan, T.H., Rosen, J.L., Somjee, L., Markovich, P.J., Stein, K., & Woods, S.W. (2002). Prospective diagnosis of the initial prodrome for schizophrenia based on the Structured Interview for Prodromal Syndromes: Preliminary evidence of interrater reliability and predictive validity. *The American Journal of Psychiatry, 159*(5), 863-865. https://doi.org/10.1176/appi.ajp.159.5.863
Y*oung Mania Rating Scale (YMRS)*	An 11-item patient self-report questionnaire to evaluate the patient's clinical condition over the last 48 hours	Lukasiewicz, M., Gerard, S., Besnard, A., Falissard, B., Perrin, E., Sapin, H., Tohen, M., Reed, C., Azorin, J.-M., & The EMBLEM Study Group. (2013). Young Mania Rating Scale: How to interpret the numbers? Determination of a severity threshold and of the minimal clinically significant difference in the EMBLEM cohort. *International Journal of Methods in Psychiatric Research, 22*(1), 46-58. https://doi.org/10.1002/mpr.1379

CONTEMPLATION QUESTIONS

1. Reflect on your experiences working or interacting with patients diagnosed with SMI.
   a) What challenges did you face during the interaction?
   b) How did you reconcile those challenges?
   c) What was the outcome of the situation?
   d) Identify one way you might address the patient or situation differently after reading this chapter.

2. Access one of the screening tools for SMI from the MD+CALC website (linked in the Chapter 6 resources list):
   a) Review the screening tool.
   b) Complete it for yourself, then total your score.
   c) Reflect on how a standardized tool for screening SMI symptoms informs your future efforts.
3. Review the SMIs in Table 7.1 and reflect on which diagnoses you are most familiar with, personally or professionally.

Use the case scenario below to answer questions 4 and 5.

Jake is an animated and talkative young man, known to his friends as the "eternal optimist." In college he could study for hours, often falling asleep at the library. He's freshly graduated and working his first "adult" job. Jake's boss values his motivation and his go-getter attitude, bragging to other department heads, "Who else has model employees like Jake that stay long after others leave and are at their desks early the next morning?" Meanwhile, Jake's colleagues refer to him as a workaholic. His mother explains Jake's behavior: "He's my Mr. Talkative. He should be excited about this job, given how hard he has worked. My Jake will set the world on fire."

His colleagues have noticed that his usual level of excitement has recently gone into hyperdrive. He brings seemingly endless energy and appears to be staying awake for days. The longer he stays awake, the loftier his ideas become. And Jake's girlfriend is getting worried. "When Jake crashes, it's not a pretty site. He withdraws for days. But he'll be back to his extroverted and wired self in no time, right?"

4. In considering a diagnosis for Jake, what might you choose, and why?
5. Use Case Management's Behavioral Health Conversation Map in Table 1.4 to script your interactions with Jake and his support system.

RESOURCES

- **National Association of Disability Representatives**
  https://www.nadr.org/
- **National Organization of Social Security Claimants' Representatives**
  https://nosscr.org/referral-service/
- **Social Security Administration**
  https://www.ssa.gov/thirdparty/

REFERENCES

- Acharya, A.B. & Sánchez-Manso, J.C. (2023). Anosognosia. [2025 Jan]. StatPearls Publishing: Treasure Island, FL. Available from: https://www.ncbi.nlm.nih.gov/books/NBK513361/
- American Psychiatric Association. (2022). *Diagnostic and Statistical Manual of Mental Disorders* (5th ed., text rev.).
- Bañón González, S.M., Ogando Portilla, N., Gamo Bravo, B., González Laynez, M.E., Sekade Gutiérrez, N., & García Sánchez, F. (2024). Schizophreniform disorder. Clinical manifestations and diagnosis. Purposely a case. *European Psychiatry 67,* S742. https://doi.org/10.1192/j.eurpsy.2024.1542. PMCID: PMC11859949.
- Bitsko, R.H., Claussen, A.H., Lichstein, J., Black, L.I., Jones, S.E., Danielson, M.L., Hoenig, J.M., Davis Jack, S.P., Brody, D.J., & Gyawali, S., et al. (2022). Mental health surveillance among children - United States, 2013-2019. *MMWR Supplements*, *71*(2), 1-42. https://doi.org/10.15585/mmwr.su7102a1
- Carolan, A., Keating, D., Strawbridge, J., & Ryan, C. (2019). Optimising prescribing for patients with severe mental illness: The need for criteria. *Evidence Based Mental Health*, *22*(4), 139-141. doi: 10.1136/ebmental-2019-300099. PMID: 31511231; PMCID: PMC10231598.
- Cather, C., Pachas, G.N., Cieslak, K.M., & Evins, A.E. (2017). Achieving smoking cessation in individuals with schizophrenia: Special considerations. *CNS Drugs*, *31*(6), 471-481. https://doi.org/10.1007/s40263-017-0438-8
- Conroy, S., Francis, M., & Hulvershorn, L.A. (2018). Identifying and treating the prodromal phases of bipolar disorder and schizophrenia. *Current Treatment Options in Psychiatry*, *5*(1), 113-128. https://doi.org/10.1007/s40501-018-0138-0
- Dickson, K.S., Stadnick, N.A., Lind, T., & Trask, E.V. (2020). Defining and predicting high cost utilization in children's outpatient mental health services. *Administration and Policy in Mental Health*, *47*(5), 655-664. https://doi.org/10.1007/s10488-019-00988-1
- Figueroa, J.F., Phelan, J., Orav, E.J., Patel, V., & Jha, A.K. (2020). Association of mental health disorders with health care spending in the Medicare population. *JAMA Network Open*, *3*(3), e201210. https://doi.org/10.1001/jamanetworkopen.2020.1210
- Forma, F., Green, T., Kim, S., & Teigland, C. (2020). Antipsychotic medication adherence and healthcare services utilization in two cohorts of patients with serious mental illness. *ClinicoEconomics and Outcomes Research*, *12*, 123-132. https://doi.org/10.2147/CEOR.S231000
- Geller, D.A., Homayoun, S., & Johnson, G. (2021). Developmental considerations in obsessive compulsive disorder: Comparing pediatric and adult-onset cases. *Frontiers in Psychiatry*, *12*, 678538. doi: 10.3389/fpsyt.2021.678538. PMID: 34248714; PMCID: PMC8269156.
- Grassi, L., McFarland, D., & Riba, M. (2023). The risk and the course of cancer among people with severe mental illness. *Clinical Practice and Epidemiology in Mental Health, 19* (Suppl-1), e174501792301032. https://doi.org/10.2174/17450179-v17-e211208-2021-HT2-1910-8

- Hua, C.L., Cornell, P.Y., Zimmerman, S., Winfree, J., & Thomas, K.S. (2021). Trends in serious mental illness in US assisted living compared to nursing homes and the community: 2007-2017. *The American Journal of Geriatric Psychiatry*, *29*(5), 434-444. https://doi.org/10.1016/j.jagp.2020.09.011
- Jerrell, J.M., & McIntyre, R.S. (2016). Factors differentiating childhood-onset and adolescent-onset schizophrenia: A claims database study. *The Primary Care Companion for CNS Disorders*, *18*(2), 10.4088/PCC.15m01901. https://doi.org/10.4088/PCC.15m01901
- Jiang, X., Cao, B., Li, C., Jia, L., Jing, Y., Cai, W., Zhao, W., Sun, Q., Wu, F., Kong, L., & Tang, Y. (2024). Identifying misdiagnosed bipolar disorder using support vector machine: Feature selection based on fMRI of follow-up confirmed affective disorders. *Translational Psychiatry*, *14*(1), 9. doi: 10.1038/s41398-023-02703-z. PMID: 38191549; PMCID: PMC10774279.
- Kelleher, I., Connor, D., Clarke, M.C., Devlin, N., Harley, M., & Cannon, M. (2012). Prevalence of psychotic symptoms in childhood and adolescence: A systematic review and meta-analysis of population-based studies. *Psychological Medicine*, *42*(9), 1857-1863. https://doi.org/10.1017/S0033291711002960
- Launders, N., Dotsikas, K., Marston, L., Price, G., Osborn, D.P.J., & Hayes, J.F. (2022). The impact of comorbid severe mental illness and common chronic physical health conditions on hospitalisation: A systematic review and meta-analysis. *PloS One*, *17*(8), e0272498. https://doi.org/10.1371/journal.pone.0272498
- Laurent, N., Bellamy, E.L., Tague, K.A., Hristova, D., & Houston, A. (2025). Ketogenic metabolic therapy for schizoaffective disorder: A retrospective case series of psychotic symptom remission and mood recovery. *Frontiers in Nutrition*, *12*, 1506304. doi: 10.3389/fnut.2025.1506304. PMID: 39990610; PMCID: PMC11844221.
- Lintunen, J., Lähteenvuo, M., Tanskanen, A., Tiihonen, J., & Taipale, H. (2023). Non-adherence to mood stabilizers and antipsychotics among persons with bipolar disorder - A nationwide cohort study. *Journal of Affective Disorders*, *333*, 403-408. https://doi.org/10.1016/j.jad.2023.04.030
- Liu, Z., & Kuai, M. (2025). The global burden of depression in adolescents and young adults, 1990-2021: Systematic analysis of the global burden of disease study. *BMC Psychiatry*, *25*(1), 767. https://doi.org/10.1186/s12888-025-07201-8
- Lu, B., Lin, L., & Su, X. (2024). Global burden of depression or depressive symptoms in children and adolescents: A systematic review and meta-analysis. *Journal of Affective Disorders, 354*, 553-562. https://doi.org/10.1016/j.jad.2024.03.074
- Luciano, A., & Meara, E. (2014). Employment status of people with mental illness: National survey data from 2009 and 2010. *Psychiatric Services*, *65*(10), 1201-1209. https://doi.org/10.1176/appi.ps.201300335
- McFarland, D.C., Voigt, L., & Alici, Y. (2021). Decisional capacity determination and serious mental illness in oncology: Implications for equitable and beneficent care. *Psycho-oncology*, *30*(12), 2052-2059. https://doi.org/10.1002/pon.5812

- Miller, M., Barbe, N., Poulsen, R.J., & Coffey, B.J. (2020). Overcoming complications in management of a difficult-to-treat adolescent with schizoaffective disorder. *Journal of Child and Adolescent Psychopharmacology, 30*(8), 526-530. https://doi.org/10.1089/cap.2020.29190.bjc
- National Alliance of Mental Illness. (2025). Supplemental Security Income (SSI) and Social Security Disability Income (SSDI). Retrieved June 15, 2025, from https://www.nami.org/advocacy/policy-priorities/supporting-community-inclusion-and-non-discrimination/supplemental-security-income-ssi-and-social-security-disability-insurance-ssdi/
- National Institute of Mental Health. (2024a). Mental Illness. Retrieved June 7, 2025, from https://www.nimh.nih.gov/health/statistics/mental-illness
- National Institute of Mental Health. (2024b). Obsessive-Compulsive Disorder: When Unwanted Thoughts or Repetitive Behaviors Take Over. Retrieved October 27, 2025, from https://www.nimh.nih.gov/health/publications/obsessive-compulsive-disorder-when-unwanted-thoughts-or-repetitive-behaviors-take-over
- National Institute of Mental Health. (n.d.) Prevalence of Bipolar Disorder for Adolescents. Retrieved June 14, 2025, from https://www.nimh.nih.gov/health/statistics/bipolar-disorder#part_2607
- Naz, B., Bromet, E.J., & Mojtabai, R. (2003). Distinguishing between first-admission schizophreniform disorder and schizophrenia. *Schizophrenia Research*, *62*(1-2), 51-58. https://doi.org/10.1016/s0920-9964(02)00332-8
- Nordentoft, M., Plana-Ripoll, O., & Laursen, T.M. (2021). Cancer and schizophrenia. *Current Opinion in Psychiatry*, *34*(3), 260-265. https://doi.org/10.1097/YCO.0000000000000697
- Olfson, M., McClellan, C., Zuvekas, S.H., Wall, M., & Blanco, C. (2024). Mental health impairment and outpatient mental health care of US children and adolescents. *JAMA Psychiatry, 81*(6), 606-610. https://doi.org/10.1001/jamapsychiatry.2024.0088
- Ramsay, S.E., Cai, Z., Sinclair, D.R., Prina, M., Osborn, D.P.J., Adamson, A.J., Kaner, E., & Adams, E.A. (2025). Inequalities at age of diagnosis of severe mental illness in England. *JAMA Network Open*, *8*(1), e2457371. https://doi.org/10.1001/jamanetworkopen.2024.57371
- Roh, D., Jang, K.W., & Kim, C.H. (2023). Clinical advances in treatment strategies for obsessive-compulsive disorder in adults. *Clinical Psychopharmacology and Neuroscience*, *21*(4), 676-685. doi: 10.9758/cpn.23.1075. PMID: 37859440; PMCID: PMC10591165.
- Shalev, D., Fields, L., & Shapiro, P.A. (2020). End-of-life care in individuals with serious mental illness. *Psychosomatics*, *61*(5), 428-435. https://doi.org/10.1016/j.psym.2020.06.003
- Sunshine, A., & McClellan, J. (2023). Practitioner review: Psychosis in children and adolescents. *Journal of Child Psychology and Psychiatry*, *64*(7), 980-988. https://doi.org/10.1111/jcpp.13777
- Vinais, T., Gellé, T., Preux, P.M., Nubukpo, P., & Lacroix, A. (2025). Cancer in severe mental illness patients: A retrospective study. *Psycho-Oncology*, *34*(5), e70183. https://doi.org/10.1002/pon.70183
- Yu, Y.H., Luo, W., He, M.X., Yang, X., Liu, B., Guo, Y., Thornicroft, G., Chan, C.L.W., & Ran, M.S. (2020). Household poverty in people with severe mental illness in rural China: 1994-2015. *BJPsych Open*, *6*(5), e111. https://doi.org/10.1192/bjo.2020.95

- Zhan, N., Sham, P.C., So, H.C., & Lui, S.S.Y. (2023). The genetic basis of onset age in schizophrenia: Evidence and models. *Frontiers in Genetics*, *14*, 1163361. doi: 10.3389/fgene.2023.1163361. PMID: 37441552; PMCID: PMC10333597.

CHAPTER 8

SUBSTANCE USE AND MISUSE

INTRODUCTION

Chapter 8 describes the current scope of one of the most convoluted domains in the DSM-5-TR. An extended list of diagnoses comprise substance-related and addictive disorders. The domain is also quite specialized. Those working in this arena should have appropriate education, training, and credentialing, such as certified substance abuse counselor or one of the many other credentials discussed in Chapter 1. When case managers identify patients with substance-related issues, they should refer the patients to specialists and treatment as available.

This chapter offers case managers the most relevant information on this domain and within the scope of their role. Emphasis will be on understanding the terms associated with severity and phasing of substance-related disorders. A high-level presentation will also address key treatment issues across diagnostic groups. The diagnostic boxes used in Chapters 4 through 7 have been omitted in lieu of expanded focus on population-specific and contextual considerations for each diagnosis. Finally, the most novel screening and assessment tools will be presented, along with critical resources and references to inform your practices.

Ethical me will add several disclaimers. First, I am not a substance use or addiction specialist, though I possess a solid working knowledge of the topic from over four decades working in healthcare. My experiences with this population span various touchpoints of care, including outpatient, community-based, ED, and acute and long-term care. Each setting has provided me a distinct perspective on patients who engage in substance use and their support systems.

My second note involves the language used in this chapter. The term *substance abuse* is dated and stigmatizing to persons who suffer from addiction, as well as their families, so I don't use it. This dated terminology also dismisses the full etiology of addiction, including neuropathophysiology contributions. Instead, this book takes the stance that *substance misuse* and *addiction* are brain disorders, for they involve functional changes to the neuropathways involved with pleasure, self-control, stress, and reward (Uhl et al., 2019). Those changes to the brain continue long after the patient has stopped using. They are also exacerbated by a person's biopsychosocial factors. Substance misuse is not a matter of patient choice, but also a biochemical response within the brain.

BEHAVIORAL LEARNING OBJECTIVES

1. Identify common terms associated with substance use and addiction
2. Explain symptoms and treatment recommendations for common DSM diagnoses
3. Analyze the incidence of substance use and addiction across life stages and populations
4. Identify current evidence-based approaches for intervening across populations
5. Recognize screening tools to assess substance use and misuse
6. Apply Case Management's Behavioral Health Conversation Map to patients and their families living with substance use disorders

ESSENTIAL TERMS

- Abstinence
- Addiction
- Alcohol
- Anxiolytics
- Benzodiazepines
- Buprenorphine
- Controlled environment
- Craving
- Dependence (physical vs. psychological)
- Hallucinogens
- Harm reduction
- Hypnotics
- Inhalants
- Intoxication
- Maintenance
- Medication-assisted treatment (MAT)
- Methadone
- Misuse
- Naloxone (Narcan)
- Nicotine
- Opioids (heroin, fentanyl, oxycodone)
- Overdose
- Perceptual disturbance
- Pharmacokinetics
- Recovery
- Relapse
- Remission (early, sustained)
- Sedatives
- Stimulants
- Substance abuse
- Substance misuse
- Substance use
- Substance use disorder (SUD)
- Synthetic drugs
- Tolerance
- Withdrawal

TERMS AND FEATURES OF SUBSTANCE USE AND ADDICTION

Case managers love jargon! It is a major accomplishment when case managers develop a working knowledge of the vast terms and definitions associated with their patients. Students and novice professionals often ask during onboarding about medical dictionaries or other resources to inform their efforts. Case managers should be proficient in the language and specifiers used in screening, assessment, and diagnosis of the population. Common terms appear in Table 8.1.

Table 8.1: *Terms associated with substance use*

Term	Definition
Abstinence	Restraint from using a substance
Addiction	A compulsive, chronic, physiological or psychological need for a habit-forming substance, behavior, or activity having harmful physical, psychological, or social effects and typically causing well-defined symptoms (such as anxiety, irritability, tremors, or nausea) upon withdrawal or abstinence (Merriam-Webster, n.d.)
Intoxication	A transient condition (and most acute phenomenon) following the administration of alcohol or other psychoactive substance, resulting in disturbances in level of consciousness, cognition, perception, affect, behavior, or other psychophysiological functions and responses (WHO, ICD-10)
Perceptual disturbances	Abnormalities in how sensory information is interpreted by the brain, leading to distortions in the perception of reality (Langguth et al., 2025)
Pharmacokinetics	What the body does to a drug or substance (whether prescribed or over-the-counter medication, or illicit) specific to the movement of a drug into, through, and out of the body—the time course of absorption, bioavailability, distribution, metabolism, and excretion (Le, 2024)
Polysubstance use	Use of two or more substances from multiple drug classes; defined by the substances involved, timing of use, and intent (Bunting et al., 2025)
Relapse	A return to previous disordered behavior; may be considered a regression or a progression in the process of recovery from substance use disorder (Moon & Lee, 2020)
Remission	A period when one stops using substances, distinguished by clear timelines (American Psychiatric Association, 2022) Early remission: No symptoms of use within a year for at least 3 months Sustained remission: No symptoms of use within a year except for a strong desire or urge to use a substance Stable remission: Sustained remission for 5 years or more
Substance use	Recurrent use or problematic use of illicit substances or the misuse of medication; the medical term for addiction (Agency for Healthcare Research and Quality, 2022)
Tolerance	A need for markedly increased amounts of a substance to achieve intoxication and the desired effect (Volkow & Blanco, 2023)
Withdrawal	Physical and mental symptoms that a person has when they suddenly stop or cut back use of an addictive substance, such as opiates and opioids, nicotine products, or alcohol (National Cancer Institute, n.d.)

Some terms are straightforward, such as the distinctions between the phases of substance use in Figure 8.1, whether use, intoxication, or withdrawal. But other terms may vary, such as when referring to a substance use disorder or non-substance related disorder. For example, the specifiers for mild, moderate, and severe substance use (Figure 8.2) are defined by the presence of a range of symptoms, independent of the substance use disorder. In contrast, the same specifiers for gambling disorder (a non-substance-related disorder) are defined by a set number of criteria that must be met for each severity level, as seen in Figure 8.3.

Figure 8.1: *Continuum of use, intoxication, and withdrawal*

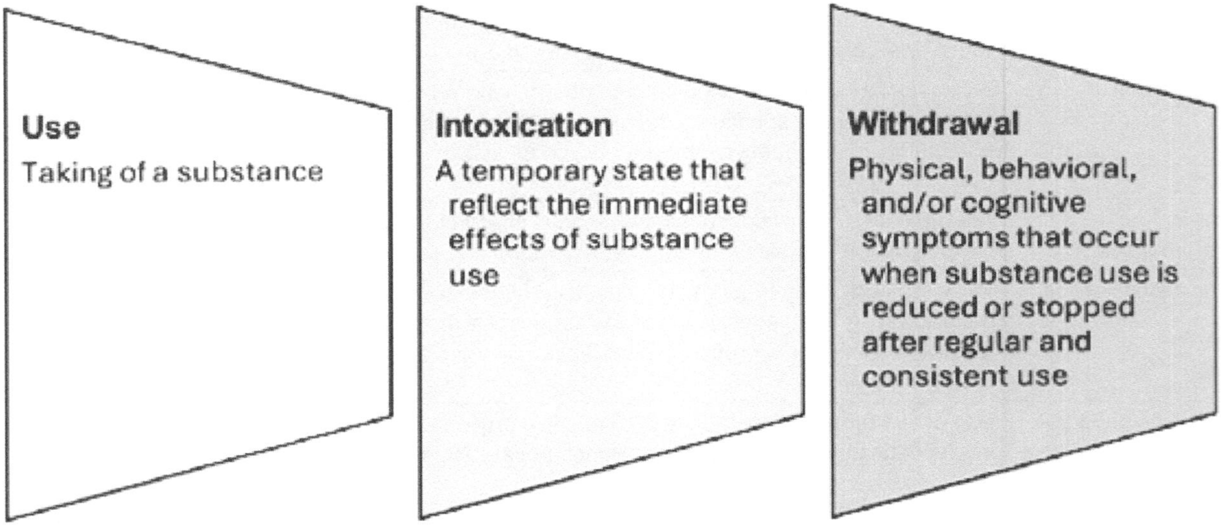

Figure 8.2: *Specifiers for severity of substance use, intoxication, and withdrawal*

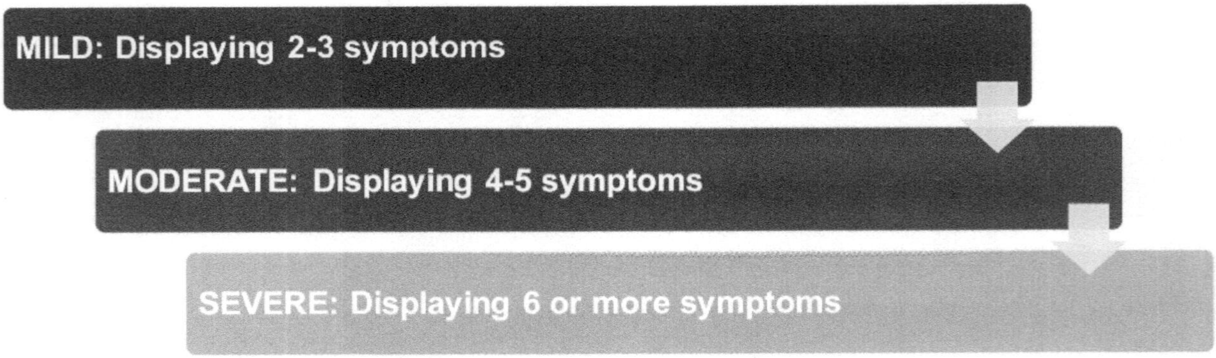

Adapted from American Psychiatric Association, 2022

Figure 8.3: *Specifiers for severity of gambling disorder*

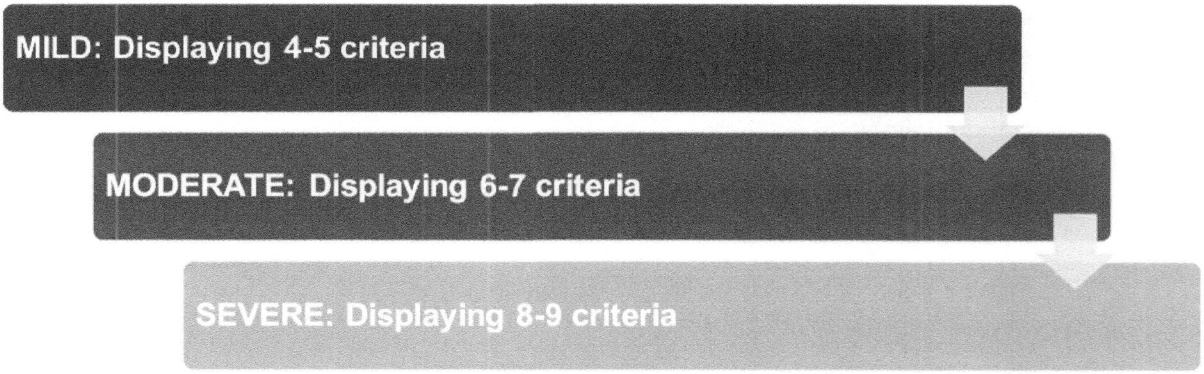

Adapted from American Psychiatric Association, 2022, p. 661

TOLERANCE

A person's body will, over time, adjust to intake of a substance, leading to a diminished response. *Tolerance* refers to the need for larger amounts of a given substance to achieve intoxication. Tolerance can occur at any point of a person's substance use journey, for it is driven by a variety of factors, including physical dynamics, such as the responsiveness of individual cells to a substance, and other neurotransmitter alterations; *pharmacokinetics,* or how the body moves, metabolizes, or breaks down substances; and genetic and psychological factors, such as a person's exposure to physical and emotional stress and psychological trauma (Volkow & Blanco, 2023).

TREATMENT

Across the diagnoses in this category, you will see the terms 'maintenance therapy' and 'controlled environment.' These specifiers appear for certain diagnoses, primarily tobacco-related disorders and Other or Unknown Substance-Related Disorders. *Maintenance therapy* refers to the phases of treatment following the acute and continuation phases (American Psychological Association, 2022). During maintenance therapy, the goal is typically to prevent relapse or reoccurrence of symptoms, to maintain stability, and to promote long-term recovery and well-being.

Controlled environments restrict access to substances and focus on supporting recovery. Such environments include acute inpatient detox or residential programs, intensive outpatient programs (IOP), or sober living houses. The American Society of Addiction Medicine (ASAM) defines a continuum of care for substance use disorder treatment, which spans early intervention to medically managed intensive inpatient care. They appear in Figure 8.4. In addition, case managers value ASAM's clinical guidelines that guide treatment management across populations and settings:

- benzodiazepine tapering
- stimulant use disorder
- opioid use disorder
- alcohol withdrawal management drug testing
- substance withdrawal in jails
- general clinical guidelines
- standards and performance measures

(American Society of Addiction Medicine, 2025)

Figure 8.4: *American Society of Addiction Medicine levels of care*

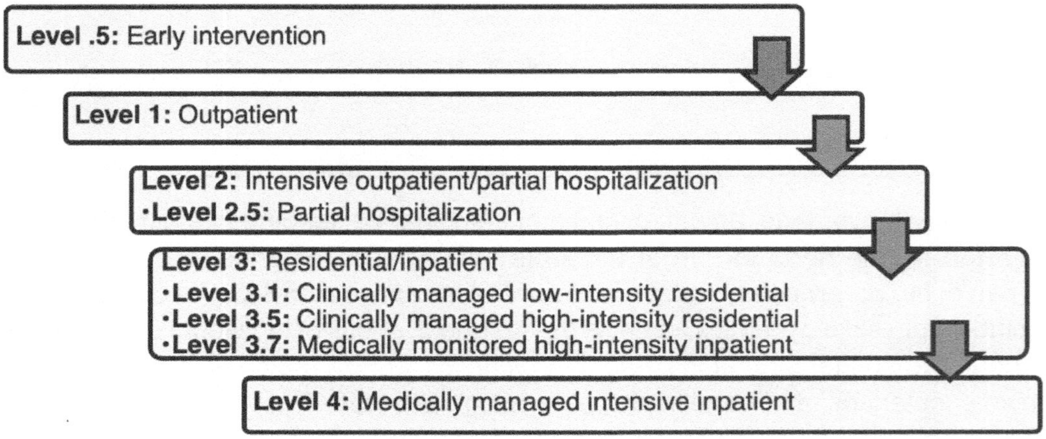

American Society of Addiction Medicine, 2025

HARM REDUCTION

Several patient-centered counseling interventions address the unpredictable treatment course for substance use. Rollnick and Miller's (2013) motivational interviewing, addressed in Chapter 12, is among the most popular treatment approaches.

A more comprehensive approach called *harm reduction* honors the autonomy and self-determination of persons who use drugs (PWUD), while simultaneously recognizing their continued use of substance(s) amid treatment. Under this approach, it is accepted that abstaining from use is not a reality all persons are ready to accept. Harm reduction prioritizes patient self-efficacy and factors in the risks and consequences faced by PWUD, acknowledging their lifestyle choices. Among these risk factors may be limited access to healthcare, unstable housing, unsafe or illegal employment, and vulnerabilities due to social inequalities of poverty, class, racism, social isolation, or other factors (Harm Reduction Coalition, 2024; Substance Abuse and Mental Health Services Administration, 2024a).

Harm reduction interventions also involve persons who have previously used drugs as part of treatment programming. These trained peers participate in planning, treatment, and evaluation of service interventions and may provide counseling through peer recovery models. The eight principles of harm reduction appear in Table 8.2. Additional information is available in the chapter resources.

The central belief of harm reduction is that persons who use drugs should be able to do so safely. This perspective is challenging for some practitioners to accept, particularly the ethical and legal implications of supporting a patient's illicit substance use and potentially unsafe lifestyle. For example, PWUD are provided resources to support safe use, including access to clean syringes, medications to reverse overdose (e.g. naloxone, aka Narcan), and information to promote the person's safety.

Many individuals engaged in sex work are exposed to drugs and use drugs (Argento et al., 2023). Their needs are also factored into the harm reduction approach, including use of psychoeducation and trauma-informed practices. The chapter resources offer additional information on this topic.

Table 8.2: *Eight principles of harm reduction*

Principle	Explanation
1	Accepts, for better or worse, that licit and illicit drug use is part of our world, and chooses to work to minimize its harmful effects rather than simply ignore or condemn people who use drugs
2	Understands drug use as a complex, multi-faceted phenomenon comprised of a continuum of behaviors (severe use to total abstinence); acknowledges that some ways of using drugs are safer than others
3	Establishes quality of individual and community life and well-being—not necessarily cessation of all drug use—as the criteria for successful interventions and policies
4	Calls for non-judgmental, non-coercive provision of services and resources to people who use drugs and the communities in which they live to assist in reducing attendant harm
5	Ensures that people who use drugs and those with a history of drug use routinely have a real voice in the creation of programs and policies designed to serve them
6	Affirms people who use drugs as the primary agents of reducing the harms of their drug use; seeks to empower them to share information and support each other in strategies which meet their actual conditions of use
7	Recognizes that the realities of poverty, class, racism, social isolation, past trauma, sex-based discrimination, and other social inequalities affect people's vulnerability to and capacity for effectively dealing with drug-related harm
8	Does not attempt to minimize or ignore the real and tragic harm and danger that can be associated with illicit drug use

Harm Reduction Coalition, 2024

PHASES OF REMISSION

Another specifier for substance use disorders addresses phases of *remission*, or when an individual stops using a particular substance. *Early remission* refers to when a patient has not had symptoms of a substance use disorder (except strong desire or urge to use a substance) for at least 3 months, up to one year. In *sustained remission*, a patient has continued without symptoms, except strong desire or urge to use a substance, for more than one year. *Stable remission* is not identified in the DSM-5-TR but is often a critical milestone for persons with substance use disorder. It refers to sustained remission for a period of 5 or more years. Figure 8.5 shows these varied phases.

Figure 8.5: *Phases of remission*

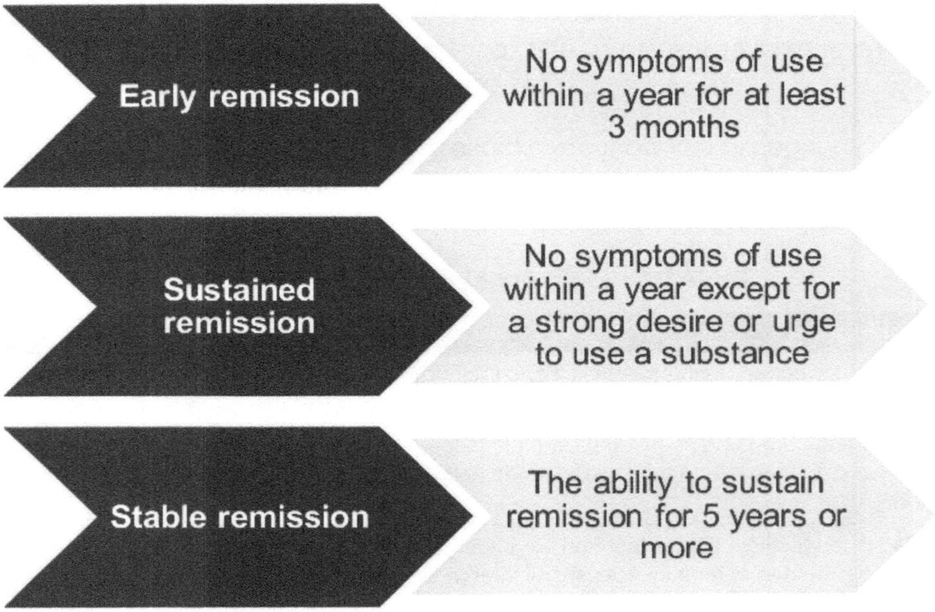

CANNABIS DISORDER

Among the most confusing aspects of cannabis disorder are the varied U.S. laws on cannabis use. Some states' laws allow for both medical and recreational marijuana use, while other states may permit only medical use. Some states restrict the dosages allowed for related products (e.g., CBD, hemp, THC). The National Conference of State Legislatures (2025) compiles a clearinghouse of U.S. legislation on cannabis use. The website is useful to case managers for many legal topics.

GAMBLING DISORDER

Gambling disorder is the only condition in the category of non-substance-related disorders. It begs for more explanation than this book allows, so I encourage you to read the criteria for diagnosis in the DSM. Individuals diagnosed with gambling disorder are entrenched in gambling for at least a year, and to the point that involvement negatively affects life, such as school performance, relationships, income, employment, and financial stability. They conceal their gambling and can become irritable when unable to participate in gambling-related activities.

The specifiers for gambling disorder's phases are episodic and persistent use, which are distinct from terms used for substance-use disorders. 'Episodic' applies to a person who meets full criteria for the diagnosis, but symptoms occasionally cease for several months. The specifier becomes 'persistent' when a person meets the full criteria consistently for consecutive years.

COMMON SUBSTANCE-RELATED DISORDERS

Table 8.3 provides the full scope of diagnoses in the substance-related disorders category. Keep in mind that the disorders and conditions associated with substance use and addiction span several diagnostic areas. Some diagnoses have appeared in prior chapters, such as substance/medication-induced anxiety disorder, which is discussed in Chapter 4 Anxiety. Substance/medication-induced bipolar and related disorders appeared in Chapter 6 Depression. Some diagnoses appear in other categories, including personality disorders and neurocognitive disorders.

Table 8.3: *DSM-5-TR substance use related disorders (page 1 of 5)*

Table 8.3: DSM-5-TR substance use related disorders			
DSM-5-TR Diagnosis	**Code**		
Alcohol-related disorders			
Alcohol use disorder	**Specify severity/remission**		
Specify: • Early or sustained remission **and if:** • In a controlled environment	Mild F10.10: Mild, 2-3 symptoms F10.11: Mild, In early remission F10.11: Mild, In sustained remission	Moderate F10.20: Moderate, 4-5 symptoms F10.21: Moderate, In early remission F10.21: Moderate, In sustained remission	Severe F10.20: Severe, > 6 symptoms F10.21: Severe, In early remission F10.21: Severe, In sustained remission
Alcohol intoxication	Code is dependent on presence of a comorbid alcohol use disorder (AUD) For yes, Mild: F10.120 or Moderate/Severe: F10.220 For No: F10.920		
Alcohol withdrawal	Code dependent on presence of comorbid AUD and presence of perceptual disturbance (PD)		

Table 8.3: DSM-5-TR substance use related disorders

DSM-5-TR Diagnosis	Code		
	For alcohol withdrawal, without PD F10.130: Mild AUD F10.230: Moderate/ Severe AUD F10.930: No AUD	For alcohol withdrawal, with PD F10.132: Mild AUD F10.232: Moderate/Severe AUD F10.932: No AUD	
Alcohol-induced mental disorders			
Unspecified alcohol-related disorder	F10.99		
Caffeine-related disorders			
Caffeine intoxication	F15.920		
Caffeine withdrawal	F15.93		
Caffeine-induced mental disorders	F15.99		
Cannabis-related disorders			
Cannabis use disorder **Specify:** • Early or sustained remission **and if:** • In a controlled environment	Mild F12.10: Mild, 2-3 symptoms F12.11: Mild, In early remission F12.11: Mild, In sustained remission	Moderate F12.20: Moderate, 4-5 symptoms F12.21: Moderate, In early remission F12.21: Moderate, In sustained remission	Severe F12.20: Severe, > 6 symptoms F12.21: Severe, In early remission F12.21: Severe, In sustained remission
Cannabis Intoxication	Code is dependent on a presence of comorbid cannabis-use disorder (CUD) and presence of PD		
	For cannabis intoxication, without PD F12.120: Mild CUD F12.220: Moderate/ Severe CUD F12.920: No comorbid CUD	For cannabis intoxication, with PD F12.122: Mild CUD F12.222: Moderate/Severe CUD F12.922: No comorbid CUD	
Cannabis withdrawal			
Cannabis-induced mental disorders			
Unspecified cannabis-related disorder	F12.99		

Table 8.3: DSM-5-TR substance use related disorders

DSM-5-TR Diagnosis	Code		
Hallucinogen-related disorders			
Phencyclidine use disorder	**Specify severity/remission**		
Specify: • Early or sustained remission **and if:** • In a controlled environment	Mild F16.10: Mild, 2-3 symptoms F16.11: Mild, In early remission F16.11: Mild, In sustained remission	Moderate F16.20: Moderate, 4-5 symptoms F16.21: Moderate, In early remission F16.21: Moderate, In sustained remission	Severe F16.20: Severe, 6 or more symptoms F16.21: Severe, In early remission F16.21: Severe, in sustained remission
Other hallucinogenic use disorder **Specify:** • Early or sustained remission **and if:** • In a controlled environment	Mild F16.10: Mild, 2-3 symptoms F16.11: Mild, In early remission F16.11: Mild, In sustained remission	Moderate F16.20: Moderate, 4-5 symptoms F16.21: Moderate, In early remission F16.21: Moderate, In sustained remission	Severe F16.20: Severe, 6 or more symptoms F16.21: Severe, In early remission F16.21: Severe, in sustained remission
Phencyclidine intoxication	Code dependent on presence of comorbid phencyclidine use disorder (PUD) F16.120: Mild comorbid PUD F16.220: Moderate/Severe comorbid PUD F16.920: No comorbid PUD		
Other hallucinogen intoxication	Code dependent on presence of comorbid hallucinogen use disorder (HUD) F16.120: Mild comorbid HUD F16.220: Moderate/Severe comorbid HUD F16.920: No comorbid HUD		
Hallucinogen persisting perception disorder	F16.983		
Phencyclidine-induced mental disorders			
Unspecified phencyclidine-related disorder	F16.99		
Hallucinogen-induced mental disorders			
Unspecified hallucinogen-related disorder	D16.99		

Table 8.3: DSM-5-TR substance use related disorders

DSM-5-TR Diagnosis	Code		
Inhalant related disorders			
Inhalant use disorder **Specify:** • Early or sustained remission **and if:** • In a controlled environment	Mild F18.10: Mild, 2-3 symptoms F18.11: Mild, In early remission F18.11: Mild, In sustained remission	Moderate F18.20: Moderate, 4-5 symptoms F18.21: Moderate, In early remission F16.81: Moderate, In sustained remission	Severe F18.20: Severe, 6 or more symptoms F18.21: Severe, In early remission F18.21: Severe, in sustained remission
Inhalant Intoxication	Code is dependent on a presence of comorbid inhalant-use disorder (IUD) F18.120: Mild comorbid IUD F16.220: Moderate/Severe comorbid IUD F16.920: No comorbid IUD		
Inhalant-induced mental disorders			
Unspecified inhalant-related disorder	F18.99		
	Code dependent on presence of comorbid hallucinogen use disorder (HUD) F16.120: Mild comorbid HUD F16.220: Moderate/Severe comorbid HUD F16.920: No comorbid HUD		
Opioid-related disorders			
Opioid use disorder	**Specify severity/remission**		
Specify: • Early or sustained remission **and if:** • In a controlled environment	Mild F11.10: Mild, 2-3 symptoms F11.11: Mild, In early remission F11.11: Mild, In sustained remission	Moderate F11.20: Moderate, 4-5 symptoms F11.21: Moderate, In early remission F11.21: Moderate, In sustained remission	Severe F11.20: Severe, 6 or more symptoms F11.21: Severe, In early remission F11.21: Severe, in sustained remission
Opioid intoxication	Code dependent on a presence of comorbid opioid-use disorder (OUD) and presence of PD		
	For Opioid Intoxication, without PD F11.120: Mild OUD F11.220: Moderate/ Severe OUD F11.920: No OUD	For opioid intoxication, with PD F11.122: Mild OUD F11.222: Moderate/Severe OUD F11.922 No OUD	
Opioid withdrawal	Code dependent on presence of comorbid opioid use disorder (OUD) F11.13: Mild comorbid HUD F11.23 Moderate/Severe comorbid HUD F11.93: No comorbid HUD		

Table 8.3: DSM-5-TR substance use related disorders

DSM-5-TR Diagnosis	Code		
Opioid-induced mental disorders			
Unspecified opioid-related disorder	F11.99		
Sedative-, hypnotic-, or anxiolytic-related disorders (SHA)			
Sedative, hypnotic, or anxiolytic use disorder **Specify:** • Early or sustained remission **and if:** • In a controlled environment	Mild F13.10: Mild, 2-3 symptoms F13.11: Mild, In early remission F13.11: Mild, In sustained remission	Moderate F13.21 Moderate, 4-5 symptoms F13.21: Moderate, In early remission F13.21: Moderate, In sustained remission	Severe F13.20: Severe, 6 or more symptoms F13.21: Severe, In early remission F13.21: Severe, in sustained remission
Sedative, hypnotic, or anxiolytic intoxication	Code dependent on presence of comorbid sedative, hypnotic, or anxiolytic use disorder (SHA-UD) F13.120: Mild comorbid SHA-UD F13.220 Moderate/Severe comorbid SHA-UD F13.920 No comorbid SHA-UD		
Sedative, hypnotic, or anxiolytic withdrawal	Code dependent on a presence of comorbid SHA-UD and presence of PD		
	For SHA-UD, without PD F13.130: Mild SHA-UD F13.230: Moderate/Severe SHA-UD F13.930: No SHA-UD	For SHA-UD, with PD F13.132: Mild SHA-UD F13.232: Moderate/Severe SHA-UD F13.932: No SHA-UD	
Sedative, hypnotic, or anxiolytic induced mental disorders			
Unspecified sedative-, hypnotic- or anxiolytic-related disorder	F13.99		
Stimulant-related disorders			
Stimulant use disorder **Specify:** • Early or sustained remission **and if:** • In a controlled environment	Mild (2-3 symptoms) F15.10: Amphetamine-type substance F14.10: Cocaine F15.10: Other/unspecified substance	Moderate (4-5 symptoms) F15.20: Amphetamine-type substance F14.20: Cocaine F15.20: Other/unspecified substance	Severe (6 or more symptoms) F15.20: Amphetamine-type substance F14.20: Cocaine F15.20: Other/unspecified substance

Table 8.3: DSM-5-TR substance use related disorders

DSM-5-TR Diagnosis	Code			
	Mild, In early remission F15.11: Amphetamine-type substance F14.11: Cocaine F15.11: Other/unspecified substance	Moderate, In early remission F15.21: Amphetamine-type substance F14.21: Cocaine F15.51: Other/unspecified substance	Severe, In early remission F15.21: Amphetamine-type substance F14.21: Cocaine F15.21: Other/unspecified substance	
	Mild, In sustained remission F15.11: Amphetamine-type substance F14.11: Cocaine F15.11: Other/unspecified substance	Moderate, In sustained remission F15.21: Amphetamine-type substance F14.21: Cocaine F15.21: Other/unspecified substance	Severe, In sustained remission F15.21: Amphetamine-type substance F14.21: Cocaine F15.21: Other/unspecified substance	
Stimulant intoxication	Code dependent on presence of comorbid stimulant use disorder (Sti-UD), specific stimulant, and presence of PD			
	Amphetamine-type substance, or other stimulant intoxication comorbid without PD Mild: F15.120 Moderate/Severe: F15:220 None: F15.920	Cocaine intoxication comorbid without PD Mild: F14.120 Moderate/Severe: F14.220 None: F14.920	Amphetamine-type substance, or other stimulant intoxication comorbid with PD Mild: F15.122 Moderate/Severe: F15:222 None: F15.922	Cocaine intoxication comorbid with PD Mild: F14.122 Moderate/Severe: F14.222 None: F14.922
Stimulant withdrawal	Code dependent on presence of comorbid Stimulant Use Disorder (Sti-UD), specific stimulant,			
	Amphetamine-type substance, or other stimulant intoxication comorbid Mild: F15.13 Moderate/Severe: F15:23 None: F15.93		Cocaine intoxication comorbid Mild: F14.13 Moderate/Severe: F14.23 None: F14.92	
Stimulant-induced mental disorders				
Unspecified stimulant-related disorder	Code dependent on type of stimulant			
	Unspecified amphetamine-type substance or other stimulant-related disorder: F15.99		Unspecified cocaine-related disorder: F 14.99	

Table 8.3: DSM-5-TR substance use related disorders

DSM-5-TR Diagnosis	Code		
Tobacco-related disorders			
Tobacco use disorder	Code based on severity and remission		
Specify: • Early or sustained remission • On maintenance therapy • In a controlled environment	Mild Z72.10: Mild, 2-3 symptoms	Moderate F17.200: Moderate: 4-5 symptoms F17.201: Moderate, In early remission F17.201: Moderate, In sustained remission	Severe F17.200: Severe: 6 or more symptoms F17.201: Severe, In early remission F17.201: Severe, In sustained remission
Tobacco withdrawal	F17.203		
Tobacco-induced mental disorders			
Unspecified tobacco-related disorder	F17.209		
Other (or unknown) substance-related disorders			
Other (or unknown) substance use disorder **Specify:** • Early or sustained remission • On maintenance therapy • In a controlled environment	Mild F19.10: 2-3 symptoms F19.11: Mild, In early remission F19.11: Mild, In sustained remission	Moderate F19.20: 4-5 symptoms F19.21: Moderate, In early remission F19.21: Moderate, In sustained remission	Severe F19.20: 6 or more symptoms F19.21: Severe, In early remission F19.21: Severe, In sustained remission
Other (or unknown) substance intoxication	Code dependent on presence of comorbid (or unknown) substance use disorder (SUD) involving the same substance and presence of PD		
	Other (or unknown) substance intoxication without PD Mild: F19.120 Moderate/Severe: F19.220 None: 19.220	Other (or unknown) substance intoxication with PD Mild: F19.122 Moderate/Severe: F19.222 None: 19.922	
Other (or unknown) substance withdrawal	Code dependent on presence of comorbid (or unknown) substance use disorder (SUD) involving the same substance and presence of PD		
	Other (or unknown) substance withdrawal without PD Mild: F19.130 Moderate/Severe: F19.230 None: 19.230	Other (or unknown) substance withdrawal with PD Mild: F19.132 Moderate/Severe: F19.232 None: 19.932	

Table 8.3: DSM-5-TR substance use related disorders

DSM-5-TR Diagnosis	Code
Other (or unknown) substance-induced mental disorders	
Unspecified other (or unknown) substance-related disorder	F19.99
Non-substance-related disorders	
Gambling disorder	F63.0
Specify if: • Episodic • Persistent and • Early or sustained remission	Mild: 4-5 criteria met Moderate: 6-7 criteria met Severe: 8-9 criteria met

American Psychiatric Association, 2022, pp. 652-661

DATA AND DEMOGRAPHICS

If you thought the list of diagnoses for substance-related disorders was vast, the data are even more expansive. This section will inform case managers of the most critical figures to support their work across populations and practice settings.

DEVELOPMENTAL LIFE STAGE

Youth

Substance-use disorders. Alcohol, cannabis, and tobacco have traditionally been the substances most used by youth globally. The average age of first experience with these substances starts in late childhood/early adolescence, ages 10-15 (Thomasius et al., 2022). Some 17 percent of all youth ages 12-17 admit to alcohol use, though researchers believe the prevalence is higher. Approximately 20 percent of youth ages 14-15 claimed to have had one drink in their lifetime, with 62 percent of those 12 and over admitting to one drink in the past year (NIH/NIAAA, n.d.; NIH/NIAAA, 2025.). Over 90 percent of adults first used alcohol during adolescence (Fadus et al., 2019).

Parental substance misuse can lead to higher likelihood of use by their children, but other factors have been cited, including biology and genetics, exposure to adverse childhood experiences (ACEs), SDoH, family income, and performance stress (Alhammad et al., 2022; Ford et al., 2020; Groenewald, 2020; Thomasius et al., 2022).

Opioid use. Opioid use, both prescribed and illicit, is a wide-ranging societal issue. Roughly 80 percent of all opioids prescribed worldwide are prescribed in the U.S., with 3.6 percent of prescriptions provided to youth for pain management (Groenewald, 2020). Despite dosing limits imposed under state laws, many youth will misuse drugs into adulthood, often progressing to fentanyl, heroin, and other illicit substances. Overdoses have risen by 49 percent in recent years for persons 15-24 years old (NIH/NIAAA, 2025). Increased use by adults has given youth greater access, too. They commonly steal pills from medicine cabinets at home or at their friends' homes. They may experiment with taking the substances or sell them to friends (Ford et al., 2020).

Non-substance-related disorders. The emergence of online gambling during the past decade has prompted a dramatic increase in gambling disorder among youth. For youth with ADHD and other impulse-control disorders (e.g., autism spectrum disorders), the convergence is even more profound. Many of these individuals use electronic and digital devices frequently, which can incite a biological pleasure-reward response in the brain. This dynamic in turn can lead to increased internet gaming, and potentially gambling (Brezing et al., 2013; Salerno et al., 2022).

Prevalence rates reveal a larger predicament, with numbers rising across youth. Gambling rates for youth are four-fold higher than for adults, and 8 percent of teens demonstrate pathological gambling behaviors, such as stealing money from relatives and friends or missing school to bet on online games (Brezing et al., 2013; Salerno et al., 2022).

Adults

Alcohol use. Eleven percent of U.S. adults (28 million people) are diagnosed with an alcohol use disorder (NIH/NIAAA, 2025). Expansive research across the U.S. reflects even rates of alcohol use by gender, as seen in Figure 8.6. For the over 224 million Americans who have used alcohol, the gender gap has narrowed over the years; 80.1 percent of females and 78.1 percent of males drink (NIH/NIAAA, 2025). Race and ethnicity breakdowns appear in Figure 8.7.

Over 178,000 deaths annually were attributed to excessive alcohol use (Centers for Disease Control and Prevention, 2024), with 2.4 million such deaths globally (Volkow & Blanco, 2023). Despite the prevalence of use and associated morbidity, less than one in ten individuals diagnosed with an alcohol use disorder (AUD) receives treatment, whether standard counseling or MAUD (medications for alcohol use disorder), which include acamprosate, disulfiram, and naltrexone (Substance Abuse and Mental Health Services Administration, 2024b). The goal of MAUD is to engage the patient in treatment and maintain recovery, but its use is very low, at only about 1.9 percent of people diagnosed with an AUD (Substance Abuse and Mental Health Services Administration, 2024b).

Opioid-use and other drug disorders. Over 10 million persons have died from opioid use. The number of deaths have risen 10-fold since 1999 (Dowell et al., 2024). Of the persons who received opioid use disorder (OUD) treatment during this timeline, barely half (45 percent) received *medication-assisted therapy* (MAT), such as methadone or buprenorphine (Dowell, et al., 2024).

In 2023, over 170,000 persons in the U.S. died from a drug overdose. Figure 8.8 shows the number of deaths by substance.

Figure 8.6: *Prevalence of lifetime drinking by gender (ages 18 and over)*

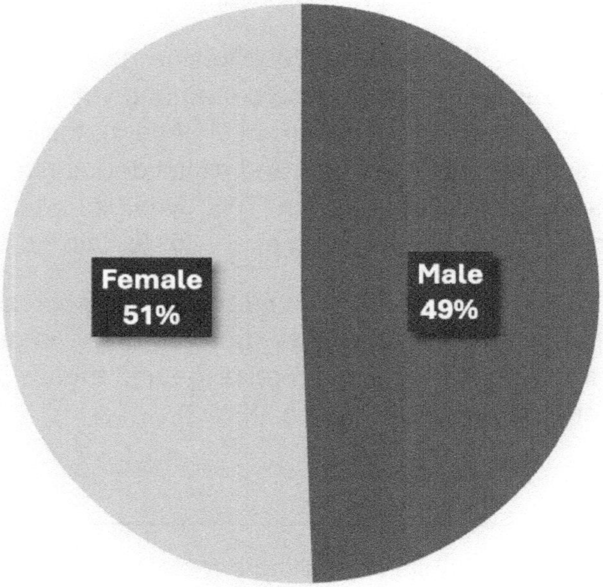

Figure 8.7: *Prevalence of lifetime drinking by race and ethnicity (ages 18 and older)*

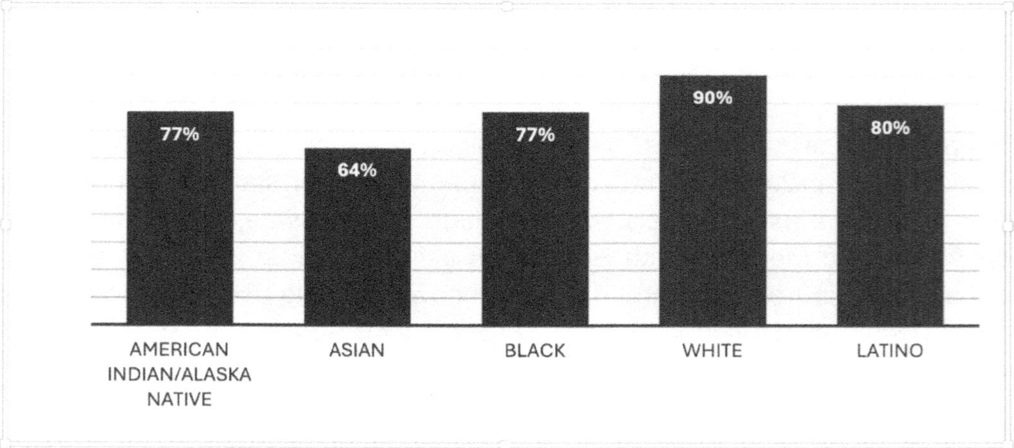

NIH/NIAAA, 2025

Note: *Data exclude Native Hawaiian/other Pacific Islanders due to limitations of the original study.*

Figure 8.8: *Overdose deaths by substance, 2023*

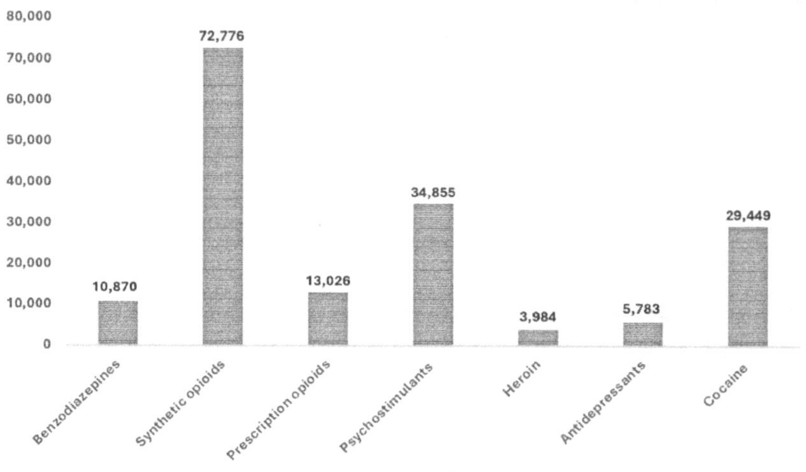

Centers for Disease Control and Prevention, 2024

Older Adults

Substance use. The data for this age group could fill volumes. Among the most startling statistics is the 190 percent increase in annual admissions to acute inpatient treatment facilities for substance use alone from 2008 to 2016 (Lin et al., 2023). The National Survey on Drug Use and Health (Substance Abuse and Mental Health Services Administration, 2025) reflects a significant rise in lifetime drugs use by older adults from 2016 to 2020, particularly a 12 percent increase in cannabis use, from 23.4 to 35.5 percent.

Figure 8.9: displays the substances most often named by older adults upon inpatient admission for substance use treatment. Alcohol continues to be the most popular substance, though increasingly opioids, sedatives, and hypnotics and other anxiolytics are noted. The increased use of illicit substances by older adults suggests practitioners should consider additional training on screening and assessment tools, short-term intervention techniques, and access to referrals for treatment.

Cannabis, polysubstance, and over-the-counter medication (OTC) use. Lin et al. (2023) identify a concerning escalation in older adults using alcohol, cocaine, opioids, and benzodiazepines, often in tandem with OTC medications. Polysubstance use by older adults puts them at grave risk, especially when combined with medications like ibuprofen, aspirin, acetaminophen, and diphenhydramine. Patients often suffer adverse drug events from mixing these assorted substances, as much as 60 percent of the time (Stone et al., 2023).

The increase in cannabis use by older adults is often attributed to the recent legality of medical marijuana and related products (e.g., CBD gummies and creams, hemp-infused snacks). But concerns for misuse remain. More than 5.7 million people over age 50 have used assorted marijuana substances, with misuse occurring in 4-5 percent of all persons older than 65 (Jacqua et al., 2022; Weber et al., 2022; White et al., 2023).

Substance sensitivity. Increased physiological sensitivity to substances is a concern in older adults. They are more sensitive to medication dosing than younger adults. Any substance use affects their physical and cognitive functioning, especially coordination and response time, and can exacerbate age-related changes in short-term memory and executive functioning (that is, organization, planning, and sequencing). When using substances, older adults are more likely to suffer falls and car accidents (White et al., 2023).

Loss of identity and gambling disorder. Older adults are vulnerable to substance use brought about by life changes like retirement or death of an intimate partner (Pollack et al., 2025). These life-stage risks appear in Box 8.1. For example, decreased socialization leads to loss of identity and diminished self-esteem. Gambling is a quick way for older adults to compensate for the shift in self-image. The emotional stimulation of gambling, whether at a casino, in a betting app, or on a gambling website, can be as appealing as any win. These are among the reasons gambling is a public health issue for older adults (Fountaine et al., 2023).

Figure 8.9: *Substance use acknowledgement upon inpatient admission for treatment*

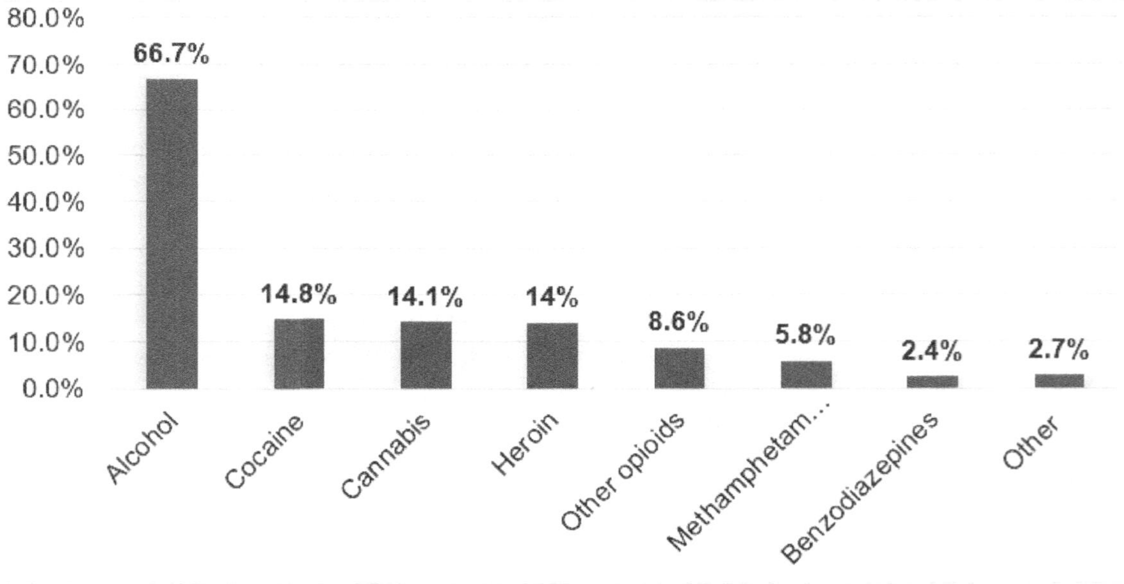

Data from Webb et al., 2022

Box 8.1: Risks for substance use and addictive behaviors in older adults

- Social isolation
- Boredom from decreased socialization and activity
- Death of intimate partners, family members, and friends
- Retirement and loss of professional identity and social standing
- Shifts in fiscal priorities (e.g., focus on saving for retirement) may transition to a "yearn to earn quickly" mentality, as a means to supplement income

POPULATION-FOCUSED MONITORING

Like many other conditions and diagnoses discussed in this text, substance-related disorders do not discriminate. It's time to explore key treatment themes across vulnerable populations.

LGBTQIA+

General substance use trends. Individuals diagnosed with gender dysphoria often have higher rates of substance use and misuse than other populations, though not consistently across all drugs (Fadus et al., 2019). Cotaina et al. (2023) researched the incidence of substance use across the trans community and found limited distinction between the population and their cisgender counterparts. Yet the authors identified slightly higher use patterns for sexual minorities with respect to tobacco, and experimentation with psychostimulants is common (Cotaina et al., 2023).

Some studies speak to increased.patterns of alcohol use for trans individuals, though other authors attribute these results to research traditionally being focused on young people. Any community within the late adolescent/young adult age group is prone to impulsive behaviors, and especially those who identify as sexual minorities.

Treatment center and population stigma. Drug detox and treatment centers are designed to serve cisgender heterosexual populations; by serving this population, they neutralize the stigma of serving the substance use community (Matsuzaka, 2018). However, this circumstance can deter sexual minorities from accessing treatment.

Non-substance-related disorders. Gambling disorder is a rising concern for the LGBTQIA+ population. Stanmyre et al. (2024) identified that the incidence of high-risk problem gambling increased with age for sexual minority individuals, while it decreased with age for heterosexuals. Upwards of 20 percent of LGBTQIA+ persons meet the full DSM-5-TR criteria for gambling disorder (Birch et al., 2015). Sexual minority women have a higher prevalence of problem gambling than their heterosexual counterparts: 20.4 percent compared to 13.5 percent (Broman et al., 2022). For men, the trend is opposite: Gay and bisexual men were less likely to engage in gambling behaviors than heterosexual men (Bush et al., 2021). A snapshot of considerations for substance-related disorders and the LGBTQIA+ community appear in Box 8.2.

Box 8.2: Substance-related disorders and LGBTQIA+

- High incidence for:
    - Stimulant use
    - Gambling disorder, especially for sexual minority women

Distinct considerations:

- Lack of access to treatment for substance use due to:
    - Prevailing stigmas related to substance use
    - Treatment centers are designed to serve cisgender communities, and thus
    - Worry for psychological safety within treatment centers, particularly inpatient
- Access to concordant care providers who respect their autonomy, gender identity, and lifestyle choices

Military members and veterans

Alcohol and drug use. The incidence and prevalence of self-medicating to manage physical and psychological trauma has been shown for every branch of the armed forces (Boden & Hoggatt, 2018; Gray et al., 2022; Hoopsick et al., 2017; Moore et al., 2023).

Boden and Hoggatt (2018) completed a national study on substance use treatment by veterans and their substances of choice. Higher use rates were identified for tobacco and alcohol than for cannabis. Hoggatt et al. (2023) expanded this research and identified a shift, with veterans increasingly using alcohol, cannabis, and stimulants combined. And the increase in opioid use across society is mirrored in the military; upwards of 72 percent of service members receive prescriptions for these substances at some point during their military career (Sparks et al., 2021).

Substance use and mortality rates. The connection between suicidality and substance use is an issue for this population. Drug overdose mortality rates for veterans have increased by 53 percent during the last decade (Bennett et al., 2022). Almost 30 percent of completed suicides have been attributed to alcohol or drug use (Teeters et al., 2017). Some 20 percent of non-combat deaths for military members and veterans have resulted from high-risk behaviors associated with substance use, often connected to polysubstance use (that is, combining alcohol, cocaine, opioids, and other stimulants) (Bennett et al., 2022).

Substance use by military family members. Substance use by military family members, especially partners, is a growing issue. Kulak et al. (2019) studied the pressures endured by military families, including frequent relocations and separations and worry for member safety during deployment. These stressors lead to increased alcohol use (29 percent of military partners) and prescription drug use—such as anxiolytics, opioids, and sedatives—at 7 percent. Roughly one-half of military spouses (47 percent) have received at least one opioid prescription in the past 2 years; they may also use remainders of their spouses' prescriptions (Sparks et al., 2021). A summary of treatments and considerations for the military and veteran communities appear in Box 8.3.

Box 8.3: Substance-related disorders and military members and veterans

High incidence for:

- Polysubstance use
    - Substance use, intoxication (alcohol, cannabis, cocaine, hallucinogens, inhalants, opioids, sedatives/hypnotics/anxiolytics, stimulants, tobacco)
    - Substance use by military family members, particularly intimate partners and spouses

High incidence for high-risk behaviors related to substance use and intoxication:

- Altercations and fights
    - Interpersonal violence
    - Sexual assault
- Increased risk of suicidal ideation and action
- Persistent addiction may lead to increased HRSNs (e.g., housing instability, social isolation, unemployment)

Distinct considerations:

- Heightened mood lability from chronic and long-term substance use and addiction
- Inconsistent and fragmented treatment access
- Access to concordant care providers who respect privacy and military identity

Persons with disabilities

Research on substance-related disorders by persons with disabilities is limited, though it is an emerging focus area. Much of the available data is specific to chronic conditions and was explored in Chapter 6. The population has higher rates of substance use and misuse for chronic conditions than persons without disabilities, with self-medication for pain being a significant driver (Reif et al., 2022).

Opioid and medical marijuana rates are higher, too, particularly for adults with multiple disabilities (Gimm et al., 2022, Hong et al., 2023). The presence of a disability has been found to increase isolation, loneliness, and alcohol use disorder (Aram et al., 2023).

Kolberg et al. (2025) identified increased use of disability benefits for consistent gambling, and a tendency to develop full-fledged gambling disorder. Few opportunities for gainful employment can drive a person to gamble, often via apps, in attempt to supplement their income (Kolberg et al., 2025). Box 8.4 shows a snapshot of the issues surrounding substance-related disorders for persons with disabilities.

Box 8.4: Substance-related disorders and persons with disabilities

High incidence for:

- Alcohol use disorder
  - Medical marijuana use: Cannabis use and intoxication disorders
  - Opioid use disorder
  - Gambling disorder to supplement disability and other income

Distinct considerations:

- Access to treatment challenges:
  - Health insurance limitations
  - Comorbid chronic pain as a factor driving self-medication

Women's health

Substance use disorders. Almost 50 million women globally live with alcohol use disorder (GBD Alcohol and Drug Use Collaborators, 2018; Webb et al., 2022). Meanwhile, mortality attributed to tobacco use is on the rise in women; 22.3 percent of women use tobacco, comprising 17.4 percent of tobacco users (Corrêa et al., 2023, World Health Organization, 2025). The intersection of tobacco use and female reproductive health yields unique concerns, per Box 8.5. Many of these issues also present with alcohol use disorder and other substance use disorders.

Box 8.5: Concerns at the intersection of tobacco use and women's reproductive health

- Female-specific cancers (e.g., cancer of the cervix)
- Coronary heart disease
- Ectopic pregnancies, miscarriage
- Impact on fertility/pregnancy, fetal development, congenital anomalies, infant mortality
- Child development challenges (e.g., low birthweight)
- Stroke and thromboembolism (increased risk with oral contraceptive use)
- Menstruation (irregular cycles and dysmenorrhea)
- Early menopause
- Osteoporosis

Corrêa et al., 2023

Shifts in addiction research. Research on addiction has primarily focused on men, though this trend is shifting. The biopsychosocial issues impacting women are vast, spreading over structural, community, interpersonal, and individual concerns. Issues span trauma exposure, human rights, access to care policies, coverage requirements, sexual orientation, role expectations, and treatment stigma (Meyer et al., 2019). The rise in domestic assault, isolation, and lack of privacy for telehealth treatment during the COVID-19 pandemic have added further barriers to substance use treatment for women.

Opioid use disorder and gender-specific treatment needs. Barbosa-Leiker et al. (2023) identified major shifts here. Of serious concern is the 649 percent increase in women's deaths from prescription opioid overdoses since 1999, compared with a 439 percent increase for men (NIH/NIDA, 2025). Of particular note are the distinct gender-specific treatment needs, particularly for co-occurring mental health issues (e.g., anxiety, depression, PTSD). The issues are embedded in women's central roles in parenting and intimate relationships (Barbosa-Leiker, et al., 2023). Emphasis on integrated care that addresses physical, mental, and psychosocial health for women is essential for overall prevention and wellness.

Gambling disorder on the rise. While gambling has traditionally appealed to men more than women, problem gambling is on the rise for women. What started as recreational gambling on vacation or weekends has escalated to behaviors that meet the full criteria for gambling disorder. Increased advertising, the enticement of quick earnings, and ease of access through apps has led to 55 percent of women meeting the criteria for pathological gambling (Matheson et al., 2021). A snapshot of the considerations for substance-related disorders in women appears in Box 8.6.

Box 8.6: Substance-related disorders and women's health

High incidence for:

- Alcohol-related disorders
  - Opioid-related disorders
  - Sedative-, hypnotic-, and anxiolytic-related disorders
  - Tobacco-related disorders
  - Gambling disorder

Distinct considerations:

- Risk of isolation
- Barriers to treatment
- Lack of comprehensive integrated care treatment
- High incidence of anxiety, depression, and PTSD, due to:
  - Parental role shifts
  - Reproductive health
    - Maternal mortality
    - Infant mortality
    - Fetal/child development
  - Trauma: Intimate partner violence, human trafficking
  - Treatment privacy

SCREENING TOOLS AND ASSESSMENT FOR SUBSTANCE-RELATED DISORDERS

A range of screening and assessment options are provided in Table 8.4 for adults and Table 8.5 for youth. Additional offerings and access points appear in the chapter resources. The lists of evidence-based offerings will provide case managers a clear starting point for interventions.

Table 8.4: *Screening tools for substance-related disorder (adults)*

Instrument	Focus	Source
Alcohol, Smoking and Substance Involvement Screening Test (ASSIST)	A comprehensive screening tool to identify substance use and related risks across varied substances (e.g. alcohol, tobacco, cannabis, cocaine, amphetamines, sedatives, hallucinogens, opioids, etc.) Assessment covers: frequency of use craving problems related to use, and injection drug use Classifies individuals into low, moderate, or high-risk categories	WHO ASSIST Working Group. (2002). The Alcohol, Smoking and Substance Involvement Screening Test (ASSIST): Development, reliability and feasibility. *Addiction, 97*(9), 1183-1194. https://doi.org/10.1046/j.13600443.2002.00185.x
Alcohol Use Disorders Identification Test (AUDIT) Alcohol Use Disorders Test-Consumption (AUDIT-C)	AUDIT: a 10-item tool to identify adults with hazardous or harmful alcohol use over the past year, including alcohol dependence Assesses: Consumption Drinking behaviors Alcohol-related problems AUDIT-C: a 3-item version focused on alcohol consumption patterns: Frequency of drinking Typical quantity consumed Frequency of heavy drinking episodes Higher scores indicate increased risk and need for further assessment or intervention	Bush, K., Kivlahan, D.R., McDonell, M.B., Fihn, S.D., & Bradley, K.A. (1998). The AUDIT alcohol consumption questions (AUDIT-C): An effective brief screening test for problem drinking. *Archives of Internal Medicine*, *158*(16), 1789-1795. https://doi.org/10.1001/archinte.158.16.1789 de Meneses-Gaya, C., Zuardi, A.W., Loureiro, S.R., & Crippa, J.A.S. (2009). Alcohol Use Disorders Identification Test (AUDIT): An updated systematic review of psychometric properties. *Psychology & Neuroscience, 2*(1), 83-97. https://doi.org/10.3922/j.psns.2009.1.12

Instrument	Focus	Source
Cut down, Annoyed, Guilty, Eye-opener (CAGE) tool Adapted version for drug use: CAGE-AID	A 4-item screening tool to assess potential problems with alcohol use primarily for those 16 years old and up Questions match the acronym: Cut down: Have you ever felt you should cut down on your drinking? Annoyed: Have people annoyed you by criticizing your drinking? Guilty: Have you ever felt bad or guilty about your drinking? Eye-opener: Have you ever had a drink first thing in the morning to steady your nerves or get rid of a hangover? The CAGE-AID queries about "drug use" in place of "drinking"	Mayfield, D., McLeod, G., & Hall, P. (1974). The CAGE questionnaire: Validation of a new alcoholism screening instrument. *The American Journal of Psychiatry, 131*(10), 1121-1123. Basu, D., Ghosh, A., Hazari, N., & Parakh, P. (2016). Use of Family CAGE-AID questionnaire to screen the family members for diagnosis of substance dependence. *The Indian Journal of Medical Research*, *143*(6), 722-730. https://doi.org/10.4103/0971-5916.191931
Drug Abuse Screen Test (DAST-10)	Self-report questionnaire of 10 (or 28) yes/no items that assesses problems related to drug use over the past 12 months (excluding alcohol and tobacco) Assesses the degree of consequences for use from 'non-severe' to 'severe'	Skinner, H.A. (1982). *Drug Abuse Screening Test (DAST)* [Database record]. APA PsycTests. https://doi.org/10.1037/t03979-000
Global Appraisal of Individual Needs (GAIN) Global Appraisal of Individual Needs: Short Screen (GAIN SS)	GAIN suite of screening tools assesses adolescents, young adults, and families for behavioral health and substance use disorders The SS-version is a 20-item self-report or interviewer-administered tool to screen adolescents likely to have behavioral health disorders, including substance use. The tool is divided into 4 sections: Internalizing disorders (e.g., depression, anxiety) Externalizing disorders (e.g., ADHD, conduct disorder) Substance use disorders Crime/violence problems	Dennis, M.L., Chan, Y.F., & Funk, R.R. (2006). Development and validation of the GAIN Short Screener (GSS) for internalizing, externalizing and substance use disorders and crime/violence problems among adolescents and adults. *The American Journal on Addictions*, *(15)1*, 80-91. https://doi.org/10.1080/10550490601006055

Instrument	Focus	Source
Opioid Risk Tool-OUD (ORT-OUD) Chart	A quick, self-report screening tool to assess a patient's risk for opioid misuse or abuse when being considered for chronic opioid therapy. The tool evaluates varied factors: personal and family history of substance abuse age history of preadolescent sexual abuse psychological conditions (e.g., ADHD, depression, bipolar disorder, schizophrenia) Scoring categorizes patients by low, moderate, or high risk to guide treatment recommendations	Cheatle, M., Compton, P., Dhingra, L., Wasser, T., O'Brien, C. (2019). Development of the revised Opioid Risk Tool to predict opioid use disorder in patients with chronic non-malignant pain. *Journal of Pain, 20*(7), 842-851.
Tobacco, Alcohol, Prescription medication, and other Substance use (TAPS)	Adapted from the NIDA quick screen for substance use during the past 12 months, comprised of a brief assessment in 2 parts: A screening component (TAPS-1) Followed by TAPS-2 Brief assessment (TAPS-2) for those who screen positive on TAPS-1. Self-report or professional-administered interview Online format A brief assessment of past 3 months of problem use	Adam, A., Schwartz, R.P., Wu, L.-T., Subramaniam, G., Laska, E., Sharma, G., Mili, S., & McNeely, J. (2019). Electronic self-administered screening for substance use in adult primary care patients: Feasibility and acceptability of the tobacco, alcohol, prescription medication, and other substance use (myTAPS) screening tool. *Addiction Science & Clinical Practice, 14,* Article 39. https://doi.org/10.1186/s13722-019-0167-z

Table 8.5: *Screening tools for substance-related disorders (youth)*

Instrument	Focus	Source
Alcohol Screening and Brief Intervention for Youth	Screening and assessment toolkit for ages 9-18, to help healthcare professionals quickly identify youth at risk for alcohol-related problems	National Institute on Alcohol Abuse and Alcoholism (NIAAA). Alcohol Screening and Brief Intervention for Youth. Retrieved from https://www.niaaa.nih.gov/alcohols-effects-health/professional-education-materials/alcohol-screening-and-brief-intervention-youth-practitioners-guide
Brief Screener for Alcohol, Tobacco, and Other Drugs (BSTAD)	Screening tool used primarily in pediatric and adolescent settings to quickly assess substance use risk in patients 12-17 years old. Asks about frequency of use in the past year for early identification of tobacco, alcohol, marijuana, and other drug use to guide appropriate intervention. Risk for use is defined by 3 domains: • No use • Occasional use • Frequent use	Kelly, S.M., Gryczynski, J., Mitchell, S.G., Kirk, A., O'Grady, K.E., & Schwartz, R.P. (2014). Validity of brief screening instrument for adolescent tobacco, alcohol, and drug use. *Pediatrics, 133*(5), 819-826. https://doi.org/10.1542/peds.2013-2346
Car, Relax, Alone, Forget, Friends/ Family, Trouble (CRAFFT)	Screens youth 12-21 years old for risky substance use and potential substance use disorders, in 2 parts: • 3 questions about alcohol and illicit drug use over the past 12 months • 6 questions assessing each letter of the CRAFFT acronym: 1. Have you ever ridden in a CAR driven by someone (including yourself) who was high or had been using alcohol or drugs? 2. Do you ever use alcohol or drugs to RELAX, feel better about yourself, or fit in? 3. Do you ever use alcohol or drugs while you are ALONE? 4. Do you ever FORGET things you did while using alcohol or drugs? 5. Do your FAMILY or FRIENDS ever tell you that you should cut down on your drinking or drug use? 6. Have you ever gotten into TROUBLE while you were using alcohol or drugs?	Oesterle, T.S., Hitschfeld, M.J., Lineberry, T.W., & Schneekloth, T.D. (2015). CRAFFT as a substance use screening instrument for adolescent psychiatry admissions. *Journal of Psychiatric Practice, 21*(4), 259-266. https://doi.org/10.1097/PRA.0000000000000083

Instrument	Focus	Source
Drug Abuse Screen Test (DAST-A) Adolescent version)*	A version of the DAST-10 adapted for adolescents, comprised of 10 yes/no items assessing drug use over the past 12 months and the degree of associated consequences	Martino, S., Grilo, C.M., & Fehon, D.C. (2000). Development of the Drug Abuse Screening Test for Adolescents (DAST-A). *Addictive Behaviors, 25*(1), 57-70. https://doi.org/10.1016/S0306-4603(99)00030-1
Modified version of the ASSIST by the National Institute of Drug Abuse (NM-ASSIST)	Brief version of the ASSIST tool (see Table 8.4) to quickly screen adolescents for multi-or poly-substance use	Oga, E.A., Mark, K., Peters, E.N., & Coleman-Cowger, V. H. (2020). Validation of the NIDA-modified ASSIST as a screening tool for prenatal drug use in an urban setting in the United States. *Journal of Addiction Medicine, 14*(5), 423-430. https://doi.org/10.1097/ADM.0000000000000614
Personal Experience Screening Questionnaire (PESQ)	40-item instrument used for youth 12-18 years old; includes a scale that measures: • severity of drinking problem • drug use history • select psychosocial problems • response distortion tendencies	Winters, K.C. (1992). *Personal Experience Screening Questionnaire (PESQ)* [Database record]. APA PsycTests. https://doi.org/10.1037/t15632-000
Screening to Brief Intervention (S2BI)	A single question about the frequency of use during the past year of 3 substances commonly used by adolescents: • tobacco • alcohol • marijuana An affirmative response prompts questions about additional types of substances used. For each substance, responses are categorized into levels of risk, from none to low or high.	Levy, S., Weiss, R., Sherritt, L., Ziemnik, R., Spalding, A., Van Hook, S., & Shrier, L.A. (2014). An electronic screen for triaging adolescent substance use by risk levels. *JAMA Pediatrics.* 168(9), 822-828. http://www.ncbi.nlm.nih.gov/pmc/articles/PMC4270364/

CONCLUSION

Substance-related disorders are complex and ever-growing. In this chapter you gained an overview of current issues. It bears repeating that a case manager's role and scope of practice may not lend itself to the specialty expertise required for intervention on substance-related disorders. It is unrealistic to expect that all case managers will be able to refer all impacted patients to relevant treatment providers. Yet my sincere hope is you now have a substantial foundation to engage in preliminary assessment and consultation with colleagues. Now we journey to Chapter 9 and the intricate, often difficult space of suicidality. Together we will explore how to assess, consider, and manage suicidal ideation, intent, and action.

CONTEMPLATION QUESTIONS

1. Consider a situation in which you experienced a person living with a substance-related disorder, then answer the following prompts:
    a) Which substance-related disorder was at issue? (If the person may have been dealing with more than one diagnosis, provide all.)
    b) How did the symptoms affect the person's social, occupational, or academic functioning?
    c) Did you intervene? If so, how? If not, why not?
    d) What is one takeaway from your experience?
2. Access any of the screening tools for substance use from Table 8.4.
    a) Review the screening tool.
    b) Complete the screening tool for a patient you are working with.
    c) Reflect on how a standardized tool for substance use screening will inform your future efforts.
3. Review the non-substance related disorders listed in Table 8.1.
    a) What is your experience with persons diagnosed with gambling disorder?
4. Reflect on the Harm Reduction model and associated principles in Table 8.3. Considering the industry controversy over this approach, answer the following questions.
    a) What are your views of the Harm Reduction model, whether positive or negative?
    b) In what circumstances is the model useful?
    c) In what circumstances might the model bring about further harm?

Use the case scenario below to answer question 5.

Danielle presented to the ED with a long history of migraines. Earlier in the year her PCP had suggested prescribing pain medications to ease her suffering. But Danielle initially declined, worried about their potential impact on her ability to care for her two children under age 5.

Danielle's spouse is in the Navy and suffered an injury last year while deployed. He was provided an opioid prescription, which he refrained from using, so the bulk of the pills remained. Danielle began to experience more frequent migraines and slowly began to use her husband's remaining pills. Her pain was considerably eased, but Danielle is now concerned about addiction.

5. Use Case Management's Behavioral Health Conversation Map in Table 1.4 to script your interactions with Danielle and her support system.

RESOURCES

- **American Society of Addiction Medicine**
  https://www.asam.org

National Conference of State Legislatures

- **State-to-State Cannabis Legislation and Policy**
  https://www.ncsl.org/health/state-cannabis-legislation-database
- **National Harm Reduction Coalition**
  https://harmreduction.org/
- **National Institute of Drug Abuse - Screening Tools and Prevention**
  https://nida.nih.gov/nidamed-medical-health-professionals/screening-tools-resources/chart-screening-tools
- **National Institute of Health/National Institute of Alcohol Abuse and Alcoholism (NIH/NIAAA)**
  https://www.niaaa.nih.gov/
- **National Problem Gambling Hotline - Interactive map of state-to-state resources**
  https://www.ncpgambling.org/help-treatment/help-by-state/
- **Substance Abuse and Mental Health Services Administration - Harm Reduction**
  https://www.samhsa.gov/substance-use/harm-reduction

REFERENCES

- Agency for Healthcare Research and Quality. (2022). Substance Use Disorders. In *2022 National Healthcare Quality and Disparities Report*. Available from: https://www.ncbi.nlm.nih.gov/books/NBK587176/
- Alhammad, M., Aljedani, R., Alsaleh, M., Atyia, N., Alsmakh, M., Alfaraj, A., Alkhunaizi, A., Alwabari, J., & Alzaidi, M. (2022). Family, individual, and other risk factors contributing to risk of substance abuse in young adults: A narrative review. *Cureus*, *14*(12), e32316. https://doi.org/10.7759/cureus.32316
- American Psychiatric Association. (2022). *Diagnostic and Statistical Manual of Mental Disorders* (5th ed., text rev.)
- American Society of Addiction Medicine. (2025). *Clinical Guidelines* (4th ed.).
- Aram, J., Slopen, N., Arria, A.M., Liu, H., & Dallal, C.M. (2023). Drug and alcohol use disorders among adults with select disabilities: The national survey on drug use and health. *Disability and Health Journal*, *16*(3), 101467. https://doi.org/10.1016/j.dhjo.2023.101467
- Argento, E., Shannon, K., Fairbairn, N., Moreheart, S., Braschel, M., & Goldenberg, S. (2023). Increasing trends and incidence of nonfatal overdose among women sex workers who use

drugs in British Columbia: The role of criminalization-related barriers to harm reduction. *Drug and Alcohol Dependence, 244*, 109789. https://doi.org/10.1016/j.drugalcdep.2023.109789

- Barbosa-Leiker, C., Campbell, A.N.C., McHugh, R.K., Guille, C., & Greenfield, S.F. (2021). Opioid use disorder in women and the implications for treatment. *Psychiatric Research and Clinical Practice, 3*(1), 3-11. https://doi.org/10.1176/appi.prcp.20190051
- Bennett, A.S., Guarino, H., Britton, P.C., O'Brien-Mazza, D., Cook, S.H., Taveras, F., Cortez, J., & Elliott, L. (2022). U.S. military veterans and the opioid overdose crisis: A review of risk factors and prevention efforts. *Annals of Medicine, 54*(1), 1826-1838. https://doi.org/10.1080/07853890.2022.2092896
- Boden, M.T., & Hoggatt, K.J. (2018). Substance use disorders among veterans in a nationally representative sample: Prevalence and associated functioning and treatment utilization. *Journal of Studies on Alcohol and Drugs, 79*(6), 853-861. https://doi.org/10.15288/jsad.2018.79.853
- Brezing, C., Derevensky, J.L., & Potenza, M.N. (2010). Non-substance-addictive behaviors in youth: Pathological gambling and problematic internet use. *Child and Adolescent Psychiatric Clinics of North America, 19*(3), 625-641. https://doi.org/10.1016/j.chc.2010.03.012
- Broman, N., Prever, F., di Giacomo, E., Jiménez-Murcia, S., Szczegielniak, A., Hansson, H., & Håkansson, A. (2022). Gambling, gaming, and internet behavior in a sexual minority perspective: A cross-sectional study in seven European countries. *Frontiers in Psychology, 12*, 707645-707645. https://doi.org/10.3389/fpsyg.2021.707645.
- Bunting, A.M., Shearer, R., Linden-Carmichael, A.N., Williams, A.R., Comer, S.D., Cerdá, M., & Lorvick, J. (2024). Are you thinking what I'm thinking? Defining what we mean by "polysubstance use". *The American Journal of Drug and Alcohol Abuse, 50*(1), 1-7. https://doi.org/10.1080/00952990.2023.2248360
- Busch, A.B., Greenfield, S.F., & Huskamp, H.A. (2025). Expanding alcohol use disorder medications in primary care. *JAMA Internal Medicine, 185(5), 489-490.* doi:10.1001/jamainternmed.2024.8325. PMID: 40029652, PMCID: PMC12070271
- Bush, R., Russell, A.M., Staiger, P.K., Waling, A., & Dowling, N.A. (2021). Risk and protective factors for the development of gambling-related harms and problems among Australian sexual minority men. *BMC Psychology, 9*(1), 1-18. https://doi.org/10.1186/s40359-021-00597-4
- Centers for Disease Control and Prevention. (2024). Drug Overdose Deaths: Facts and Figures. Retrieved July 14, 2025, from https://nida.nih.gov/research-topics/trends-statistics/overdose-death-rates#Fig9
- Corrêa, P.C.R.P., Sales, R.K.B., Knorst, M.M., Pinto, S.R.H.L., Ragnini, L.F.Q., Tourinho, C.A.P., Storrer, K.M., Scuarcialupi, M.E.C.A., Castellano, M.V.C.O., Albuquerque Neto, A.A., & Ravara, S.B. (2023). The challenge of tobacco and nicotine use among women. *Revista da Associacao Medica Brasileira, 69*(suppl 1), e2023S124. https://doi.org/10.1590/1806-9282.2023S124
- Cotaina, M., Peraire, M., Boscá, M., Echeverria, I., Benito, A., & Haro, G. (2022). Substance use in the transgender population: A meta-analysis. *Brain Sciences, 12*(3), 366. https://doi.org/10.3390/brainsci12030366

- Dowell, D., Brown, S., Gyawali, S., Hoenig, J., Ko, J., Mikosz, C., Ussery, E., Baldwin, G., Jones, C.M., & Olsen, Yngvild et al. (2024). Treatment for opioid use disorder: Population estimates — United States, 2022. *Morbidity and Mortality Weekly Report*, *73*, 567-574. doi: http://dx.doi.org/10.15585/mmwr.mm7325a1.
- Fadus, M.C., Squeglia, L.M., Valadez, E.A., Tomko, R.L., Bryant, B.E., & Gray, K.M. (2019). Adolescent substance use disorder treatment: An update on evidence-based strategies. *Current Psychiatry Reports*, *21*(10), 96. https://doi.org/10.1007/s11920-019-1086-0
- Fontaine, M., Lemercier, C., Bonnaire, C., Giroux, I., Py, J., Varescon, I., & Le Floch, V. (2023). Gambling and aging: An overview of a risky behavior. *Behavioral Sciences, 13*(6), 437. https://doi.org/10.3390/bs13060437
- Ford, J.A., Pomykacz, C., Szalewski, A., Esteban McCabe, S., & Schepis, T.S. (2020). Friends and relatives as sources of prescription opioids for misuse among young adults: The significance of physician source and race/ethnic differences. *Substance Abuse*, *41*(1), 93-100. https://doi.org/10.1080/08897077.2019.1635955
- GBD 2016 Alcohol and Drug Use Collaborators. (2018). The global burden of disease attributable to alcohol and drug use in 195 countries and territories, 1990-2016: A systematic analysis for the Global Burden of Disease Study 2016. *The Lancet Psychiatry*, *5*(12), 987-1012. https://doi.org/10.1016/S2215-0366(18)30337-7
- Gray, J.C., Larson, M.J., Moresco, N., Ritter, G.A., Dufour, S., Milliken, C.S., & Adams, R.S. (2021). The association of engagement in substance use treatment with negative separation from the military among soldiers with post-deployment alcohol use disorder. *Drug and Alcohol Dependence, 221*, 108647. https://doi.org/10.1016/j.drugalcdep.2021.108647
- Gimm, G., Parekh, T., & Kitsantas, P. (2023). Assessing the prevalence and risk factors of marijuana use in adults with disabilities. *Addictive Behaviors*, *138*, 107559. https://doi.org/10.1016/j.addbeh.2022.107559
- Groenewald, C.B. (2019). Opioid-prescribing patterns for pediatric patients in the United States. *The Clinical Journal of Pain*, *35*(6), 515-520. https://doi.org/10.1097/AJP.0000000000000707
- Harm Reduction Coalition. (2024). Harm Reduction Principles. Retrieved July 20, 2025, from https://harmreduction.org/about-us/principles-of-harm-reduction/
- Hoggatt, K.J., Chawla, N., Washington, D.L., & Yano, E.M. (2023). Trends in substance use disorder diagnoses among veterans, 2009-2019. *The American Journal on Addictions*, *32*(4), 393-401. https://doi.org/10.1111/ajad.13413
- Hong, Y.R., Xie, Z., Yadav, S., Tanner, R., Striley, C., & Marlow, N.M. (2023). Opioid use behaviors among people with disability in the United States: An analysis of the National Survey on Drug Use and Health. *Journal of Addiction Medicine*, *17*(1), e27-e35. https://doi.org/10.1097/ADM.0000000000001031
- Hoopsick, R.A., Fillo, J., Vest, B. M., Homish, D.L., & Homish, G.G. (2017). Substance use and dependence among current reserve and former military members: Cross-sectional findings from the National Survey on Drug Use and Health, 2010-2014. *Journal of Addictive Diseases*, *36*(4), 243-251. https://doi.org/10.1080/10550887.2017.1366735

- Jaqua, E.E., Nguyen, V., Scherlie, N., Dreschler, J., & Labib, W. (2022). Substance use disorder in older adults: Mini review. *Addiction & Health*, *14*(1), 62-67. https://doi.org/10.22122/ahj.v14i1.1311
- Judkins, J.L., Smith, K., Moore, B.A., & Morissette, S.B. (2022). Alcohol use disorder in active duty service members: Incidence rates over a 19-year period. *Substance Abuse*, *43*(1), 294-300. https://doi.org/10.1080/08897077.2021.1941512
- Kolberg, E., Smith, O.R.F., Leino, T., Pallesen, S., Griffiths, M.D., Mentzoni, R.A., & Syvertsen, A. (2025). Disability benefit and gambling disorder: A longitudinal study based on national registry data. *Journal of Gambling Studies (41),* 1349-1360. https://doi.org/10.1007/s10899-024-10368-6
- Kulak, J.A., Fillo, J., Homish, D.L., Kahn, L., & Homish, G.G. (2019). Substance use and mental health among military spouses and partners. *Military Behavioral Health*, *7*(3), 257-267. https://doi.org/10.1080/21635781.2019.1591314
- Langguth, B., Landgrebe, M., & De Ridder, D. (2025). Perceptual disturbances and disorders in the ICD-11: An overview and a proposal for systematic classification. *Brain Sciences*, *15*(1), 81. https://doi.org/10.3390/brainsci15010081
- Le, J. (2024). Pharmacokinetics. In *Merck Manual Professional Version*. Retrieved July 13, 2025, from https://www.merckmanuals.com/professional/clinical-pharmacology/pharmacokinetics/overview-of-pharmacokinetics
- Lin, J., Arnovitz, M., Kotbi, N., & Francois, D. (2023). Substance use disorders in the geriatric population: A review and synthesis of the literature of a growing problem in a growing population. *Current Treatment Options in Psychiatry*, 1-20. Advance online publication. https://doi.org/10.1007/s40501-023-00291-9
- Matheson, F.I., Dastoori, P., Hahmann, T., Woodhall-Melnik, J., Guilcher, S.J.T., & Hamilton-Wright, S. (2022). Prevalence of problem gambling among women using shelter and drop-in services. *International Journal of Mental Health and Addiction*, *20*(4), 2436-2447. https://doi.org/10.1007/s11469-021-00524-z
- Matsuzaka S. (2018). Transgressing gender norms in addiction treatment: Transgender rights to access within gender-segregated facilities. *Journal of Ethnicity in Substance Abuse*, *17*(4), 420-433. https://doi.org/10.1080/15332640.2016.1264338
- Merriam-Webster. (n.d.). Addiction, definition. Retrieved July 12, 2025, from https://www.merriam-webster.com/dictionary/addiction
- Meyer, J.P., Isaacs, K., El-Shahawy, O., Burlew, A.K., & Wechsberg, W. (2019). Research on women with substance use disorders: Reviewing progress and developing a research and implementation roadmap. *Drug and Alcohol Dependence*, *197*, 158-163. https://doi.org/10.1016/j.drugalcdep.2019.01.017
- Moon, S.J.E., & Lee, H. (2020). Relapse to substance use: A concept analysis. *Nursing Forum*, *55*(3), 523-530. https://doi.org/10.1111/nuf.12458

- Moore, M.J., Shawler, E., Jordan, C.H. et al. (2023). Veteran and Military Mental Health Issues. [Updated 2023 Aug 17]. StatPearls Publishing: Treasure Island, FL. Available from https://www.ncbi.nlm.nih.gov/books/NBK572092/
- National Cancer Institute. (n.d.). Withdrawal, definition. Retrieved July 12, 2025, from https://www.cancer.gov/publications/dictionaries/cancer-terms/def/withdrawal
- National Conference of State Legislatures. (2025). State Medical Cannabis Laws. Retrieved July 15, 2025, from https://www.ncsl.org/health/state-medical-cannabis-laws
- NIH/NIDA (National Institute of Health/National Institute on Drug Abuse). (2025). Drug Overdose Deaths: Facts and Figures. Retrieved July 15, 2025, from https://nida.nih.gov/research-topics/trends-statistics/overdose-death-rates
- NIH/NIAAA (National Institute of Health/National Institute on Alcohol Abuse and Alcoholism). (2025). Alcohol Treatment Facts in the United States, January 2025. Retrieved July 14, 2025, from https://www.niaaa.nih.gov/alcohols-effects-health/alcohol-topics/alcohol-facts-and-statistics
- NIH/NIAAA (National Institute of Health/National Institute on Alcohol Abuse and Alcoholism). (n.d.). Get the Facts About Underage Drinking. Retrieved July 14, 2025, from https://www.niaaa.nih.gov/publications/brochures-and-fact-sheets/underage-drinking
- Pinedo, M., Zemore, S., Beltrán-Girón, J., Gilbert, P., & Castro, Y. (2020). Women's barriers to specialty substance abuse treatment: A qualitative exploration of racial/ethnic differences. *Journal of Immigrant and Minority Health*, *22*(4), 653-660. https://doi.org/10.1007/s10903-019-00933-2
- Pollack, H., Mackiewicz, M. Sinha, S. (2025). Invisible and overlooked (again): Older adults, ageism, and substance misuse. *Milbank Quarterly* Opinion. March 31, 2025. https://doi.org/10.1599/mqop.2025.0331
- Reif, S., Karriker-Jaffe, K.J., Valentine, A., Patterson, D., Mericle, A.A., Adams, R.S., & Greenfield, T.K. (2022). Substance use and misuse patterns and disability status in the 2020 US National Alcohol Survey: A contributing role for chronic pain. *Disability and Health Journal*, *15*(2S), 101290. https://doi.org/10.1016/j.dhjo.2022.101290
- Salerno, L., Becheri, L., & Pallanti, S. (2022). ADHD-gaming disorder comorbidity in children and adolescents: A narrative review. *Children*, *9*(10), 1528. https://doi.org/10.3390/children9101528
- Sparks, A.C., Radakrishnan, S., Corry, N.H., McDonald, D., Carlson, K., Carballo, C.E., & Stander, V. (2021). Associations between spouse and service member prescriptions for high-risk and long-term opioids: A dyadic study. *Addictive Behaviors Reports*, *14*, 100364. https://doi.org/10.1016/j.abrep.2021.100364
- Stone, J.A., Lester, C.A., Aboneh, E.A., Phelan, C.H., Welch, L.L., & Chui, M.A. (2017). A preliminary examination of over-the-counter medication misuse rates in older adults. *Research in Social & Administrative Pharmacy*, *13*(1), 187-192. https://doi.org/10.1016/j.sapharm.2016.01.004
- Substance Abuse and Mental Health Services Administration. (2024a). Harm Reduction. Retrieved July 14, 2025, from https://www.samhsa.gov/substance-use/harm-reduction

- Substance Abuse and Mental Health Services Administration. (2024b). Medications, Counseling, and Related Conditions: Substance Use Disorders. Retrieved July 14, 2025, from https://www.samhsa.gov/substance-use/treatment/options/medications
- Substance Abuse and Mental Health Services Administration. (2025). National Survey on Drug Use and Health. Retrieved July 14, 2025, from https://www.samhsa.gov/data/data-we-collect/nsduh-national-survey-drug-use-and-health
- Thomasius, R., Paschke, K., & Arnaud, N. (2022). Substance-use disorders in children and adolescents. *Deutsches Arzteblatt International, 119*(25), 440-450. https://doi.org/10.3238/arztebl.m2022.0122
- Uhl, G.R., Koob, G.F., & Cable, J. (2019). The neurobiology of addiction. *Annals of the New York Academy of Sciences, 1451*(1), 5-28. https://doi.org/10.1111/nyas.13989
- Uscher-Pines, L., Lin, K. & Busch, A.B. (2024). Expanding treatment options for alcohol use disorder. *JAMA Health Forum, 5*(8), e242184. https://doi.org/10.1001/jamahealthforum.2024.2184
- Volkow, N.D. & Blanco, C. (2023). Substance use disorders: A comprehensive update of classification, epidemiology, neurobiology, clinical aspects, treatment and prevention. *World Psychiatry: Official Journal of the World Psychiatric Association, 22*(2), 203-229. https://doi.org/10.1002/wps.21073
- Webb, L., Fox, S., Skårner, A., & Messas, G. (2022). Editorial: Women and substance use: Specific needs and experiences of use, others' use and transitions towards recovery. *Frontiers in Psychiatry, 13*, 1078605. https://doi.org/10.3389/fpsyt.2022.1078605
- White, A.M., Orosz, A., Powell, P.A., & Koob, G.F. (2023). Alcohol and aging - An area of increasing concern. *Alcohol, 107*, 19-27. https://doi.org/10.1016/j.alcohol.2022.07.005
- World Health Organization. (2015). ICD-10: *International Statistical Classification of Diseases and Related Health Problems* (10th revision, 5th ed.).
- World Health Organization. (2025). *Global Report on Trends in Prevalence of Tobacco Use 2000-2024 and Projections 2025-2030* (6th ed.). Retrieved October 10, 2025, from https://www.who.int/publications/i/item/9789240116276

CHAPTER 9

SUICIDAL IDEATION

INTRODUCTION

There has been one constant over my 40-plus years as a clinical social worker: discomfort when patients present with suicidal ideation or intent. This distress is a given, no matter the depth of one's expertise or the years of experience. Most behavioral health practitioners feel the same discomfort.

The distress stems in part from the tragic possibility of missing life-saving signs or cues. Sometimes a person's mood improves and reports feeling well again. Sometime later, though, you get a call, email, or text from the person's family: The patient has died by suicide. I wish I could promise that the content in this chapter will spare you this reality.

Those misses cause practitioners to question or even doubt their suicidality assessments. As a clinician, you hope your assessment skills haven't missed anything, *but sometimes your clinical gut will scream for you to be cautious.* You consult with a psychiatrist about your doubts, and she confirms the patient does not need inpatient treatment. *Do you believe it?* The family tells you they can provide support and supervision, *but will this be enough to keep the patient safe once he leaves your treatment space?* You screen for signs of suicide, and the tool scores the patient as low risk for self-harm, *but do you have faith in the results with unquestioning certainty?* The discrepancies between what we assess and the patient's true intent aren't always as clear as we would hope. This chapter contains the foundation to successfully navigate this difficult domain.

BEHAVIORAL LEARNING OBJECTIVES

1. Identify common terms and definitions associated with suicidality
2. Explain symptom presentation for related diagnoses in the DSM
3. Identify new diagnoses related to suicide for future versions of the DSM
4. Analyze the incidence of suicide across life stages and populations
5. Identify general considerations for suicidality across populations

6. Recognize screening tools used to assess for suicidal ideation, intent, and foreseeable and imminent self-harm
7. Apply Case Management's Behavioral Health Conversation Map when intervening with patients (and their support systems) dealing with suicidality

ESSENTIAL TERMS

- Altruistic suicide
- Anomic suicide
- Clustering
- Contagion
- Cutting
- Ego integrity versus despair
- Egoistic suicide
- Fatalistic suicide
- Foreseeable harm
- Imminent harm
- Injurious behaviors
- Narrative crisis model of suicide
- Non-self-injurious behaviors
- Nonsuicidal self-injury
- Nonsuicidal self-injurious behavior (NSSI)
- Protective factors
- Self-harm
- Self-inflicted
- Suicidal ideation
- Suicidality
- Suicide attempt
- Suicide behavioral disorder
- Suicide crisis
- Suicide crisis syndrome (SCS)
- Suicide plan
- Survivor

TERMS AND FEATURES OF SUICIDALITY

To lay the foundation for suicidality knowledge, we will cover guiding theories, frameworks, and professional perspectives on suicide. Attention will be paid to shifting diagnoses related to suicidality in the DSM and ICD.

THE SUICIDALITY CONTINUUM

Case managers often must assess patients for the presence and severity of *suicidal ideation* (SI). Are the patient's thoughts random and fleeting in nature? Or are they occurring with more frequency and consistency, such as multiple times over the course of one day, or even every day? The assessment should consider whether the patient is experiencing passive or active suicidal ideation (PSI or ASI).

Imagine the student who despairingly discloses to her teacher, "My parents put more pressure on me than I can handle; I'm just done." It was a one-and-done conversation, and the student quickly recanted. "I'm just kidding. I get stressed but would never hurt myself." Several months later, another teacher engages in similar conversations with the student, which are occurring with greater frequency and with concern for the student self-harming. Based on the conversations, the teacher detects a real possibility for harm to occur in the near future, known as *imminent* or *foreseeable harm,* so he contacts the school social worker to meet with the student. The student admits she brought a bottle of pills to school and thought about taking them after lunch. The student has detailed a plan with a specific timeframe and an identifiable means of harm, known as a *suicidal plan*: specific thoughts about a self-initiated action that facilitates self-harming behavior or a suicide attempt.

Over the past few weeks, the student's thoughts have advanced through the suicidality continuum, which ranges from occasional or fleeting thoughts of ending one's life to those occurring more consistently. Ultimately, the person develops a viable plan that is enacted, resulting in an established suicide attempt. *Completed suicide* is when a death is caused by self-directed injurious behavior, with the person intending to die as a result of their actions. A revised rendering of the *suicidality continuum* developed by Cai et al. (2021) appears in Figure 9.1.

Figure 9.1: *Suicidality continuum*

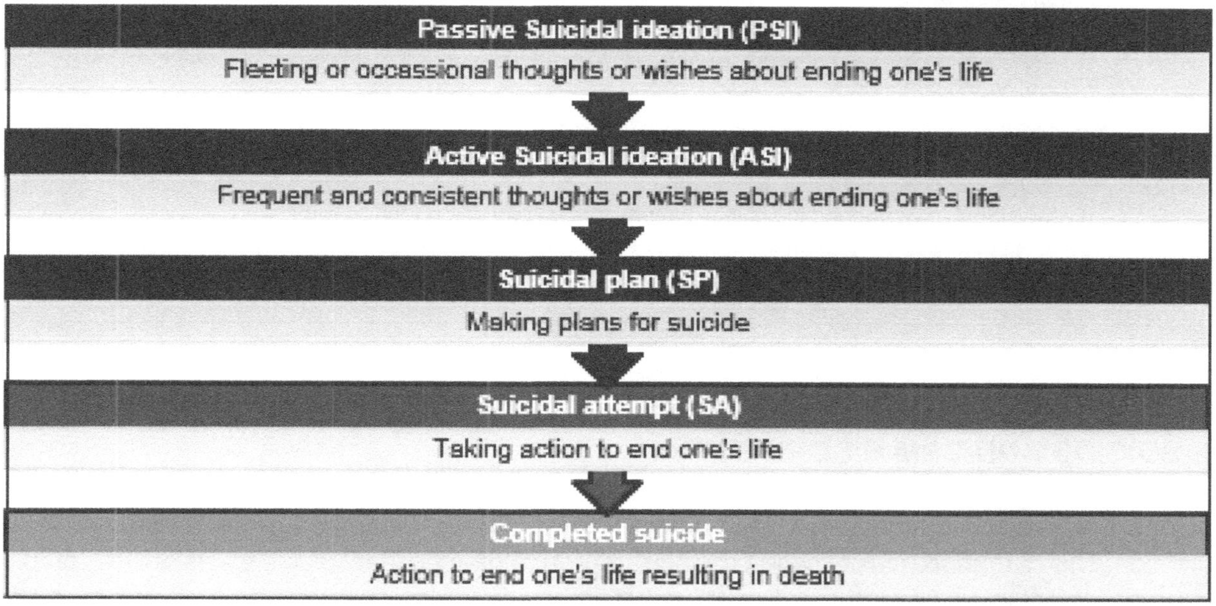

Adapted from Cai et al., 2021

DURKHEIM'S FOUR TYPES OF SUICIDE

Among early professional theories on suicide were those by Emil Durkheim, a sociologist interested in the relationships between individuals and society. Durkheim associated the tendency to commit suicide with societal integration; the more socially integrated and connected a person was to society, the less likely he or she would be to commit suicide (Mueller et al., 2021). Durkheim identified four types of suicide that are aligned with a person's level of social integration. His seminal model appears in Table 9.1, along with examples for each type.

Table 9.1: *Durkheim's four types of suicide*

Types	Explanation and Example
Altruistic suicide	Occurs when a person is overly integrated into a social group and sacrifices themself for the perceived benefit of the group or a cause they believe in Characterized by a strong sense of obligation or duty to the collective Examples: soldiers sacrificing in battle, suicide for political or religious causes
Anomic suicide	Occurs when there is a lack of social regulation or a breakdown of social norms and values, as in periods of rapid social or economic change or instability People face moral confusion and disorientation, struggling to find their place and purpose within society, leading to feelings of disappointment and hopelessness Examples: suicide during economic downturns or mass disasters, or amid sudden gains in wealth and then struggling with expectations and aspirations
Egoistic suicide	Occurs when a person has weak social ties and feels isolated and detached from their community or social groups Characterized by feelings of meaninglessness Examples: Couples or individuals experiencing infertility who feel a weak sense of belonging to family and community
Fatalistic suicide	Occurs when a person experiences excessive social regulation and oppression, which leads to feelings of powerlessness and despair Individuals feel trapped in societal circumstances and see no future without suffering Examples: Prisoners sentenced for life, where death presents the only escape from a life without agency or meaning

Adapted from Mueller et al., 2021

SUICIDE AND DSM DISORDERS

Despite the societal attention given to suicide, the DSM contains no formal diagnosis for the condition. This diagnostic classification (or lack thereof) reinforces that suicide exists due to complex biopsychosocial interconnections. The DSM-5-TR does include a section, Other Conditions That May Be a Focus of Clinical Attention, that describes assorted psychosocial and environmental circumstances that may prompt a person to need treatment, one of which is suicidal behavior. Other situations on the list are relationship or marital tension, job stress, economic pressures, and difficulties adjusting to particular life stages (e.g., transition to college, divorce, retirement). These conditions often drive individuals, couples, and families to seek counseling and are shown in Box 9.1. They may also be identified during treatment for other mental health conditions, and they can influence the course of treatment.

The DSM does contain two conditions related to suicide: *suicidal behavior* and *nonsuicidal self-injury* (NSSI). Suicidal behavior diagnoses use the T codes from ICD-10, where the sixth character is coded as shown in Table 9.2.

Box 9.1: DSM-5-TR section on 'Other conditions that may be a focus of clinical attention'

1. Suicidal behavior: Encompasses self-injurious behavior with at least some intent to die, and nonsuicidal self-injury (intentional self-inflicted damage to the body in the absence of suicidal intent)
2. Relational problems: Includes parent-child relational problems, sibling relational problems, relationship distress with a spouse or intimate partner, disruption of a family by separation or divorce, and high expressed emotion levels within the family
3. Abuse and neglect: Encompasses child physical abuse (confirmed or suspected), child sexual abuse (confirmed or suspected), child neglect (confirmed or suspected), child psychological abuse (confirmed or suspected), spouse or partner violence (physical, sexual, psychological, or neglect), and adult abuse by a non-spouse or non-partner
4. Educational problems: Illiteracy or low-level literacy, schooling unavailable or unattainable, failed school exams, and underachievement in school
5. Occupational problems: Unemployment, change of job, threat of job loss, stressful work schedule, discord with boss or colleagues
6. Housing and economic problems: Includes homelessness, inadequate housing, discord with a neighbor, lodger, or landlord, insufficient social insurance or welfare support, and other unspecified housing or economic problems
7. Problems related to the social environment: Includes phase of life problems, problems related to living alone, acculturation difficulty, social exclusion or rejection, and being the target of (perceived) adverse discrimination or persecution
8. Problems related to crime or interaction with the legal system: Includes being a victim of crime, conviction in civil or criminal proceedings without imprisonment, imprisonment or other incarceration, problems related to release from prison, and other legal circumstances
9. Problems related to access to medical and other health care: Includes unavailability or inaccessibility of health care facilities and unavailability or inaccessibility of other helping agencies
10. Circumstances of personal history: Includes other personal history of psychological trauma, personal history of self-harm, personal history of military deployment, or other personal risk factors
11. Other health service encounters for counseling and medical advice: Used when the individual seeks counseling related to sex education, sexual behavior, sexual orientation, sexual attitudes, others' sexual behavior or orientation, sexual enjoyment, or any other sex-related issue
12. Additional conditions or problems that may be a focus of clinical attention: A broad category of conditions such as malingering, uncomplicated bereavement, adult antisocial behavior, child or adolescent antisocial behavior, religious or spiritual problems, nonadherence to medical treatment, overweight or obesity, and wandering associated with a mental disorder

American Psychiatric Association, 2022, pp. 821-836

Table 9.2: *Suicidal behavior and nonsuicidal self-injury diagnoses*

DSM-5-TR Diagnosis	Code
Suicidal behavior: Individual has engaged in potentially self-injurious behavior with at least some intent to die as a result of the act. Evidence may be explicit (e.g., a formal letter, phone call, email, social media post) or inferred from the behavior or circumstance (e.g., carrying pills intended for self-harm, possessing a weapon intended for self-harm, general comments about self-harm). **A (Initial encounter):** the patient is receiving active treatment for the condition (e.g., ED encounter, evaluation and treatment by a new clinician), or D (Subsequent encounter): The patient has received treatment for the condition or is receiving routine care for the condition during a healing or recovery phase (e.g., medication adjustment, aftercare, follow-up visits) History of suicidal behavior: If suicidal behavioral has occurred in a person's lifetime	T14.91XA T14.91XD Z91.51
Nonsuicidal self-injury: Individual has engaged in intentional self-inflicted damage to their body, of type likely to induce bleeding, bruising, or pain (e.g., cutting, burning, stabbing, hitting, excessive rubbing) in the absence of suicidal intent. **Current nonsuicidal self-injury:** If nonsuicidal self-injurious behavior is part of the clinical presentation History of nonsuicidal self-injury: If nonsuicidal self-injurious behavior has occurred during the individual's lifetime	R45.88 Z91.52

American Psychiatric Association, 2022, pp. 920, 923

Both suicidal behavior and nonsuicidal self-injury are independently being considered for inclusion as unique disorders in a future version of the DSM. A diagnosis covering formal criteria has been developed for each condition, with both in the process of rigorous, multi-step vetting by the American Psychiatric Association, involving review of the latest research and scientific evidence, assorted field trials, and solicitation of public comment. The decision will made public with the next edition of the DSM. The proposed criteria for suicidal behavior disorder and nonsuicidal self-injurious disorder appear in Boxes 9.2 and 9.3.

Box 9.2: Signs and symptoms of proposed suicidal behavior disorder Proposed DSM criteria:

Patients must meet all five of the following diagnostic criteria:

Criterion A. Within the last 24 months, the individual has made a suicide attempt.

- A suicide attempt is defined as "a self-initiated sequence of behaviors by an individual who, at the time of initiation, expected that the set of actions would lead to his or her own death."

Criterion B. The act does not meet criteria for non-suicidal self-injury
Criterion C. The diagnosis is not applied to suicidal ideation or to preparatory acts
Criterion D. The act was not initiated during a state of delirium or confusion
Criterion E. The act was not undertaken solely for a political or religious objective

Includes two specifiers:

1. Current: not more than 12 months since the most recent attempt
2. In early remission: 12-24 months since the most recent attempt

American Psychiatric Association, 2022, p. 920

Box 9.3: Signs and symptoms of proposed nonsuicidal self-injury disorder (NSSID)

Proposed DSM criteria:

Criterion A: Individual engages in NSSI on 5 or more days in the past year

Criterion B: Individual expects that NSSI will relieve negative thoughts or feelings, resolve interpersonal difficulties, or induce a positive emotional state

Criterion C: The NSSI is associated with at least one of the following:

- Negative thoughts or feelings (e.g., anxiety, sadness, self-criticism) immediately before the self-injury
- Interpersonal difficulties (e.g., conflicts with others) before the self-injury
- A strong urge to self-injure that is difficult to resist
- Preoccupation with thoughts about self-injury

Criterion D: The behavior is not socially sanctioned (e.g., part of a religious ritual) or restricted to minor self-injurious behaviors (e.g., nail biting)
Criterion E: The NSSI causes clinically significant distress or impairment in social, occupational, or other important areas of functioning
Criterion F: The NSSI does not occur exclusively during psychosis, delirium, or substance use/withdrawal and is not better explained by another mental disorder

American Psychiatric Association, 2022, p. 923

Both disorders significantly affect society; over 10 million adults have considered suicide, of whom more than 3 million have made formal plans, and 1.4 million have made attempts (Ivey-Stephenson et al., 2022). In addition, one in five individuals have presented with NSSI (Dierickx et al., 2023). As attention on both disorders rises, their identification as formal diagnoses could have major clinical and fiscal implications for treatment outcomes and revenue capture.

NONSUICIDAL SELF-INJURY

Also known as *cutting*, the purpose of NSSI is to relieve intense and internalized emotional discomfort or psychological distress by providing a mechanism for release and regulation (Klonsky, 2009). Family members and other individuals in a patient's support system can struggle to understand this level of physical destruction on the body without SI or other suicidal intent.

Multiple methods are commonly used, such as heating small objects (e.g., cigarettes, ends of safety pins or other metal) to burn the skin, scratching oneself (e.g., with fingernails, razors, scissors, writing utensils), or banging or hitting a body part to prompt pain or bruising. The marks may be superficial but often run deep emotionally. Tattoos and body piercings can be forms of self-mutilation, but neither are viewed as self-harm behaviors unless that is their deliberate intent (Adilah & Setiawati, 2025). Youth who engage in NSSI are likely to advance to suicidal attempts, particularly as they move into adolescence and young adulthood (Predescu & Sipos, 2023).

Even the most experienced professionals can feel overwhelmed when a person presents with NSSI. Can we have full confidence the person will not engage in more advanced self-harm? The quick answer is *no,* which means case managers should always assess and refer patients who present with cutting behaviors for immediate evaluation by licensed mental health professionals who can render treatment recommendations.

SUICIDE CRISIS SYNDROME

The rising incidence of suicide has prompted urgency among professionals to expand assessment frameworks and diagnoses. As many as 75 percent of people who completed suicide explicitly denied SI at their final meeting with a health professional (Berman & Silverman, 2020). Other research notes that almost 20 percent of persons who make a suicide attempt do not have a diagnosable mental disorder (Oquendo et al., 2024).

One promising framework for assessing suicidality is the *narrative crisis model* of suicide (NCM), which reflects four stages of suicidal progression from acute or imminent risk to less-urgent, chronic suicidal risk (Galynker at al., 2024). Stage 4 of the model is *suicide crisis syndrome* (SCS), which has also been suggested for inclusion in the DSM. The NCM is shown in Figure 9.2, and the proposed criteria for suicide crisis syndrome appear in Box 9.4.

Figure 9.2: *Narrative crisis model of suicide*

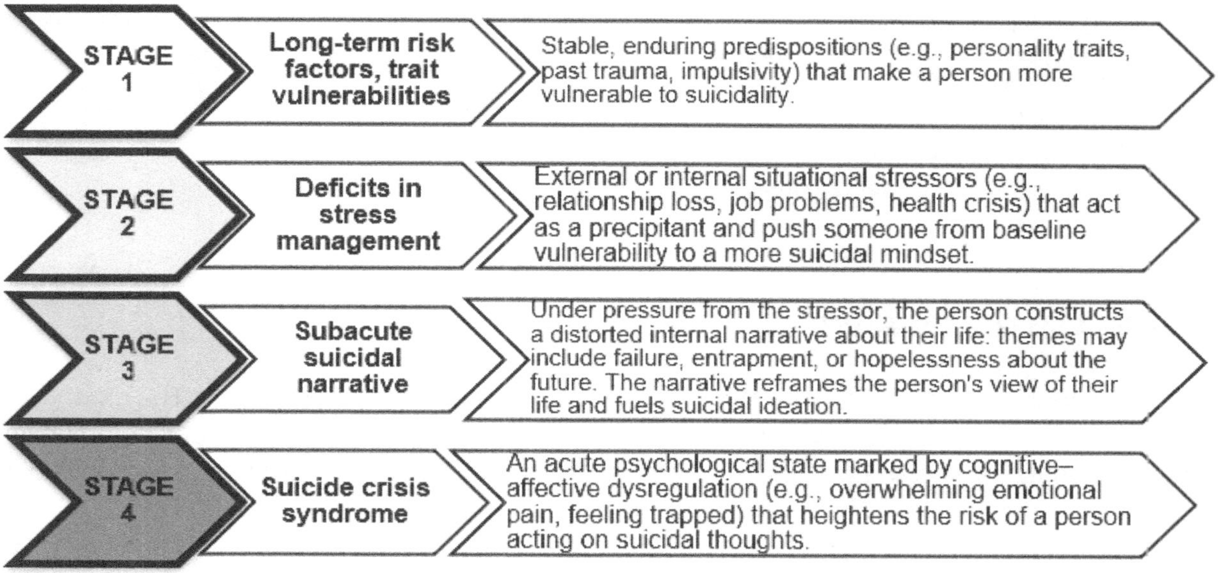

Galynker et al., 2024

Box 9.4: Criteria for proposed suicide crisis syndrome

Proposed DSM criteria:

Must meet criterion A and have at least one symptom from each of criteria B1-B4.

Criterion A: Features a persistent and intense feeling of frantic hopelessness, in which the individual feels trapped in a situation experienced both as intolerable and inescapable

Criterion B: Includes four distinct dimensions

- **B1** Affective disturbance, manifests itself through:
    1) emotional pain
    2) depressive turmoil
    3) extreme anxiety with unusual physical sensations; and

  4) acute anhedonia
- **B2** Loss of cognitive control involves:
    1) ruminations
    2) cognitive rigidity
    3) failed thought suppression; and
    4) ruminative flooding, which is the loss of control over thoughts, accompanied by headaches or head pressure

- **B3** Hyperarousal involves:
  1) agitation/restlessness
  2) hypervigilance (e.g., an intense and exaggerated responsiveness to sensory inputs)
  3) irritability; and
  4) insomnia
- **B4** Social withdrawal involves:

  Avoidance of social engagements and evasive communication with others

Galynker et al., 2024

DATA AND DEMOGRAPHICS

Suicide is a public health priority; it ranks among the top global contributors to death. The urgency for action is amplified by its emotional and traumatic impact on *survivors,* the persons and communities left behind: family, friends, colleagues, teachers, students, and broader social groups, even including social media connections.

GENERAL RISK FACTORS

Patients with depressive disorders, particularly those diagnosed with MDD, are at greatest risk of suicide. Upwards of 90 percent of people with MDD complete suicide (Cai et al., 2021). Suicide and the quality of one's life experiences go hand in hand. With over 800,000 persons dying annually from suicide in the U.S., providers and practitioners wrestle with the best means to assess suicidality and detect its myriad presentations. Countless studies have identified the individual, relational, community, and societal risk factors that can put human beings at greater risk of suicide. A list of suicide risk factors appears in Box 9.5.

Protective factors

Another way to evaluate for suicide risk is to assess and account for the opposite of risk factors—protective factors (Cai et al., 2021). *Protective factors* are life experiences that reduce suicide risk, the aspects of upbringing that shield people from the harm of risk factors. They are biological, psychological, or psychosocial factors that promote personal and psychological safety in individuals. Ki et al. (2024) found that protective factors inversely impact suicidal ideation and suicidality; the more protective factors one gathers over his or her lifetime, the less likely he or she will be to experience SI. The authors identified a series of protective factors, shown in Box 9.6.

Box 9.5: Risk factors associated with suicide

Individual risk factors

- Previous suicide attempt
- History of depression and other mental illnesses
- Serious illness, such as chronic pain
- Criminal/legal problems
- Job loss or financial problems
- Impulsive or aggressive tendencies
- Substance use
- Current or prior history of adverse childhood experiences
- Sense of hopelessness
- Violence victimization and/or perpetration

Relationship risk factors

- Bullying
- Family/loved one's history of suicide
- Loss of relationships
- High conflict or violent relationships
- Social isolation

Community risk factors

- Lack of access to healthcare
- Suicide cluster in the community
- Stress of acculturation
- Community violence
- Historical trauma
- Discrimination

Societal risk factors

- Easy access to lethal means
- Unsafe media portrayals of suicide

Centers for Disease Control and Prevention, 2024

Box 9.6: Protective factors against suicidality

- Coping
- Hope
- Life satisfaction
- Mattering (to self or others)
- Perceived control
- Positive relationships
- Purpose in life
- Religiosity (spirituality)
- Resilience
- Self-regulation
- Sense of belonging
- Social connectedness
- Social participation
- Social support
- Well-being and quality of life

Ki et al., 2024

Clustering and contagion

Social media elevates attention to suicides through quick, mass exposure, and often in graphic detail. Public coverage may include details about the method and location, which garners curiosity and attracts positive attention to the victim. Yet even before the advent of social media, sociologists identified concerning trends associated with suicide, such as *clustering* (Hawton et al., 2020). This term relates to a statistically unusual or unexpected event of three or more suicide attempts or completed suicides occurring in a common geographical location and within a short time frame. Institutional settings (e.g., schools, universities, and psychiatric units) are common community locations for clustering events. Approximately 5 percent of adolescent suicides occur in clusters (Walling, 2021).

Clusters are attributed to the *Werther effect*, also called *contagion* (Phillips, 1974). The terms refer to the process by which exposure to a suicidal attempt or completed suicide by one person prompts suicidal behaviors in others. Contagion occurs via direct or indirect exposure. A direct exposure occurs when, for example, a high school community experiences a death by suicide, then several students later engage in their own suicide attempts. An indirect exposure often comes from public coverage like a news broadcast or a social media post that focuses, for example, on increased suicides in response to high unemployment. A direct connection can be made between sensationalized reporting, normalization of suicidal behavior as an escape from a challenging reality, and subsequent suicide attempts.

DEVELOPMENTAL LIFE STAGE

Every age group is presenting with an increased frequency and intensity of suicide behaviors, including an increase in hangings and use of firearms. This reality enjoins case managers to be familiar with the latest data for the populations they care for.

Youth

Family members, teachers, practitioners, and providers are on high alert for suicidality in this age group. Suicide is the second most common cause of death in youth 10-14 years of age—6.5 out of every 100,000 suicides in the U.S. (Hink et al., 2022). Suicide prevalence for preteens (ages 8-12) has risen by 8 percent in the past decade (Ruch et al., 2024). Prior attempts are the strongest indicator for a future attempt: a prior attempt increases the likelihood of another attempt 4.3-fold for children and 5.4-fold for young adults (Ong et al., 2021).

Data from the U.S. Preventive Services Task Force (USPSTF) speak to compelling need for early and proactive assessment of SI in younger children (U.S. Preventive Services Task Force et al., 2022). Even though the USPSTF recommends screening all children 12 years and older for depression and all children 8 and older for anxiety, SI is not consistently screened. The data emphasize a compelling need for youth screening, and in younger populations.

Youth ages 10-18 who identified as female and completed suicide were more likely than their male counterparts to have a mental health treatment history and a history of SI with prior suicide attempts. They more frequently left a suicide note or shared with someone (e.g., a therapist or a friend) when interpersonal and intimate partner problems contributed to their suicide (Lee & Wong, 2020).

Suicide rates for youth rose significantly during the COVID-19 pandemic. Yard et al. (2021) identified the shift as a response to mandatory home schooling, limited socialization, and increased isolation. Researchers identified a leap in ED visits for youth 12-17 years old for suicide attempts; a 50.6 percent increase for girls and a 3.7 percent increase for boys. Suicide attempts also rose 28 percent across students of color who identified as non-Hispanic White, non-Hispanic Black, and American Indian or Alaskan Native (Yard et al., 2021).

Methods. The most common methods of suicide for youth are firearms, overdose and poisoning, and hanging and suffocation, with Figure 9.3 showing the incidence by method.

Recent data reveal a troubling increase in use of firearms for suicide by youth. Almost half (48 percent) of the suicide events reported for ages 15-19 involved a gun; 38 percent in ages 10-14 (Bhatt et al., 2023). For families that legally own firearms, access to the weapons is a critical point for analysis. Data reflect contradictory views between parents and children about ease of access to weapons. Almost 39 percent of parents who reported that their children did not know the location of household guns were challenged on that information by a child. The 22 percent of parents who reported that their children had never handled a gun were also mistaken. When teachers and clinicians screen for SI or a suicidal plan, researchers suggest they also focus on firearm availability and access (Bhatt et al., 2023).

Figure 9.3: *Leading methods for suicide in youth*

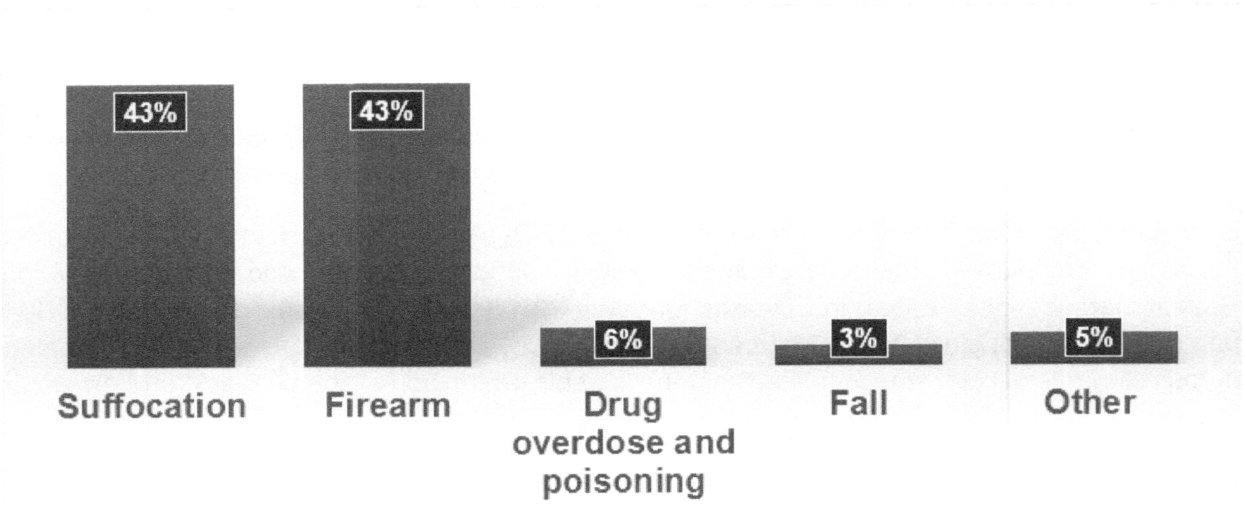

Data from Hink et al., 2022

Cutting and NSSI. NSSI is on the rise. Seminal research by Barrocas et al. (2012) revealed trends based on gender orientation and age. Figure 9.4 shows a greater prevalence of cutting and carving behaviors in females, while males tend to hit themselves by their own hand or objects. Figure 9.5 shows the primary behaviors by age groups. Younger children are more often engaged in hitting, while those children ages 14 and older tend to carve their skin.

Research by DeCamp and Bakken (2016) reveals that adolescents who identify as sexual minorities engage in NSSI more (as shown in Figure 9.6), and a high percentage of those individuals experienced active SI. Roughly 13 percent of the research respondents used this behavior as a coping strategy, with 47 percent of the study's more than 7,000 randomly selected students admitting to active SI in the past. This issue continues to be a focus of research, as practitioners wrestle with determining when those who engage in NSSI may have intent for suicidal self-harm.

Figure 9.4: *Primary NSSI behaviors by gender*

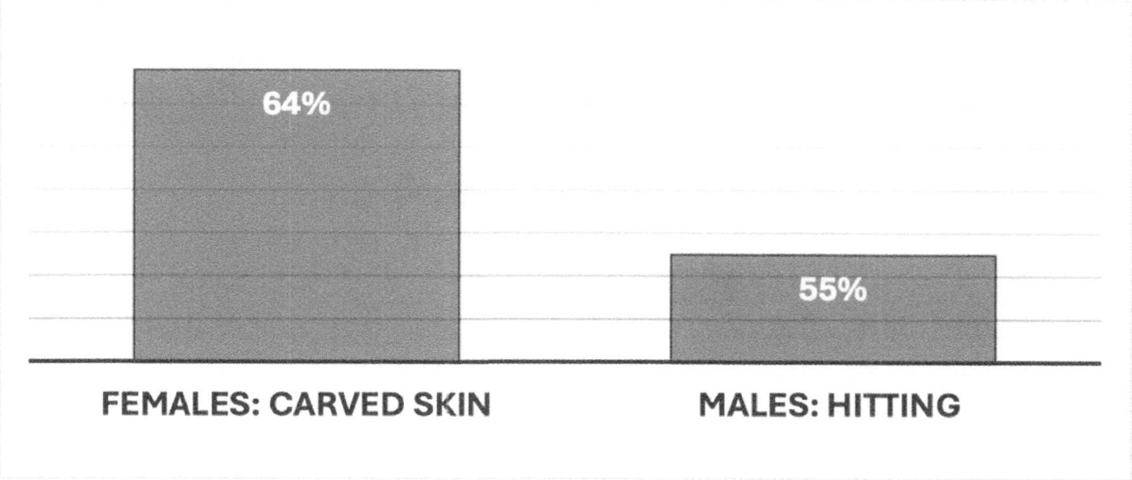

Data from Barrocas et al., 2012

Figure 9.5: *Primary NSSI behaviors by age*

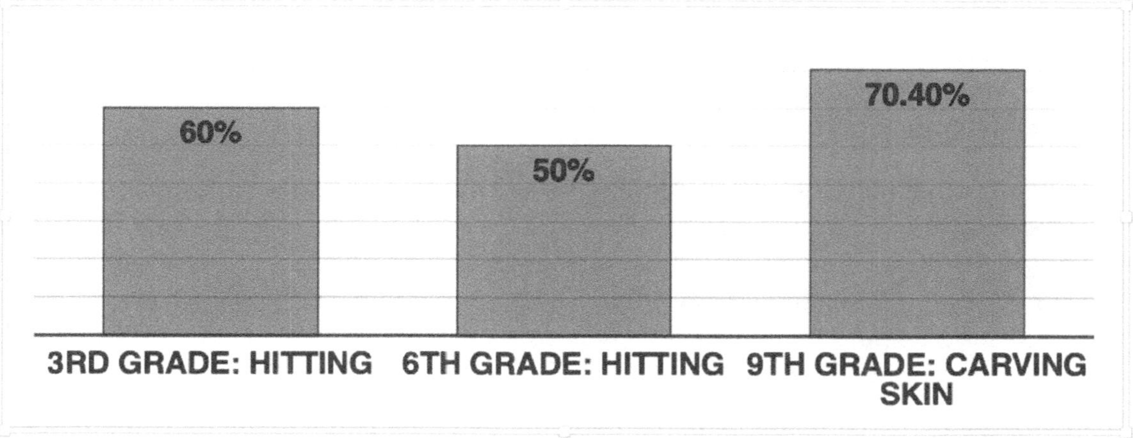

Data from Barrocas et al., 2012

Figure 9.6: *Incidence of NSSI among heterosexual and sexual minority adolescents*

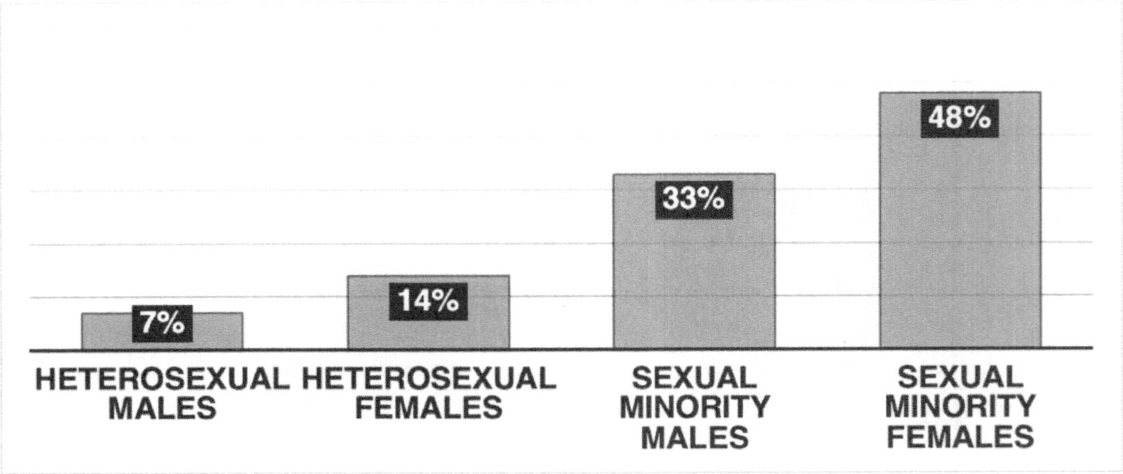

Data from DeCamp & Bakken, 2016

Adults

The numbers for adult suicides are also staggering. For each suicide attempt by an adult, two additional individuals contemplate suicide or make suicidal plans, and another 7 persons have active suicide ideation. For each completed suicide, 35 are attempted (Harmer et al., 2024). These are alarming numbers, especially to those in healthcare professions.

Other pertinent numbers to chew on: Suicide is the second leading cause of death for adults 25-34 years of age. (Unintentional injuries and accidents are the top cause.) It is the fourth leading cause of death for adults 35-44, behind unintentional injuries, heart disease, and malignant neoplasms. Adult males 55-64 showed the largest percent increase in suicide rates over recent decades, reaching 29.5 suicides per 100,000. In comparison, women 45-64 have the highest rate of suicide among all women, 8.6 suicides per 100,000 (CDC, n.d.; Garnett et al., 2023).

The CDC maintains the Web-based Injury Statistics Query and Reporting System (WISQARS) Fatal Injury Data, which provides national, regional, and state-level data on fatal injuries in the U.S. Just over 16 percent of all events listed in the WISQARS are suicides (Centers for Disease Control and Prevention, n.d.). An interactive map offers a look at the number of suicides state-to-state. It shows the U.S. Midwest has a high concentration of states with 20 or more suicides per every 100,000 persons.

Older adults

Prior chapters have detailed how age-related changes in physical and cognitive functioning can worsen mental health. It is no coincidence that older adults have among the highest suicide rates. The eighth stage of Erikson's eight stages of psychosocial development (Orenstein & Lewis, 2022) was aptly named *ego integrity versus despair.* Older adults feel either contentment about their personal and professional accomplishments over their lives, or they feel disdain for or regret about what they could not attain. Greater regret and disdain lead to a higher rate of suicide, with physical illness, family issues, financial issues, and hopelessness also contributing to increase suicide rates (Dhole et al., 2023).

Recent research by Garnett et al. (2023) noted elevated rates of suicide, particularly for men 85 years and older: 55.7 deaths per 100,000 of the population. Women 65-74 years of age have experienced a 44 percent rise in suicide since 2001, though still represent fewer total deaths annually: 5.6 per 100,000 (Garnett et al., 2023). Methods for suicide vary within the demographic group. Persons in their 60s, 70s, and 80s prefer non-violent means to end their lives with differing methods prioritized, as shown in Figure 9.7.

Access to firearms has become a concerning factor for this age group over the past decade. DeLeo and Gianotti (2021) noted that when older adults have a gun in the home, the risk of self-harm is tripled. A narrative review by Price and Khubchandani (2021) identified that upwards of 70 percent of all older adult suicides are the result of a firearm, especially those occurring in rural communities.

Figure 9.7: *Non-violent methods of suicide by older adults*

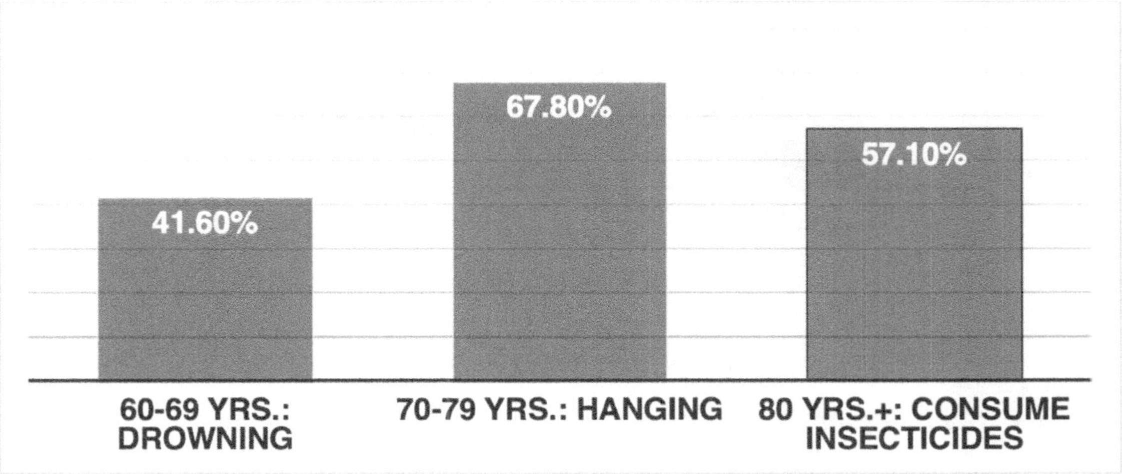

Data from Crimmins, 2015

POPULATION-FOCUSED MONITORING

LGBTQIA+

The sexual minority population is at greater risk of suicide than most populations, across all age groups. Individuals may consider suicide a way to escape a reality they think will never match their hopes. They're also subjected to more negative life experiences due to others questioning their identity or not welcoming their gender orientation.

Youth and young adults. Upwards of 40 percent of LGBTQIA+ young people seriously consider suicide annually, with 12 percent attempting self-harm. The population is more than four times more likely to attempt suicide compared to their sexual majority peers. Figure 9.8 shows that sexual minority teens (ages 13-17) are far more likely to engage in suicide behaviors than young adults (ages 18-24) (Nath et al., 2024).

Figure 9.8: *LGBTQIA+ suicidal behaviors in the past year*

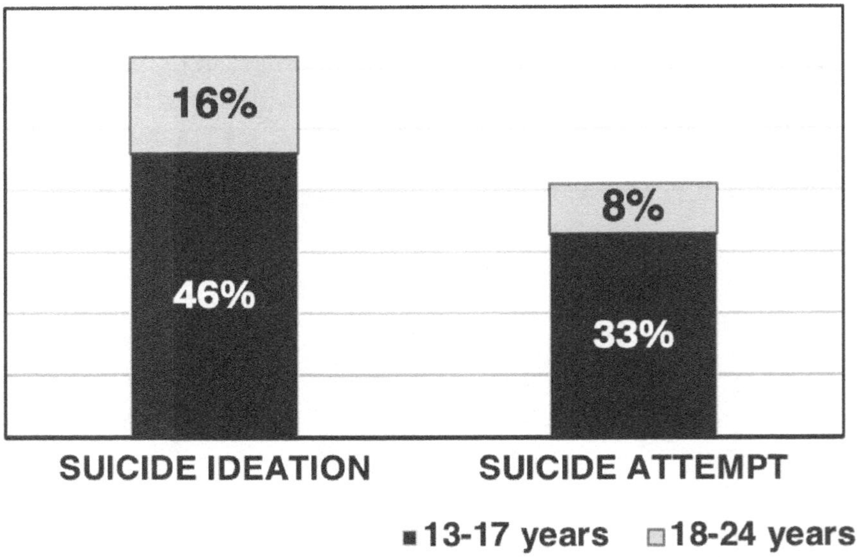

Data from Nath et al., 2024

The sociopolitical climate. The current, global sociopolitical climate is impacting suicidality rates for sexual minorities. Researchers are exploring how these dynamics affect the community, especially for people who identify as transgender, are amid gender-affirming treatments, or are seeking access to them. Current data is limited on SI, intent, or action tied to the sociopolitical climate, but anecdotal experience shines a light on the scope of impact. My colleagues, friends, and family members have shared personal and professional perspectives that convey an increase in suicidal behaviors in response to executive orders and state laws that impede access to treatment and the autonomy to make personal choices.

Middle and older adults. Sexual minority adults in middle and older age also experience elevated risk for suicide compared to heterosexuals (Capistrant & Nakash, 2019). Persons 50 and older were 17 percent more likely to engage in suicidal planning compared with heterosexuals of the same age group. Contributing factors are quality of social supports, having an intimate partner or similar relationship, and overall quality of life. Several familiar factors add stress and influence suicidality in this population, such as social stigma, discrimination, and rejection by family of origin, peers, or social networks (e.g., employers, religious, spiritual). A summary of issues around suicidality and the LGBTQIA+ community is in Box 9.7.

Box 9.7: Suicidality and LGBTQIA+

High incidence for:

- Suicidal ideation and action in adolescents
- Suicide planning in adults over 50

Distinct considerations:

- Heightened suicide risk from:
    - Bullying by peers in youth
    - Concealment of sexual identity, increasingly for youth and young adults
    - Abandonment and rejection by family members and friends, or fear of it
    - Worries by trans and non-binary individuals of limited access to gender-affirming care, and the ability to live an authentic life
    - Worry about the policy and legal climate and its impact on autonomy
- Access to concordant care providers who respect their autonomy

Military members and veterans

Data for this community are as distressing as for other populations. There is more to report than this chapter allows for, but I'll summarize pertinent data and treatment considerations. The suicide rate among the U.S. armed forces has more than doubled in the past 15 years. The overall suicide rate for the total force is 25.6 per 100,000 service members (Department of Defense, 2024). The breakdown among active duty, reservists, and National Guard appears in Figure 9.9.

Suicide prevalence for service personnel is influenced by geography, age, race and ethnicity, marital status, education, military experiences, mental health history, and exposure to firearms. Common stressors contributing to suicide are shown in Figure 9.10 (Department of Defense, 2024; Griffin et al., 2021).

Veterans. The suicide rate per 100,000 veterans is 32.0 persons, almost twice as high as the rate for nonveterans, at 17.2 (Ramchand, 2022). Most veterans who die by suicide are 55-74 years old. Among veteran women, the suicide rate is also double that of nonveteran women: 14.8 persons out of 100,000, compared to 7.6. For women 18-34, the rate of suicide is three times higher in veterans than in nonveterans: 21.8 individuals per 100,000, compared to 6.8.

Military spouses and partners. A significant number of spouses and dependents of military members died by suicide in 2022, as shown in Figure 9.11. Common causes were hanging, asphyxiation, or firearms. Most spouses were female and under age 40. Most dependents were male and under 18 years of age (Department of Defense, 2024). Box 9.8 provides a snapshot of issues involving suicide for military members, veterans, and their spouses and partners.

Figure 9.9: *Suicide rate for active component service members (based on 100,000)*

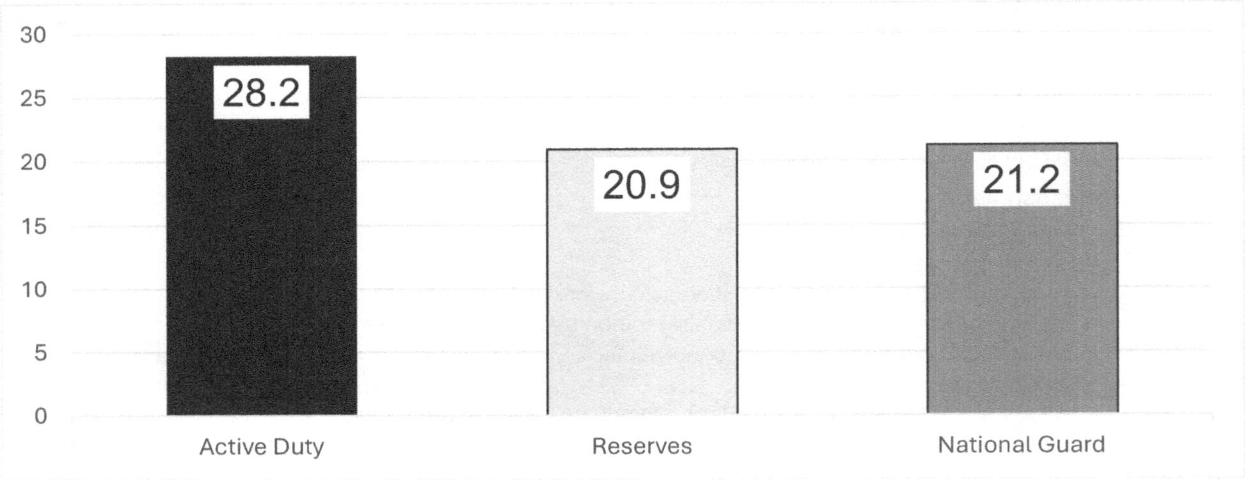

Data from Department of Defense, 2024

Figure 9.10: *Health and life stressors experienced by service members who died by suicide*

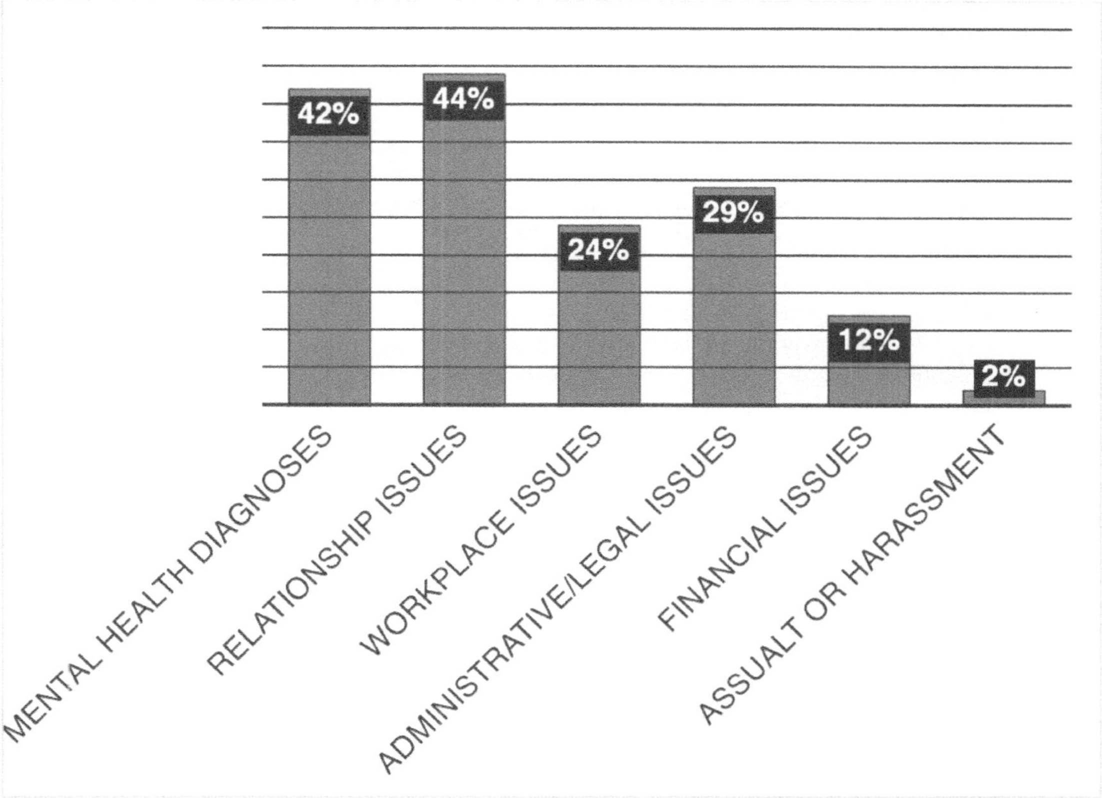

Data from Department of Defense, 2024

Figure 9.11: *Military family members who died by suicide in 2022*

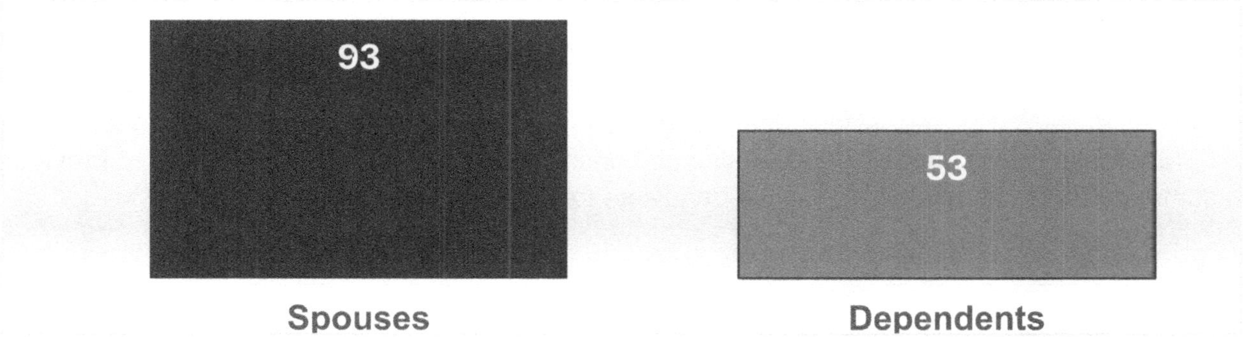

Date from Department of Defense, 2024

Box 9.8: Suicidality and military members, veterans, and spouses/partners

High incidence for:

- Suicidal ideation and action by:
  - Military members, including active-duty, reservists, and National Guard
  - Veterans, especially female veterans
  - Spouses and dependents of military members

Distinct considerations:

- Heightened risk due to:
  - Administrative and legal issues
  - Deployments and social isolation (for member and family)
  - Frequent moves and readjustment to schools, peers, and employment (for family)
  - Financial stressors
  - Exposure to harassment and sexual assault
  - Mental health diagnoses
  - Relationship issues
  - Unmet mental health needs

Persons with disabilities

Of adults who engaged in SI, suicide planning, and suicide attempts, close to 20 percent had a disability (Marlow et al., 2021), and most had one or more functional disabilities (e.g., physical, cognitive, vision). The presence of more disabilities aligned with a greater incidence of suicidal behaviors. Literature shows universal themes contribute to suicidality in this group, as shown in Box 9.9. These themes validate the difference protective factors can make for all populations. (Protective factors were previously displayed in Box 9.6.)

Invisible disabilities. A growing area of concern is the rise in suicide by persons with invisible disabilities, examples of which appear in Box 9.10. 'Invisible disabilities' refers to any chronic physical, mental, or neurological condition that is not readily apparent to others but can significantly limit or challenge a person's functionality and quality of life (Invisible Disability Association, n.d.; Pederson et al., 2017). The list includes autoimmune disorders, chronic illnesses, and long COVID. All SMI presented in Chapter 7 should also be considered invisible disabilities. Box 9.11 provides a summary of issues related to suicidal behaviors for persons with disabilities.

Box 9.9: Global themes contributing to risk of suicide for persons with disabilities

- Clinical anger
- Congenital disabilities
- Depressive symptoms
- Emotional reliance
- Experienced stigma
- Fearlessness about death
- High levels of social stress
- Low income
- Low levels of social support
- Perceived burdensomeness
- Severity of physical disability
- Thwarted belongingness

Kumar et al., 2024

Box 9.10: Invisible disabilities (including, but not limited to, the following)

- Autoimmune disorders
- ADHD (attention-deficit/hyperactivity disorder)
- Autism spectrum disorder (high-functioning presentations)
- Brain injuries (mild traumatic brain injury, concussion syndromes)
- Chronic fatigue syndrome (myalgic encephalomyelitis)
- Chronic pain conditions (e.g., fibromyalgia)
- Crohn's disease
- Diabetes (Type 1 and Type 2)
- Dysautonomia (including postural orthostatic tachycardia syndrome, aka POTS)
- Dyslexia and learning disabilities
- Epilepsy (except during seizures)
- Hearing impairments (partial hearing loss)
- Heart conditions (e.g. arrhythmias)
- Irritable bowel syndrome (IBS)
- Long COVID
- Lupus
- Lyme disease (chronic presentations)
- Migraine disorders
- Multiple sclerosis (early or mild stages)
- Rheumatoid arthritis (when not visibly joint deforming)
- Severe mental illness (e.g., bipolar, MDD, OCD, PTSD, schizophrenia, etc.)
- Sickle cell disease
- Sleep disorders (e.g., narcolepsy)
- Thyroid disorders (hypothyroidism, hyperthyroidism)

Box 9.11: Suicidality and persons with disabilities

High incidence for:

- Suicidal behaviors across age groups
- Suicide by those with greater numbers of functional disabilities
- Suicidality for persons with invisible disabilities

Distinct considerations:

- **Heightened risk due to psychosocial stressors:**
  - Accessible housing
    - Chronic health issues
    - Employment instability
    - Fearlessness and impulsivity (e.g., associated with traumatic brain injury and other cognitive issues)
    - Isolation
    - Lack of family and peer support
    - Limited finances
    - Pain management
    - Perception of increased dependence
    - Thwarted belongingness

Women's health

Considerable research demonstrates that women consistently have higher rates of SI, planning, and attempts than men. However, the rate of death by suicide for men is four- to five-fold higher than for women (Carretta et al., 2023).

Traditional roles, emotional release, and communication styles. Women are 1.78 times more likely to attempt suicide than men, according to self-reported lifetime attempts (Bommersbach et al., 2022). Mental health disorders are one factor, as women are diagnosed with MDD twice as often as men. Women are also more likely to internalize emotions around both positive and negative life experiences (Bommersbach et al., 2022).

Debates over traditional gender roles in marital and intimate relationships may also be at play. Women are less likely to verbalize distress or frustration, which can lead to a need to release pent-up emotions using self-harming behaviors (e.g., deep cutting, driving while intoxicated, overdose on prescription or OTC meds). Carretta et al. (2023) identified that women are more prone to binging on alcohol or other substances (e.g., cannabis), which may reduce control over their impulses and further prompt suicidal behaviors.

Suicides by middle-aged women have risen steadily during the past several decades, by as much as 30 percent; the number has risen over 40 percent for female older adults (CDC, n.d.; Garnett et al., 2022; Tsai et al, 2015). Studies have attributed this shift to the presence (or absence) of social networks. The greater one's social integration, the less incidence of suicide (Tsai et al., 2015).

Maternal mortality and suicide. Much attention has focused on behavioral health during the perinatal period, especially the rising incidence of self-harm. Perinatal suicide deaths have been considered pregnancy-related or been included in formal maternal mortality reviews only for the past decade (Chin et. al., 2022). In 2012 the ICD for Maternal Mortality (ICD-MM) began to identify suicides in pregnancy as direct obstetric deaths up to 12 months postpartum (Howard & Khalifeh, 2020). Passage of the Preventing Maternal Deaths Act in 2018 led to standardization of definitions for maternal mortality. There was also increased funding for state maternal mortality review committees, to enhance tracking of maternal deaths across the states, including by self-harm.

The adjusted average maternal mortality rate in 48 of the U.S. states was estimated to have risen 27 percent from 2000 to 2014: 18.8 to 23.8 per 100,000 live births. There is also high incidence of SI during the perinatal period, over 20 percent in some geographic regions. Data show worldwide prevalence of suicide attempts by pregnant and postpartum women at 680 attempts per 100,000. These numbers demonstrate a need to advance the assessment, identification, and treatment of women at risk (Chin et al., 2022). Box 9.12 provides a summary of key points for case managers in this domain.

Box 9.12: Suicidality and women's health

High incidence for:

- Diagnosis of MDD and other depressive disorders
    - SI and suicidal attempts across all age groups, compared to males
    - Suicidal behaviors during the perinatal period
    - Suicidal behaviors during middle age related to socialization and social integration

Distinct considerations:

- Challenges imposed by traditional marital and relationship roles
    - Discomfort in communication and expression of needs, wants, and emotions
    - Increased use of self-harm to express emotions
- Increased social networks and social integration reduce incidence of SI
- Increased attention for funding, legislation, assessment, and intervention to address increased maternal mortality rates related to suicide

SCREENING TOOLS AND ASSESSMENT FOR SUICIDE

The importance of screening tools to assess for suicidality cannot be overstated. In fact, it is why Phase 2 of Case Management's Behavioral Health Conversation Map includes a prompt for completion of screening tools. Every time PCPs and other front-line clinicians don't proactively perform preventive screening for suicide, it's a missed opportunity. Some 80 percent of suicide victims had seen a PCP within one year of their death, while only 25 to 30 percent had seen psychiatric clinicians in that timeframe (Harmer et al., 2024).

The list of tools to assess suicidality is lengthy. Table 9.3 provides instruments for assessing suicidality in adults. Table 9.4 includes tools for children and adolescents. Many practitioners and settings use the PHQ-9 and PHQ-A (for adolescents) to screen for suicidal ideation and intent. They are found in Chapter 6, Table 6.3 with screening tools for depression.

Table 9.3: *Screening tools for suicide (youth and adults)*

Instrument	Focus	Source
Beck Hopelessness Scale (BHS)	A 20-item true/false self-report inventory used in clinical settings to measure a patient's negative outlook • feelings about the future • loss of motivation • expectations Higher score indicates greater level of hopelessness	Beck, A.T., Weissman, A., Lester, D., & Trexler, L. (1974). The measurement of pessimism: The Hopelessness Scale. Journal of Consulting and Clinical Psychology, 42(6), 861865. https://doi.org/10.1037/h0037562
Beck Scale for Suicide Ideation (BSS) (for adolescents to adults)	A 21-item clinician-administered or self-report tool used to assess the severity of suicidal ideation in individuals Evaluates intensity, frequency, and characteristics of a person's thoughts, plans, and attitudes toward suicide during the past week. The first 19 items focus on specific suicidal thoughts and intentions, and the final 2 items assess previous suicide attempts. Higher scores indicate greater suicide risk.	Beck, A.T., Kovacs, M., & Weissman, A. (1979). Scale for Suicide Ideation. (SSI) [Database record]. APA PsycTests. https://doi.org/10.1037/t01299-000
Columbia-Suicide Severity Scale (C-SSRS) (for adults)	This tool evaluates SI and aligned behaviors. The Screener version is used in primary care and EDs for quick assessments, and it contains 6 items covering suicidal ideation severity and behavior. Structured as an interview with sections, the number of questions asked varies according to an individual's responses. The full assessment includes: • 5 core questions on SI severity • Added questions on SI intensity, with 5 sub-items on suicidal behavior: actual attempts, aborted attempts, interrupted attempts, preparatory behavior, and lethality	Posner, K. (2007). Columbia-Suicide Severity Rating Scale (C-SSRS) [Database record]. APA PsycTests. https://doi.org/10.1037/t52667-000

Instrument	Focus	Source
MINI International Neuropsychiatric Interview	A short, structured diagnostic interview to assess major psychiatric disorders per DSM and ICD-10 criteria. Administration takes 15-30 minutes and covers mood disorders, anxiety disorders, substance use disorders, psychotic disorders, and suicidality.	Lecrubier, Y., Sheehan, D.V., Weiller, E., Amorim, P., Bonora, I., Sheehan, K. H., Janavs, J., & Dunbar, G.C. (1997). Mini International Neuropsychiatric Interview. [Database record]. APA PsycTests. https://doi.org/10.1037/t18597-000
Patient Safety Screener-3 (PSS-3)	Brief, 3-item screening tool used mostly in EDs to assess suicide risk and psychiatric distress in adults. Focus is on: • Depression symptoms and active SI over the past 2 weeks • Lifetime suicide attempt history If an item is positive, further suicide risk assessment is indicated.	Boudreaux, E.D., Jaques, M.L., Brady, K.M., Matson, A., & Allen, M.H. (2015). The patient safety screener: Validation of a brief suicide risk screener for emergency department settings. *Archives of Suicide Research*, *19*(2), 151-160. https://doi.org/10.1080/13811118.2015.1034604
SAD PERSONS Scale	Tool based on a 10-word mnemonic: • Sex • Age • Depression • Previous suicide attempt • Excess alcohol or substance use • Rational thinking loss • Separated or single • Organized plan • No social support • Sickness	Patterson, W.M., Dohn, H. H., Bird, J., & Patterson, G. A. (1983). SAD PERSONS Scale [Database record]. APA PsycTests. https://doi.org/10.1037/t29953-000
Suicide Assessment Five-Step Evaluation and Triage (SAFE-T)	A 5-step clinical framework to assess and manage suicide risk then define treatment planning 1. Identify risk factors: psychiatric disorders, substance use, history of attempts 2. Identify protective factors: coping skills, social support 3. Conduct suicide inquiry: assess ideation, plans, behaviors, and intent 4. Determine risk level and intervention: low, moderate, and high risk with corresponding actions 5. Document: assessment, risk level, and treatment plan	Fowler, J.C. (2012). Suicide risk assessment in clinical practice: Pragmatic guidelines for imperfect assessments. *Psychotherapy, 49*(1), 81-90. https://doi.org/10.1037/a0026148

Instrument	Focus	Source
Suicide Crisis Inventory (SCI) Suicide Crisis Inventory-Short Form (SCI-2)	A self-report measure to assess the intensity of suicidal crisis states rather than suicidal ideation alone Evaluation of cognitive and emotional symptoms aligned with imminent suicide risk: feelings of entrapment affective disturbance loss of cognitive control hyperarousal social withdrawal The SCI captures the acute psychological state preceding suicidal behavior.	Galynker, I., Yaseen, Z.S., Cohen, L.J., Benhamou, L., Hawes, S., & Briggs, J. (2017). Validation of the Suicide Crisis Inventory. *Journal of Affective Disorders, 295*, 1280-1291 De Luca, G.P., Parghi, N., El Hayek, R., Bloch-Elkouby, S., Peterkin, D., Wolfe, A., Rogers, M.L., & Galynker, I. (2024). Machine learning approach for the development of a crucial tool in suicide prevention: The Suicide Crisis Inventory-2 (SCI-2) Short Form. *PLoS One, 19*(5), e0299048. https://doi.org/10.1371/journal.pone.0299048
Suicide Narrative Inventory (SNI)	A 38-item self-report questionnaire (with 8 subscales) that assesses elements of the suicidal narrative: a cognitive and emotional state that precedes a suicide attempt Focus is on understanding the meaning, context, and subjective experience of SI and SA by eliciting detailed accounts of these experiences. SNI assesses themes, such as: The person's story and meaning-making around their suicidality Events leading up to suicidal crises Cognitive, emotional, and interpersonal factors involved The perceived function or purpose of suicidal thoughts or acts	Menon, V., Bafna, A.R., Rogers, M.L., Cohen, L.J., Richards, J., & Galynker, I. (2023). Factor structure and validity of the suicidal narrative inventory among Indian adults. *Crisis, 44*(5), 371-379. https://doi.org/10.1027/0227-5910/a000884

Table 9.4: *Screening tools for suicide (youth)*

Instrument	Focus	Source
Ask Suicide Screening Questions (ASQ) Toolkit (for 10-24 years old)	A brief tool to quickly identify patients at risk for suicide • 5 yes/no screening questions target recent suicidal ideation and lifetime suicide attempts • Final question assesses for acute risk if any of initial 4 answers are affirmative The ASQ Toolkit provides: • Scripts for administration • Guidance for interpreting results • Follow-up assessment protocols • Versions tailored for pediatric and adult patients in medical settings (e.g., ED, inpatient, outpatient) Designed for use by non-psychiatric clinicians in under 2 minutes	Horowitz, L.M., Bridge, J.A., Teach, S.J., Ballard, E., Klima, J., Rosenstein, D.L., Wharff, E.A., Ginnis, K., Cannon, E., Joshi, P., & Pao, M. (2012). Ask Suicide-Screening Questions. *Archives of Pediatrics & Adolescent Medicine, 166*(12), 1170-1176. https://doi.org/10.1001/archpediatrics.2012.1276
Child-Columbia Suicide Severity Rating Scale (7-18 years old)	The youth version contains 11 items and uses developmentally appropriate language	Posner, K., Brent, D., Lucas, C., Gould, M., Stanley, B., Brown, G., Fisher, P., Zelazny, J., Burke, A., Oquendo, M., & Mann, J. (2008). Columbia-Suicide Severity Rating Scale (C-SSRS) Children's Baseline/Screening. The Research Foundation for Mental Hygiene, Inc.
Reynolds Adolescent Depression Scale-2	30-item self-report screening instrument used with 11-20 year-olds	Reynolds, W.M. (2004). The Reynolds Adolescent Depression Scale-Second Edition (RADS-2). In M.J. Hilsenroth & D.L. Segal (Eds.), *Comprehensive Handbook of Psychological Assessment, Vol. 2. Personality Assessment* (pp. 224-236). John Wiley & Sons, Inc.
Risk of Suicide Questionnaire	Brief 4-item screening for pediatric EDs and related settings	Horowitz, L.M., Wang, P.S., Koocher, G.P., Burr, B.H., Smith, M.F., Klavon, S., & Cleary, P.D. (2001). Detecting suicide risk in a pediatric emergency department: Development of a brief screening tool. *Pediatrics, 107*(5), 1133-1137. https://doi.org/10.1542/peds.107.5.1133

Instrument	Focus	Source
Suicide Ideation Questionnaire SIQ-Adolescent (15-18 years old) SIQ-JR (pediatric version, 12-14 years old)	A 30-item self-report assessment tool used in clinical and school settings to measure the severity and frequency of SI in youth Each item is rated on a 7-point scale ranging from, "I never had this thought" to "Almost every day." A brief 15-item version (SIQ-JR) for younger adolescents or quick screening. The SIQ is widely used in clinical and school settings to identify youth at risk for suicide and to guide intervention decisions.	Reynolds, W.M. (1991). Adult Suicidal Ideation Questionnaire [Database record]. APA PsycTests. https://doi.org/10.1037/t03904-000 Reynolds, W.M., & Mazza, J.J. (1999). Assessment of suicidal ideation in inner-city children and young adolescents: Reliability and validity of the Suicidal Ideation Questionnaire-JR. *School Psychology Review, 28*(1), 17-30.

CONCLUSION

Suicide is a complex, sensitive, and often taboo topic. All case managers will likely experience some phase of the suicidality continuum with a patient or family member during the course of their careers. Their role with the patient will be based on the practice setting, their discipline of origin, and their scope of practice. The knowledge gained here will bolster their ability to navigate this difficult domain.

CONTEMPLATION QUESTIONS

1. Case managers experience an array of feelings when intervening with patients who have thoughts of self-harm. Review the Suicidality Continuum in Figure 9.1, then imagine a patient with SI is referred to you for assessment.
   a) What concerns do you have about working with patients who present with SI?
   b) How might you manage these concerns in the moment?
   c) If you have previously intervened with a patient who has SI or who engaged in a suicide attempt, reflect on that experience.
      i. How did you intervene?
      ii. What was one takeaway from the experience?
2. Review the proposed diagnoses for suicide behavior disorder, nonsuicidal-self injurious disorder, and suicide crisis syndrome found in Boxes 9.2, 9.3, and 9.4.
   a) What are your thoughts about formal integration of these disorders in the DSM?
   b) What do you believe are the pros and cons of their implementation?
3. Review the chapter content on risk and protective factors. Pick any 5 of the protective factors identified in Box 9.6. For each factor:

   a) Identify ways you have seen it reduce suicide risk for a particular patient or the population you work with.
   b) Consider other protective factors you might add to the list and why you view them as important.

4. Access two screening tools for suicide from Tables 9.3 and 9.4. Choose tools that are least unfamiliar to you.
   a) Review the screening tool.
   b) Complete the screening tool for a patient you are working with.
   c) Reflect on how use of a standardized tool for suicide screening will inform your future efforts.
5. As the case manager for a federally qualified health center, you are case managing Gina, a 30-year-old patient with recurrent thoughts of suicide and a 15-year history of NSSI, specifically cutting. Gina has appeared this day with her usual array of superficial cuts, but this time also a few deeper cuts.

Use Case Management's Behavioral Health Conversation Map in Table 1.4 to script your interactions with Gina and her support system. Carefully consider what screening tools you might use to assess Gina's SI in Phase 2.

RESOURCES

- **988 Suicide and Crisis Lifeline**
  https://988lifeline.org/

Centers for Disease Control and Prevention

- **WISQARS (Web-based Injury Statistics Query and Reporting System): Fatal injury data**
  https://www.cdc.gov/injury/wisqars/fatal.html
- **Centre for Suicide Prevention**
  https://www.suicideinfo.ca/
- **Health.mil Official Website of the Military Health System: Military Suicide**
  https://www.health.mil/Military-Health-Topics/Mental-Health/Mental-Health-Topics/Suicide-Prevention
- **International Association for Suicide**
  https://www.iasp.info/suicidalthoughts/
- **Invisible Disabilities Association**
  https://invisibledisabilities.org
- **National Alliance for Suicide Prevention**
  https://theactionalliance.org/veteran-and-military-suicide-prevention-resources

- **Stop Soldier Suicide**
  https://stopsoldiersuicide.org
- **Suicide Prevention Resource Center**
  https://sprc.org
- **The Trevor Project**
  https://www.thetrevorproject.org
- **Veteran Crisis Line**
  https://www.veteranscrisisline.net
- **Veteran Suicide Prevention**
  https://www.va.gov/health-care/health-needs-conditions/mental-health/suicide-prevention/

REFERENCES

- Adhilah, N., & Setiawati, Y. (2025). Current phenomenon of self-harm in children and adolescents. *Journal of the Korean Academy of Child and Adolescent Psychiatry, 36*(2), 47-53. https://doi.org/10.5765/jkacap.250003
- American Psychiatric Association. (2022). *Diagnostic and Statistical Manual of Mental Disorders* (5th ed., text rev.).
- Barrocas, A.L., Hankin, B.L., Young, J.F., & Abela, J.R. (2012). Rates of nonsuicidal self-injury in youth: Age, sex, and behavioral methods in a community sample. *Pediatrics, 130*(1), 39-45. https://doi.org/10.1542/peds.2011-2094
- Berman, A.L., & Silverman, M.M. (2020). Near term suicide risk assessment: A commentary on the clinical relevance of protective factors. *Archives of Suicide Research: Official Journal of the International Academy for Suicide Research, 24*(sup2), S370-S380. https://doi.org/10.1080/13811118.2019.1612804
- Bhatt, A., Gonzales, H., Pallin, R., & Barnhorst, A. (2023). Rising rates of adolescent firearm suicide and the clinician's role in addressing firearms. *Journal of the American Academy of Child and Adolescent Psychiatry, 62*(6), 614-617. https://doi.org/10.1016/j.jaac.2022.07.820
- Bommersbach, T.J., Rosenheck, R.A., Petrakis, I.L., & Rhee, T.G. (2022). Why are women more likely to attempt suicide than men? Analysis of lifetime suicide attempts among US adults in a nationally representative sample. *Journal of Affective Disorders, 311*, 157-164. https://doi.org/10.1016/j.jad.2022.05.096
- Cai, H., Xie, X.M., Zhang, Q., Cui, X., Lin, J.X., Sim, K., Ungvari, G.S., Zhang, L., & Xiang, Y.T. (2021). Prevalence of suicidality in major depressive disorder: A systematic review and meta-analysis of comparative studies. *Frontiers in Psychiatry, 12*, 690130. https://doi.org/10.3389/fpsyt.2021.690130
- Capistrant, B.D., & Nakash, O. (2019). Suicide risk for sexual minorities in middle and older age: Evidence from the National Survey on Drug Use and Health. *The American Journal of Geriatric Psychiatry, 27*(5), 559-563. https://doi.org/10.1016/j.jagp.2018.12.023

- Carretta, R.F., McKee, S.A., & Rhee, T.G. (2023). Gender differences in risks of suicide and suicidal behaviors in the USA: A narrative review. *Current Psychiatry Reports*, *25*(12), 809-824. https://doi.org/10.1007/s11920-023-01473-1
- Centers for Disease Control and Prevention. (2024). Suicide Prevention. Risk and Protective Factors for Suicide. Retrieved July 18, 2025, from https://www.cdc.gov/suicide/risk-factors/index.html
- Centers for Disease Control and Prevention. (n.d.). WISQARS (Web-based Injury Statistics Query and Reporting System). Fatal Injury Data. National Center for Injury Prevention and Control, CDC. Retrieved July 21, 2025, from https://wisqars.cdc.gov
- Chin, K., Wendt, A., Bennett, I.M., & Bhat, A. (2022). Suicide and maternal mortality. *Current Psychiatry Reports*, *24*(4), 239-275. https://doi.org/10.1007/s11920-022-01334-3
- Cole, R., Cowan, R.G., Pearce, E., Quintana, T., & Ren, X. (2025). Investigation of military spouse suicide. *Military Medicine, (190)*3-4, e717-e723. https://doi.org/10.1093/milmed/usae524
- Crimmins E.M. (2015). Lifespan and healthspan: Past, present, and promise. *The Gerontologist*, *55*(6), 901-911. https://doi.org/10.1093/geront/gnv130
- DeCamp, W., & Bakken, N.W. (2016). Self-injury, suicide ideation, and sexual orientation: Differences in causes and correlates among high school students. *Journal of Injury & Violence Research*, *8*(1), 15-24. https://doi.org/10.5249/jivr.v8i1.545
- De Leo, D., & Giannotti, A.V. (2021). Suicide in late life: A viewpoint. *Preventive Medicine*, *152*(Pt 1), 106735. https://doi.org/10.1016/j.ypmed.2021.106735
- Department of Defense. (2024). Annual Report on Suicide in the Military. Retrieved July 22, 2025, from https://www.dspo.mil/Portals/113/2024/documents/annual_report/ARSM_CY23_final_508c.pdf
- Dierickx, S., Claes, L., Buelens, T., Smits, D., & Kiekens, G. (2023). DSM-5 non-suicical self-injury disorder in a community sample: Comparing NSSI engagement, recency and severity among emerging adults. *Frontiers in Psychiatry*, *14*, 1251514. https://doi.org/10.3389/fpsyt.2023.1251514
- Dhole, A.R., Petkar, P., Choudhari, S.G., & Mendhe, H. (2023). Understanding the factors contributing to suicide among the geriatric population: A narrative review. *Cureus*, *15*(10), e46387. https://doi.org/10.7759/cureus.46387
- Galynker, I., Bloch-Elkouby, S., & Cohen, L.J. (2024). Suicide crisis syndrome: A specific diagnosis to aid suicide prevention. *World Psychiatry*, *23*(3), 362-363. https://doi.org/10.1002/wps.21229
- Garnett, M.F., Spencer, M.R., & Weeks, J.D. (2023). Suicide among adults age 55 and older, 2021. *NCHS Data Brief* (*483*), 1-8. PMID: 38051033.
- Griffin, B.A., Grimm, G.E., Smart, R., Ramchand, R., Jaycox, L.H., Ayer, L., Leidy, E.N., Davenport, S., Schell, T.L., & Morral, A.R. (2021). Comparing the Army's suicide rate to the general U.S. population: Identifying suitable characteristics, data sources, and analytic approaches. *Rand Health Quarterly*, *9*(2), 8.

- Harmer, B., Lee, S., Rizvi, A., & Saadabadi, A. (2024). Suicidal Ideation. StatPearls Publishing: Treasure Island, FL.
- Hawton, K., Hill, N.T.M., Gould, M., John, A., Lascelles, K., & Robinson, J. (2020). Clustering of suicides in children and adolescents. *The Lancet Child & Adolescent Health*, *4*(1), 58-67. https://doi.org/10.1016/S2352-4642(19)30335-9
- Hink, A.B., Killings, X., Bhatt, A., Ridings, L.E., & Andrews, A.L. (2022). Adolescent suicide–Understanding unique risks and opportunities for trauma centers to recognize, intervene, and prevent a leading cause of death. *Current Trauma Reports*, *8*(2), 41-53. https://doi.org/10.1007/s40719-022-00223-7
- Howard, L.M., & Khalifeh, H. (2020). Perinatal mental health: A review of progress and challenges. *World Psychiatry, 19*(3), 313-327. https://doi.org/10.1002/wps.20769
- Invisible Disability Association. (n.d.). About. Retrieved July 22, 2025, from https://invisibledisabilities.org
- Ivey-Stephenson, A.Z., Crosby, A.E., Hoenig, J.M., Gyawali, S., Park-Lee, E., & Hedden, S.L. (2022). Suicidal thoughts and behaviors among adults aged ≥18 years — United States, 2015-2019. *Morbidity and Mortality Weekly Report Surveillance Summaries*, *71*(1), 1-19. http://dx.doi.org
- Ki, M., Lapierre, S., Gim, B., Hwang, M., Kang, M., Dargis, L., Jung, M., Koh, E.J., & Mishara, B. (2024). A systematic review of psychosocial protective factors against suicide and suicidality among older adults. *International Psychogeriatrics*, *36*(5), 346-370. https://doi.org/10.1017/S104161022300443X
- Klonsky, E.D. (2009). The functions of self-injury in young adults who cut themselves: Clarifying the evidence for affect-regulation. *Psychiatry Research*, *166*(2-3), 260-268. https://doi.org/10.1016/j.psychres.2008.02.008
- Kumar, S., Lata, S., Verma, S., & Anupriya. (2024). Associated factors of suicidal behavior among persons with physical disability: A systematic review. *Indian Journal of Psychological Medicine*, *46*(4), 298-304. https://doi.org/10.1177/02537176231209513
- Marlow, N.M., Xie, Z., Tanner, R., Jo, A., & Kirby, A.V. (2021). Association between disability and suicide-related outcomes among U.S. adults. *American Journal of Preventive Medicine*, *61*(6), 852-862. https://doi.org/10.1016/j.amepre.2021.05.035
- Melzer, L., Forkmann, T., & Teismann, T. (2024). Suicide Crisis Syndrome: A systematic review. *Suicide and Life-Threatening Behavior*, *54*(3), 556-574. https://doi.org/10.1111/sltb.13065
- Mueller, A.S., Abrutyn, S., Pescosolido, B., & Diefendorf, S. (2021). The social roots of suicide: Theorizing how the external social world matters to suicide and suicide prevention. *Frontiers in Psychology*, *12*, 621569. https://doi.org/10.3389/fpsyg.2021.621569
- Nath, R., Matthews, D.D., DeChants, J.P., Hobaica, S., Clark, C.M., Taylor, A.B., Muñoz, G. (2024). 2024 U.S. National Survey on the Mental Health of LGBTQ+ Young People. Retrieved October 10, 2025, from www.thetrevorproject.org/survey-2024

- Ong, M.S., Lakoma, M., Gees Bhosrekar, S., Hickok, J., McLean, L., Murphy, M., Poland, R.E., Purtell, N., & Ross-Degnan, D. (2021). Risk factors for suicide attempt in children, adolescents, and young adults hospitalized for mental health disorders. *Child and Adolescent Mental Health*, *26*(2), 134-142. https://doi.org/10.1111/camh.12400
- Oquendo, M.A., Wall, M., Wang, S., Olfson, M., & Blanco, C. (2024). Lifetime suicide attempts in otherwise psychiatrically healthy individuals. *JAMA Psychiatry*, *81*(6), 572-578. https://doi.org/10.1001/jamapsychiatry.2023.5672
- Orenstein, G.A., & Lewis, L. Erikson's Stages of Psychosocial Development. [Updated 2022 Nov 7]. StatPearls Publishing: Treasure Island, FL. Available from https://www.ncbi.nlm.nih.gov/books/NBK556096
- Paceley, M.S., Dikitsas, Z.A., Greenwood, E., McInroy, L.B., Fish, J.N., Williams, N., Riquino, M.R., Lin, M., Birnel Henderson, S., & Levine, D.S. (2023). The perceived health implications of policies and rhetoric targeting transgender and gender diverse youth: A community-based qualitative study. *Transgender Health*, *8*(1), 100-103. https://doi.org/10.1089/trgh.2021.0125
- Pederson, C.L., Gorman-Ezell, K., & Hochstetler-Mayer, G. (2017). Invisible illness increases risk of suicidal ideation: The role of social workers in preventing suicide. *Health & Social Work*, *42*(3), 183-186. https://doi.org/10.1093/hsw/hlx029
- Phillips, D.P. (1974). The influence of suggestion on suicide: Substantive and theoretical implications of the Werther effect. *American Sociological Review*, *39*(3), 340-354.
- Price, J.H., & Foh, E.P. (2024). Descriptive epidemiology of female suicides by race and ethnicity. *Journal of Community Health*, *49*(6), 1054-1061. https://doi.org/10.1007/s10900-024-01368-z
- Price, J.H., & Khubchandani, J. (2021). Firearm suicides in the elderly: A narrative review and call for action; *Journal of Community Health*, *46*(5), 1050-1058. https://doi.org/10.1007/s10900-021-00964-7
- Ramchand, R. (2022). Suicide among veterans: Veterans' issues in focus. *Rand Health Quarterly*, *9*(3), 21.
- Ruch, D.A., Horowitz, L.M., Hughes, J.L., Sarkisian, K., Luby, J.L., Fontanella, C.A., Bridge, J. A. (2024). Suicide in U.S. preteens aged 8 to 12 years, 2001-2022. *JAMA Network Open*, *7*(7), e2424664.
- Tsai, A.C., Lucas, M., & Kawachi, I. (2015). Association between social integration and suicide among women in the United States. *JAMA Psychiatry*, *72*(10), 987-993. https://doi.org/10.1001/jamapsychiatry.2015.1002
- U.S. Preventive Services Task Force, Mangione, C.M., Barry, M.J., Nicholson, W.K., Cabana, M., Chelmow, D., Coker, T.R., Davidson, K.W., Davis, E.M., & Donahue, K.E. et al. (2022). Screening for depression and suicide risk in children and adolescents: U.S. Preventive Services Task Force Recommendation Statement. *JAMA*, *328*(15), 1534-1542. https://doi.org/10.1001/jama.2022.16946
- Walling, M.A. (2021). Suicide contagion. *Current Trauma Reports*, *7*(4), 103-114. https://doi.org/10.1007/s40719-021-00219-9

- Yard, E., Radhakrishnan, L., Ballesteros, M.F., Sheppard, M., Gates, A., Stein, Z., Hartnett, K., Kite-Powell, A., Rodgers, L., & Adjemian, J. et al. (2021). Emergency department visits for suspected suicide attempts among persons aged 12-25 years before and during the COVID-19 Pandemic — United States, January 2019-May 2021. *Morbidity and Mortality Weekly Report*, *70*(24), 888-894. https://doi.org/10.15585/mmwr.mm7024e1

CHAPTER 10

TRAUMA EXPOSURE

INTRODUCTION

Trauma's influence on poor health outcomes has been identified across every population and is among case management's most pressing priorities. The fiscal toll alone is massive. Costs for persons with post-traumatic stress disorder in the U.S. are over $232 billion, or $19,630 per person (Davis et al., 2022). Globally, over 70 percent of the population may experience trauma at some point in their life, with a fiscal tally in the trillions (World Health Organization, 2024).

Trauma is also tied to healthcare worker burnout—long an occupational hazard of the industry. Workforce retention rates are historically low, with burnout incidence impacting more than 60 percent of the healthcare labor force. Costs associated with workplace trauma in the U.S. exceed hundreds of billions of dollars annually due to increased turnover, reduced work hours, and patient safety incidents (Mohr et al., 2025).

Trauma affects all aspects of health: physical and behavioral health, the quality of intimate and social relationships, success in education and employment, and overall engagement in activities of life. It is also a reality of the human experience—thus why assessing for it lands on case managers' radar. Case management's standards of practice emphasize the importance of patient and family assessment, so accounting for trauma is an extension of this professional responsibility.

Chapter 10 provides fundamental knowledge on trauma and the DSM category of trauma and stressor-related disorders. The content within these pages will advance your understanding of key terminology, common diagnoses, and prevalence across age groups and populations. Material on general risk factors and trauma's impact on distinct populations is integrated in the developmental life stage content, rather than in individual sections to leave room for treatment approaches, trauma-informed care, and the CUES model for physical and sexual assault. Like the other chapters in Section 2, screening and assessment instruments are also included.

BEHAVIORAL LEARNING OBJECTIVES

1. Identify common terms and definitions associated with trauma
2. Explain symptoms and treatment recommendations for DSM diagnoses
3. Analyze the incidence of trauma across life stages and populations
4. Identify screening tools used to assess trauma- and stressor-related disorders
5. Apply the elements of trauma-informed care
6. Apply Case Management's Behavioral Health Conversation Map when intervening with patients (and their support systems) experiencing trauma

ESSENTIAL TERMS

- ACE pyramid
- Acute stress disorder
- Acute stress response
- Acute trauma
- Adjustment disorder
- Adverse childhood experiences (ACEs)
- Allostatic load
- Big-T and little-t traumas
- Chronic trauma
- Compassion fatigue
- Complex trauma
- CUES model
- Developmental trauma
- Event trauma
- Experiential trauma
- Fight or flight response
- Historical trauma
- Intergenerational trauma
- Interpersonal violence (IPV)
- Persistent complex bereavement disorder
- Post-traumatic stress disorder (PTSD)
- Psychological safety
- Relational trauma
- Retraumatization
- Trauma
- Trauma-informed care
- Type I and Type II traumas
- Weathering

TERMS AND FEATURES OF TRAUMA

Trauma is any deeply distressing or disturbing experience that overwhelms a person's ability to cope (Van Der Kolk, 2014). Since case managers work directly with the human condition, its characteristics, challenges, and promises, including trauma, are part of it. Trauma may refer to a firsthand experience of a one-and-done event, such as a motor vehicle accident. It can also refer to a series of incidents experienced over a longer period of time, by individuals, groups, or communities, during which those involved feel physically or emotionally at risk. Examples include bullying, harassment, or discrimination of a person or group. Key vocabulary appears in Table 10.1.

Secondhand exposure to trauma can be as devastating as a firsthand experience, and it's an occupational hazard for case managers. Imagine you witness a horrific car accident. The image may be buried among other memories such that your brain cannot fully process the intense emotional impact—a dynamic due to how the brain processes and stores memories under inordinate stress or traumatic conditions (Van der Kolk, 2014). The memory may be suddenly triggered and recalled later, however—perhaps by experiencing a similar event. Or you may relive it frequently and repeatedly through flashbacks or other emotional or somatic releases. Trauma practitioners emphasize that once a person sees a traumatic event, it becomes difficult to "unsee" it. This is why recognizing and processing trauma is important.

Case managers are subject to profound *compassion fatigue* as the rigors of the role and the psychological cost of caring for others accumulate. Compassion fatigue is a type of trauma, defined as a state of emotional, physical, and mental fatigue that can occur over time in individuals who work with or care for people who experience trauma, suffering, or distress (Merriam-Webster, 2025). Case managers witness heartbreaking reactions from patients and families, observe tense dynamics in abuse situations, and encounter death and dying. The tumult of emotions tax a case manager's emotional reserve, over time leading to the compassion fatigue trauma response, and burnout.

Trauma's adverse effects on an individual's emotional and psychological functioning intensify depression, anxiety, and suicidal ideation. Any trauma pushes the body out of homeostasis, forcing compensation. The added burden of adaptation stress increases a person's *allostatic load,* or wear and tear on the body due to chronic stress. The strain causes changes in metabolism, damages body systems and organs, and stimulates onset or exacerbation of chronic illness (Pfatz & Schnyder, 2023).

Table 10.1: *Terms associated with trauma*

Term	Definition	Example
Acute stress response	An immediate short-term physiological and psychological response to a stressful event; a transient disorder in response to a stressful event (Maercker & Eberle, 2022)	A patient is trapped in an elevator and experiences sudden shortness of breath, a racing heartbeat, and becomes lightheaded.
Burnout	An occupational phenomenon characterized by chronic workplace stress comprised of exhaustion, cynicism on the job, and reduced professional efficacy (World Health Organization, 2019)	A case manager has more patients than usual due to staff shortages. He is chronically exhausted and reacts to patients with sarcasm. His patients experience increased length of stay across all units.
Collective trauma	Cultural, historical, social, political, and structural traumas that impact individuals and communities across generations (Hirschberger, 2018)	Following the terrorist attacks on 9/11, a profound and traumatic grief and loss response was experienced not only by those persons directly impacted (e.g., victims, their families, first responders, members of neighboring communities) but also across the population.

Term	Definition	Example
Collective occupational trauma	A dynamic where healthcare professionals experience the same reality as their patients, families, and support systems; professional boundaries become blurred, leading to high levels of emotional vulnerability that can prompt development of more pervasive psychopathology (Fink-Samnick, 2022)	During the COVID-19 pandemic, nurses treated high numbers of patients. Professional boundaries that traditionally supported their coping were hampered because all nurses were enduring similar experiences, as well as personal losses due to the virus.
Fawn	A trauma response characterized by people-pleasing and appeasing others to avoid conflict and ensuring safety (Schlote, 2023)	A person exposed to child abuse is unable to confront an abusive boss about aggressive behaviors toward staff. Instead, the person limits interaction with the boss and simply does what is asked.
Fight or flight	The body's automatic response or reaction to a perceived threat (Dhabhar, 2009)	A person asked to present at a staff meeting develops dry mouth, is worried about passing out, and forgets the focus of their presentation. With little explanation, the person darts from the conference room.
Freeze	A survival mechanism that occurs when a person feels trapped or overwhelmed by a perceived threat. It is an automatic involuntary state to protect the person from accompanying stressors (Hagenaars et al., 2012)	A person has been in a car accident but is not hurt and could escape from the vehicle but cannot move due to intense fear.
Hyperarousal	A state of increased physiological and psychological activation marked by agitation, increased alertness and vigilance, difficulty concentrating, emotional reactivity, and physical symptoms (Brzozowska & Grabowski, 2025)	A person loses their footing and falls in a busy hotel lobby, then experiences rapid heartbeat, shortness of breath, and difficulty breathing.
Hypervigilance	An increased state of alertness and sensitivity to one's surroundings, and a key symptom of hyperarousal (Brzozowska & Grabowski, 2025)	A person with a history of domestic violence seeks medical assistance at a local urgent care center. The person is guarded, presents as agitated, and has trouble following conversations with the treatment team.

TYPES OF TRAUMAS

Professionals classify traumas in multiple ways. One model, which frames trauma as *acute, chronic*, or *complex,* appears in Table 10.2. Acute trauma has a clear, single cause. Chronic and complex trauma both involve prolonged exposure to traumatic events, but they differ in the nature of the events and their impact. Chronic trauma usually involves repeated exposure to similar traumatic events, such as domestic abuse or neglect. In contrast, complex trauma involves exposure to multiple and varied traumatic events, often interpersonal in nature, occurring particularly during the formative years, such as childhood abuse or neglect (Ferriante & Sharma, 2023). Trauma can also be understood by the circumstances that drive it, as shown in Table 10.3.

Table 10.2: *Types of traumas*

Type	Explained	Examples
Acute	A single, discrete event that causes significant distress or harm	Firsthand experience or secondhand exposure: Motor vehicle accident Natural disaster Mass casualty event Witness to a violent assault or loved one having a medical emergency
Chronic	Repeated and prolonged exposure to traumatic events	Firsthand experience or secondhand exposure: Adverse childhood experiences (ACEs) Bullying, gaslighting Domestic violence or intimate partner violence Adult or child neglect Long-term, life-limiting chronic illness Human trafficking
Complex	Exposure to multiple traumatic events, often within the context of interpersonal relationships	Firsthand experience or secondhand exposure: Adverse childhood experiences (ACEs) Bullying Child or adult abuse, exploitation, and neglect Intimate partner violence

Adapted from Ferriante & Sharma, 2023

Table 10.3: *Drivers of trauma*

Developmental trauma	Distress experienced by persons due to early and chronic trauma, often involving neglect or abuse in childhood (e.g., ACEs) (Cruz et al., 2022)
Experiential trauma	How a traumatic event is processed and stored in an individual's mind and body; the subjective and often unconscious impact of the event
Event trauma	A specific event or circumstance that results in physical, emotional, and/or life threatening harm
Historical trauma	A specific type of multigenerational, collective, and cumulative trauma due to systematic oppression or massive group trauma (Borda Bohigas et al., 2015)
Intergenerational trauma	A broad term for emotional, psychological, and social distress passed down through generations; it can stem from individual or collective experiences (e.g., the Holocaust, child physical or sexual abuse, growing up in home with domestic or interpersonal violence (Bove et al., 2025)
Relational	Psychological harm from unhealthy relationships, often involving abuse, neglect, or betrayal, within close or immediate relationships, and particularly those in positions of power or authority (e.g., adult, boss, parent, intimate partner, spouse) (Lannert et al., 2014)

'BIG-T' AND 'LITTLE-T' TRAUMAS

'Big-T' traumas are major life events that cause severe distress, such as motor vehicle or other serious accidents, sexual or physical assaults, or natural and other disasters. Chronic stressors, on the other hand, cause *'little-t' traumas,* such as bullying, gaslighting, teasing, or other interpersonal dynamics. The cumulative effect over time wears on self-esteem and resilience.

'Little-t' traumas can be as impactful as any single 'big-T'. Yet there is a discrepancy among the trauma community about this distinction. Trauma is relative, in that its psychological toll is unique for everyone. What impacts one person severely may have little effect on another. Thought leaders view the difference between big-T and little-t as less significant than how a person perceives the traumatic event (or series of events).

TYPE I AND TYPE II TRAUMAS

Type I and *type II traumas* focus on the severity and duration of an event through the lens of individual self-evaluation and perception (Wang et al., 2023). Type I traumas are single, isolated events that are overwhelming to those who experience them. The events are perceived as life-threatening: for example, near-death accidents or medical emergencies like anaphylactic allergic reactions.

Type II traumas are more enduring. They are repeated, ongoing events that can be psychologically demanding and contribute to allostatic overload, such as child or adult physical or sexual abuse, neglect, exploitation, or interpersonal violence. Complex PTSD is classified as a type II trauma, as the intense attacks strain a person's health over time. *Weathering,* a public health priority, is another example; it occurs when the chronic stress of discrimination, systemic racism, and poverty combined cause premature aging and increased health disparities for marginalized populations and communities (Geronimous et al., 2006). Poor health outcomes are a direct result of type I and II traumas, which is why they are a priority for case managers everywhere. Table 10.4 summarizes the two traumas.

Table 10.4: *Type I and Type II traumas*

Type I Trauma	Type II Trauma
Single, unexpected, and life-threatening event that is clearly defined	Chronic and sustained exposure to highly stressful situations, often interpersonal in nature
Examples: Natural disaster (flood, earthquake) Traumatic accident (motor vehicle, boating, swimming) Medical emergency (severe allergic reaction, heart attack) Violent attack, as victim or witness (assault, mugging)	Examples: Chronic abuse, neglect, exploitation A chronic or terminal illness Domestic or interpersonal violence Living in a war-torn region

Anomie and type I and type II traumas. Mass disaster events like earthquakes, floods, hurricanes, wildfires, and wars devastate life, property, and community infrastructure. Normalcy is disrupted, and people who lived in the impacted region become emotionally disoriented. They lose the sense of belonging or purpose that comes from living in a community, with its norms of functioning. Anomie describes this state of normlessness or loss of identity that emerges during periods of rapid social change, crisis, or cultural upheaval (Teymoori et al., 2016).

As mentioned in Chapter 9, Durkheim identified a correlation between the trauma of social upheaval and loss of social identity with anomic suicide (Kar and Singh, 2023). This dynamic presents globally at sites of sociopolitical unrest. It can impact any case manager's patient population and should be a consideration within the biopsychosocial assessment.

ADVERSE CHILDHOOD EXPERIENCES (ACES)

The original Adverse Childhood Experiences (ACE) study was completed by the Centers for Disease Control and Prevention and Kaiser Permanente from 1995 to 1997. The research provided critical information on the influence of stressors associated with abuse, neglect, and household dysfunction—or *adverse childhood experiences* (ACEs)—on development, namely disease emergence, morbidity, and patient mortality. Over 17,000 members of Kaiser Permanente health plans in southern California completed confidential surveys during their annual physical on the topic of childhood experiences and current health status and behaviors. The study is among the largest investigations into the impact of childhood abuse and neglect on later-life health and well-being and found that ACEs can impact pathophysiology, psychopathology, and neuropathophysiology over the life course.

An ACE score tallied the number of adverse childhood experiences reported by respondents in their first 18 years of life. Scores could range from 0 to 10, with a higher score putting patients at greater risk of poor health outcomes. Figure 10.1 shows the 10 ACEs, divided into three domains. Some 75 percent of all participants reported at least one ACE, while 1 in 5 reported three or more. The original survey demographics invited further exploration, since most respondents were White, middle-class, college-educated, and employed. Researchers realized that if the ACEs were so prevalent in that population, then vulnerable communities would likely show higher ACE scores. The concern was validated by further research.

The ACE Pyramid is a representation for how traumatic and stressful life events impact a person from birth to death. The position of ACEs at the base of the pyramid is a reminder of their influence on development. A higher ACE score is associated with chronic health and mental health conditions, which manifest in new ways as one moves up the pyramid. Increased illness morbidity and early mortality is at the top to demonstrate the correlation between exposure to ACEs and physical, behavioral, neurodevelopmental, and psychosocial functioning. The ACE Pyramid is found in Figure 10.2.

The original ACE study findings are available through the CDC. Many versions of the original questionnaire have been developed for distinct populations. They are accessible through sources in the chapter resources list.

Figure 10.1: *Adverse childhood experiences*

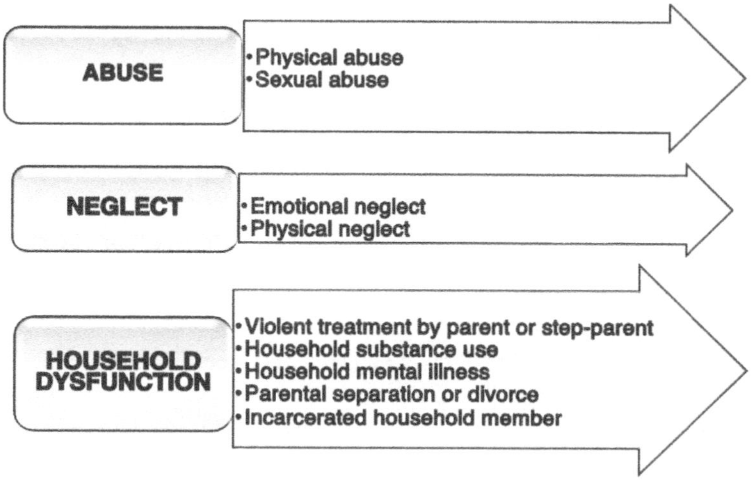

Centers for Disease Control and Prevention, 2021; Felitti et al., 1998

Figure 10.2: *The ACE Pyramid*

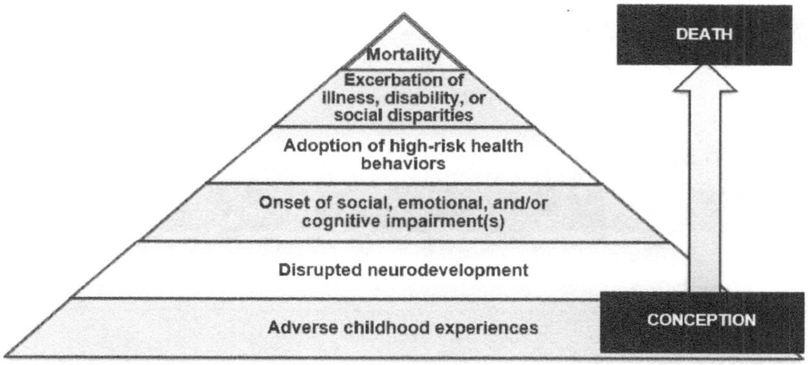

Adapted from Centers for Disease Control and Prevention, 2021

PSYCHOLOGICAL SAFETY

Psychological safety describes when a person can openly express his thoughts and feelings about a topic without fear of retribution, excessive scrutiny, or need for self-censorship (Edmonson & Bransby, 2023). Its alignment with trauma-informed practices has made it a popular focus in healthcare, and it influences patient safety, interprofessional collaboration, quality improvement, and reporting of adverse events in risk management (Ito et al., 2022).

Psychological safety can be operationalized in assorted ways. It may relate to supporting patients who feel vulnerable in the care setting. Cultural views of power play out in the treatment process and can leave patients and their families reluctant to ask questions, seek clarification, or inquire about treatment, discharge planning, or their options.

Psychological safety is also applied to team functioning in the workplace. Imagine you are doing care coordination rounds and are about to present on a patient. Suddenly, you are frozen by fear of critique or personal attack by colleagues. Prioritizing psychological safety means paying attention to operations in healthcare settings, such as teamwork, comfort with seeking help and support, and speaking up (Edmonson & Bransby, 2023).

TRAUMA- AND STRESSOR-RELATED DISORDERS

The DSM-5 introduced a dedicated category for *trauma- and stressor-related disorders.* Trauma-specific conditions were included in prior DSM versions but organized in other diagnostic categories areas. Post-traumatic stress disorder (PTSD) had been placed with anxiety disorders, and adjustment disorders were placed in a standalone category. The new, dedicated category acknowledges trauma as a critical factor in the diagnosis of mental illness. This section will detail only those disorders that case managers encounter with frequency, namely PTSD, acute stress disorder, adjustment disorders, and prolonged grief disorder. See Table 10.5. Note: Acute stress disorder is sometimes abbreviated as ASD. Since that abbreviation is also commonly used for autism spectrum disorder, to avoid confusion, I will use the full name here.

Table 10.5: *DSM-5-TR trauma- and stressor-related disorders*

DSM-5-TR Diagnosis	Code
Reactive attachment disorder	F94.1
Disinhibited social engagement disorder	F94.2
Post-traumatic stress disorder (PTSD) **Specify with:** Dissociative symptoms Depersonalization: Persistent or recurrent experiences of feeling detached from one's mental processes or body, as if one were an outside observer Derealization: Persistent or recurrent experiences of unreality of surroundings **Specify if:** With delayed expression: If full diagnostic criteria is not met until at least 6 months after the event **Note:** Distinct symptoms present for children 6 years and younger	F43.10
Acute stress disorder	F43.0

DSM-5-TR Diagnosis	Code
Adjustment disorders Specify if: Acute Persistent (chronic)	F43.21: With depressed mood F43.22: With anxiety F43.23: With mixed anxiety and depressed mood F43.24: With disturbance of conduct F43.25: With mixed disturbance of emotions and conduct F43.20: Unspecified
Prolonged grief disorder	F43.8
Other specified trauma- and stressor-related disorder	F43.8
Unspecified trauma- and stressor-related disorder	F43.9

American Psychiatric Association, 2022

Post-traumatic stress disorder (PTSD)

Post-traumatic stress disorder is among the most common trauma diagnoses encountered by case managers. Symptoms can be missed in our fast-paced practice settings, and so should be considered during every assessment. Studies validate the importance of early identification of PTSD. Over 25 percent of patients appearing in the ED for a severe medical episode or accident developed PTSD symptoms and depression post-visit (Jaramillo et al., 2019). Even in patients who are discharged home, continuing symptoms commonly associated with trauma's initial *fight or flight response* can present. Patients may perseverate about the initial event or experience *hyperarousal*—that is, extreme sensitivity to one's circumstances post-trauma—which can exacerbate their symptoms or their perception that the condition is worsening. These concerns increase the likelihood of readmission. Proactive assessment for PTSD allows case managers to give care marked by empathy for individual circumstances. Box 10.1 provides a summary of the common signs, symptoms and treatment of PTSD.

PTSD and children. PTSD can be challenging to diagnose in youth. Children 6 and younger may present with unique PTSD symptoms, as well as symptoms reflective of acute stress disorder. Children are easily overwhelmed by a trauma experience. Their verbal expressions can become limited or stunted. A child may dissociate if he or she is unable to process the enormity of the experience. PTSD impairment can be affected by the child's age at the time of the event as well as their emotional development.

For example, consider a child who witnesses the sudden and violent death of a parent. Such children commonly develop selective mutism or sit as if in a trance. The child may present regressive behaviors, such as bedwetting, night terrors, or agitation when in unfamiliar surroundings. The child might reenact the event during interactions with friends or family, which often evokes worry and concern in adults. Screening and assessment by informed and knowledgeable providers are critical in situations of PTSD in children. Box 10.2 provides these unique nuances.

Box 10.1: Signs, symptoms, and treatment of post-traumatic stress disorder (PTSD)

DSM-5-TR criteria:

Patients must have been exposed to a traumatic event and have symptoms from each of the four categories below for a period ≥ 1 month, whether:

- Directly experiencing the event
- Witnessing the event in person
- Learning the event occurred to a close family member or friend. When actual or threatened death of the person is at issue, the event must have been violent or accidental.
- Experiencing repeated or extreme exposure to aversive details of the event (e.g., first responder accounts of child or adult abuse, neglect, exploitation, or collection of human remains)

Note: Exposure via social media, television, movies, or pictures is excluded unless the exposure is work-related

- **Intrusion symptoms** (≥ 1 of the following):
  - a. Recurrent, involuntary, intrusive, or disturbing memories
  - b. Recurrent, disturbing dreams (i.e., nightmares) of the event
  - c. Feeling as if the event were happening again (e.g., flashbacks, losing awareness of surroundings)
  - d. Feeling intense psychological or physiologic distress when reminded of the event (e.g., on its anniversary, hearing sounds or smelling odors similar to those experienced during the event)
- **Avoidance symptoms** (≥ 1 of the following):
  - e. Avoiding thoughts, feelings, or memories associated with the event
  - f. Avoiding activities, places, conversations, or people that trigger memories of the event

A. **Negative effects on cognition and mood** (≥ 2 of the following):
- Memory loss for significant parts of the event (dissociative amnesia)
- Persistent and exaggerated negative beliefs or expectations about oneself, others, or the world
- Persistent distorted thoughts about the cause or consequences of the trauma that lead to blaming self or others
- Persistent negative emotional state (e.g., anger, fear, guilt, horror, or shame)
- Markedly diminished interest or participation in important activities
- Feeling detached or estranged from others
- Consistent inability to experience positive emotions (e.g., empathy, happiness, or loving feelings)

B. **Altered arousal and reactivity** (≥ 2 of the following):
- Difficulty sleeping
- Irritability or angry outbursts
- Reckless or self-destructive behavior
- Problems concentrating
- Increased startle response
- Hypervigilance

- In addition:
  - Symptoms must cause significant distress or impairment in social or occupational functioning, and

- Symptoms must not be attributable to the physiologic effects of substance use or another medical disorder

Treatments:

- Medication:
  - Anti-depressants
  - Close monitoring of sedatives, anti-psychotics, or mood stabilizers
  - Practitioner-approved and -guided use of psychedelics (e.g., ketamine, MDMA, psilocybin)
- Alternative and complementary interventions:
  - Acupuncture
  - Hypnosis
  - Massage therapy
  - Reiki
  - Tai-Chi
  - Yoga
- Psychotherapy:
  - Cognitive behavioral therapy (trauma-informed)
  - Eye movement desensitization and reprocessing (EMDR) (Note: not until 3 months post-trauma)
  - Expressive art therapies
  - Mindfulness
  - Psychoeducation
  - Relaxation therapies
  - Somatic experiencing

American Psychiatric Association, 2022, pp. 301-303; Korovynskyi et al., 2025; Kwon et al., 2023; Strauss et al. (n.d.)

Box 10.2: Signs, symptoms, and treatment of post-traumatic stress disorder and acute stress disorder in children 6 years and younger

Intrusion symptoms:

- Recurrent, involuntary, and distressing memories or dreams of the traumatic event
- Dissociative reactions: often in the form of flashbacks where patients reexperience the trauma
- Note: young children may reenact the event in play
- Distress at internal or external cues that resemble some aspect of the trauma (e.g., seeing a dog or someone who resembles a perpetrator)

Avoidance symptoms:

- Persistent avoidance of memories, feelings, or external reminders of the trauma

Negative effects on cognition and/or mood:

- Inability to remember important aspects of the traumatic event
- Distorted thinking about the causes and/or consequences of the trauma (e.g., feeling they are to blame or could have avoided the event by certain actions)
- A decrease in positive emotions or an increase in negative emotions like fear, guilt, sadness, shame, or confusion
- Overall lack of interest, social withdrawal, or feeling numb, with foreshortened expectation of the future (e.g., thinking "I will not live to see 20")

Altered arousal and/or reactivity:

- Aggressive or reckless behavior
- Disrupted sleep (e.g., nightmares)
- Irritable behavior with angry outbursts
- Jitteriness, exaggerated startle response, difficulty relaxing, difficulty concentrating

Dissociative symptoms:

- Feeling detached from one's body, as if in a dream or feeling the world is unreal

Treatments:

- Self-care:
  - Personal safety
  - Physical health
  - Mindfulness
- SSRIs: Anti-depressants and anti-anxiolytics with close monitoring
- Psychotherapy:
  - Cognitive behavioral therapy (trauma-informed)
  - Eye movement desensitization and reprocessing (EMDR)
  - Expressive art therapies

American Psychiatric Association, 2022, p. 304

ACUTE STRESS DISORDER

Case managers may note similarities between acute stress disorder and PTSD. However, like other disorders in the DSM, the most significant distinction involves the timing of onset and presentation of symptoms. With PTSD, individuals typically present symptoms immediately following the traumatic event, and they last from several days to 1 month. To illustrate PTSD symptoms, imagine a patient who arrives at urgent care for recurrent nightmares. She was hit by someone riding a scooter the week prior. She relates, "I was out walking my dog as I do every morning, then BOOM....that idiot came out of nowhere! Those scooters are a menace and should be outlawed. Since then, I can't sleep and feel like I'm only watching myself go through the day rather than being an active participant. I tried to go out walking yesterday but couldn't bring myself to leave the house. I had to get a friend to drive me here for our appointment, and that was a whole production. This can't continue."

Acute stress disorder can be considered an escalation of PTSD. Imagine this patient's symptoms have continued for 3 days and have now intensified. She reports chronic thoughts about the accident being her fault. "I always move too fast and can't stop thinking that I didn't look both ways before stepping off that curb. This constant crying is so not me. I had to take a leave of absence from work, and I'm worried I'll lose my job. I tried working from home but am too distracted! These symptoms keeping getting worse, not better." Patients may see their symptoms become chronic and appear reflective of an SMI. Box 10.3 provides readers a view of the signs, symptoms, and treatment intervention for acute stress disorder.

Box 10.3: Signs, symptoms, and treatment of acute stress disorder

DSM-5-TR criteria:

Patients must have been exposed directly or indirectly to a traumatic event, and have ≥ 9 of the following symptoms from any of the 5 categories for 3 days to 1 month following the event:

- **Intrusion symptoms**
  - Recurrent, involuntary, and intrusive distressing memories of the event
  - Recurrent distressing dreams of the event
  - Dissociative reactions (e.g., flashbacks in which patients feel as if the traumatic event is reoccurring)
  - Intense psychological or physiologic distress when reminded of the event (e.g., by entering a similar location, by sounds similar to those heaard during the event)
- **Negative mood**
  - Persistent inability to experience positive emotions (e.g., happiness, satisfaction, or loving feelings)
- **Dissociative symptoms**
  - An altered sense of reality (e.g., feeling in a daze, time slowing, altered perceptions)
  - Inability to remember an important part of the traumatic event
- **Avoidance symptoms**
  - Efforts to avoid distressing memories, thoughts, or feelings associated with the event

- Efforts to avoid external reminders (people, places, conversations, activities, objects, or situations) associated with the event
- **Arousal symptoms**
  - Sleep disturbance
  - Irritability or angry outbursts
  - Hypervigilance
  - Difficulty concentrating
  - Exaggerated startle response

In addition:

- Symptoms must cause significant distress or significantly impair social or occupational functioning, and
- Symptoms should not be attributable to the physiologic effects of a substance-related or other medical disorder

Treatments:

- Self-care:
  - Personal safety
  - Physical health
  - Mindfulness, relaxation strategies, sleep hygiene
- SSRIs:
  - Anti-depressants
  - Close monitoring of sedatives
  - Practitioner-approved and -guided use of psychedelics (e.g., ketamine, MDMA, psilocybin)
- Alternative and complementary interventions:
  - Acupuncture
  - Hypnosis
  - Massage therapy
  - Reiki
  - Tai-Chi
  - Yoga
- Psychotherapy:
  - Trauma-focused cognitive behavioral therapy (Note: for trauma-focused, not until at least 2 weeks post-event)
  - Eye movement desensitization and reprocessing (EMDR)
  - Debriefing: Within 72 hours of the event
  - Crisis-intervention
  - Play and expressive therapies (e.g., art, bibliotherapy, music)
  - Support groups

American Psychiatric Association, 2022, pp. 313-315

ADJUSTMENT DISORDER

Imagine you are case managing a patient who experienced an acute, unexpected, negative outcome from a medical procedure. The patient had what was supposed to be a routine lower back surgery. The neurosurgeon met with the patient prior to the procedure for an informed consent discussion on risks, benefits, and potential consequences of the planned surgery. After the procedure, the patient experiences onset of new nerve pain and increased numbness in one leg. She becomes upset and regrets having the procedure.

Moodiness and emotional lability ensue and continue over the next several months. The patient's anger is a direct response to an identifiable stressor and the unanticipated consequences of her surgery. An assessing practitioner might diagnose this patient with an *adjustment disorder*.

Adjustment disorders can be misunderstood by practitioners; they're often considered a general condition that is nonspecific and relatively mild, rather than a response to a traumatic event. This is one reason (of several) that the DSM-5-TR task force moved adjustment disorders to the trauma-related disorders and stressors category. The action also highlights the importance of identifying and assessing each person's response to trauma.

Adjustment disorders typically begin within days of a stressful event and resolve within 6 months of the termination of the stressor or its consequences. Let's say our angry lumbar surgery patient has seen a reduction in post-surgical swelling and positive results from physical therapy. She subsequently experiences a full resolution of her behavioral health symptoms, too. The issue triggering the patient's emotions has been settled, and her adjustment disorder resolved. In some cases, however, symptoms may persist and become chronic in nature. This fact speaks to the importance of therapeutic intervention to address a patient's initial stressors and adjustment response for their ongoing treatment and recovery.

Case managers should note the three categories of adjustment disorder symptoms: depressed mood, anxiety, and conduct disturbance. Patients can present with one symptom (e.g., isolation, agitation, increased volatility) or a combination. Our lumbar surgery patient was depressed, and perhaps she also began to lash out at visitors, throwing a coffee mug or cell phone out of frustration. Such conduct disturbance would also be specified. Box 10.4 provides information on adjustment disorders.

Box 10.4: Signs, symptoms, and treatment of adjustment disorders

DSM-5-TR criteria:

- Patients must have emotional or behavioral symptoms within 3 months of exposure to the stressor.
- Symptoms must be clinically significant and appear as marked distress that is out of proportion to the stressor. Note: Cultural and other factors must be accounted for in diagnosing.
- The symptoms significantly impair social, occupational, or other important areas of functioning.

Treatments:

- Assessment and evaluation for psychopharmacological management of specific symptoms in collaboration with a provider (e.g., anxiolytics, mood stabilizers, sleep enhancement)

Note: Caution with benzodiazepines, which can lead to dependence rather than addressing underlying symptoms and their root causes (i.e., the traumatic event)

- Psychotherapy:
    - Trauma-focused cognitive behavioral therapy
    - Eye movement desensitization and reprocessing (EMDR)
    - Mindfulness, relaxation strategies, and sleep hygiene
    - Psychodynamic approaches
    - Support groups

American Psychiatric Association, 2022, pp. 319-320

PROLONGED GRIEF DISORDER (PGD)

Prolonged grief disorder (PGD) is one of healthcare's newest diagnoses, but grief, mourning, and bereavement have long been a diagnostic focus of the DSM. Prior to formalizing PGD, persons experiencing a strong response to a death that occurred at least 12 months prior for adults and 6 months prior for children were diagnosed with *persistent complex bereavement disorder.* The condition was characterized by an intense and ongoing grief that impacted an individual's social, occupational, or other areas of functioning (American Psychiatric Association, 2013). Although any death is distressing for loved ones, PGD is often associated with unexpected, violent, or traumatic deaths, rather than deaths from natural causes (Glickman, 2021). Box 10.5 displays a snapshot of considerations for persons experiencing prolonged grief disorder.

Persons dealing with grief-related depression for 6 months or more have commonly, but inappropriately, been diagnosed with MDD. As a result, patients might be provided psychopharmacological medication management rather than bereavement counseling. The true source of a patient's depressed state might not be appropriately identified, leaving unaddressed the longer-term issues, such as decreased socialization, inability to focus, or avoidance of the loss.

Box 10.5: Signs, symptoms, and treatment of prolonged grief disorder

DSM-5-TR criteria:

Patient must have experienced the loss of a loved one:

- For adults: at least one year prior
- For youth: at least 6 months prior

The grieving individual must have experienced at least 3 of the following symptoms nearly every day for at least the last month prior to diagnosis:

- Identity disruption, such as feeling that a part of oneself has died
- Marked sense of disbelief about the death
- Avoidance of reminders that the person is dead
- Intense emotional pain, whether anger, bitterness, or sorrow, related to the death
- Difficulty with reintegration; problems engaging with friends, pursuing interests, or planning for the future
- Emotional numbness: absence or marked reduction of emotional experience
- Feeling that life is meaningless
- Intense loneliness or feeling alone or detached from others
- Bereavement lasts longer than expected based on social, cultural, or religious norms

Treatments:

- SSRIs: anti-depressants
- Psychotherapy:
    - Bereavement support groups
    - Trauma-focused cognitive behavioral therapy
    - Complicated grief treatment
    - Eye movement desensitization and reprocessing (EMDR)
    - Mindfulness, relaxation strategies, sleep hygiene

American Psychiatric Association, 2022, pp. 322-23

DATA AND DEMOGRAPHICS

This section will provide a synopsis of statistics on trauma across each age group. Organizations rely on this research to plan for population health programming and employee training.

DEVELOPMENTAL LIFE STAGE

It can be difficult to fathom trauma's full impact on human functioning through the life course. Research now identifies human exposure to trauma starting in utero and spanning all developmental life stages. These details still may not represent the full scope of trauma's wrath: After all, in some populations, considerable stigma exists about even acknowledging trauma.

Youth

Almost 70 percent of all children experience at least one traumatic event in their lives (Frawley et al., 2023). Figure 10.3 shows exposure by gender. Female children are more than twice as likely to witness or experience trauma compared to male children. These numbers align with ACE data and validate the need for assessment and intervention.

Roughly 15 percent of youth who are exposed to traumatic events go on to develop PTSD (National Center for PTSD, 2025a). Over 14 percent of children with PTSD are later diagnosed with acute stress disorder (Meiser-Steadman et al., 2017). Causes of PTSD in youth vary, with the findings shown in Figure 10.4.

By age 16, most adolescents have dealt with some type of trauma (Lawrence-Sidebottom et al., 2024). Research by Swedo et al. (2024) reveals that over 80 percent of teens have experienced one ACE, and over 22 percent experienced 4 or more. The data also highlights increased exposure to ACEs for youth of color and those who identify as members of the LGBTQIA+ community. Figure 10.5 shows prevalence by key ACE areas. Figure 10.6 shows the distinct cultural contexts for youth exposed to 4 or more ACEs.

Exposure to grief and PGD. Even though PGD is a new diagnosis, the research engine is working overtime. The vast numbers of youth who experienced sudden and traumatic deaths of family members during the COVID-19 pandemic has provided a large population to draw from, along with youth who have lost relations from gang violence and mass disasters. Van Dijk et al. (2023) found that as many as 10 percent of youth who deal with bereavement and grief display symptoms of PGD. A new generation of screening tools are also being developed to assess and proactively respond to PGD, including the Trauma Grief Inventory-Kids, which appears in Table 10.9.

Figure 10.3: *Prevalence of trauma exposure in youth by gender*

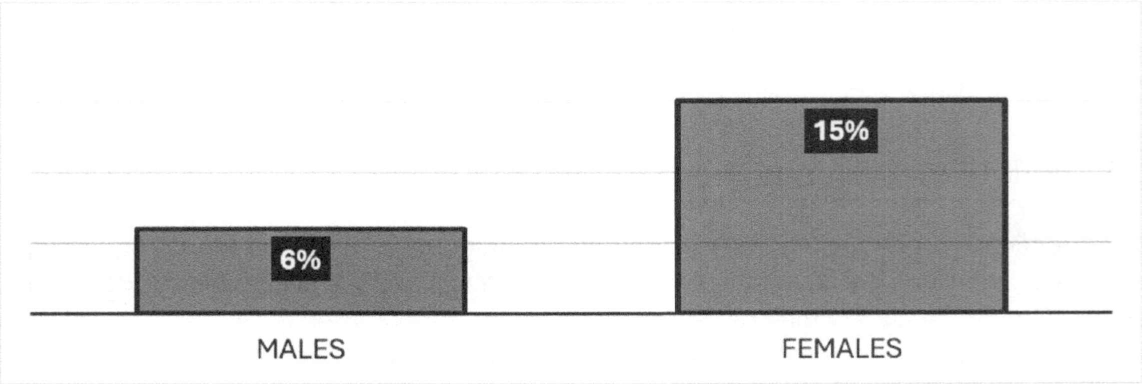

Data adapted from the National Center for PTSD, 2025a

Figure 10.4: *Common causes of PTSD in children*

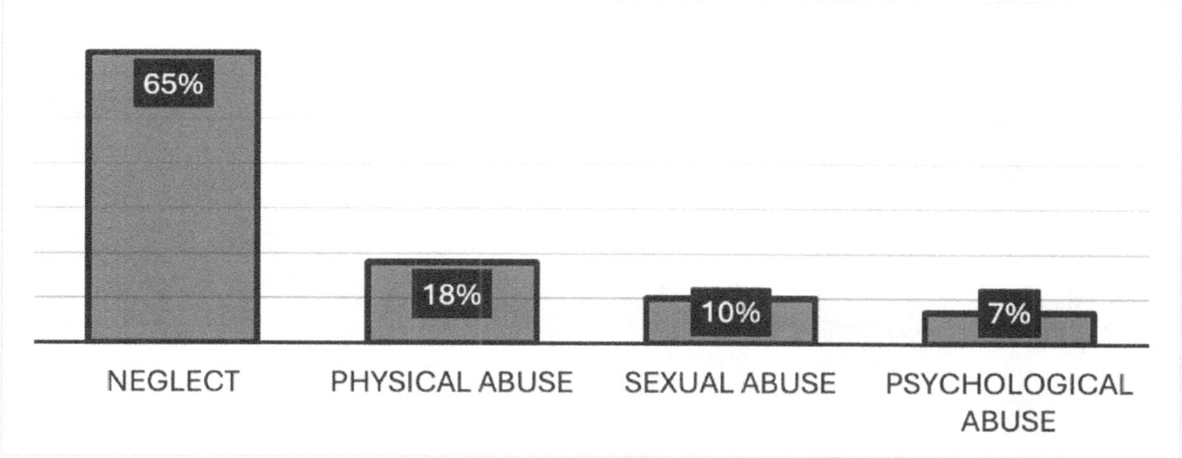

Data adapted from the National Center for PTSD, 2025a

Figure 10.5: *Adolescent ACE exposure*

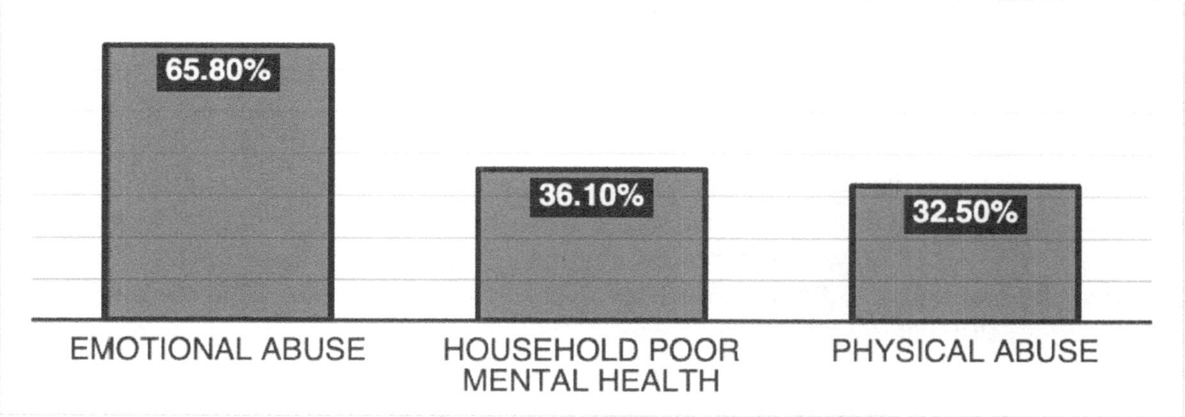

Adapted from Swedo et al., 2024

Figure 10.6: *Adolescent exposure to 4 or more ACEs by cultural context*

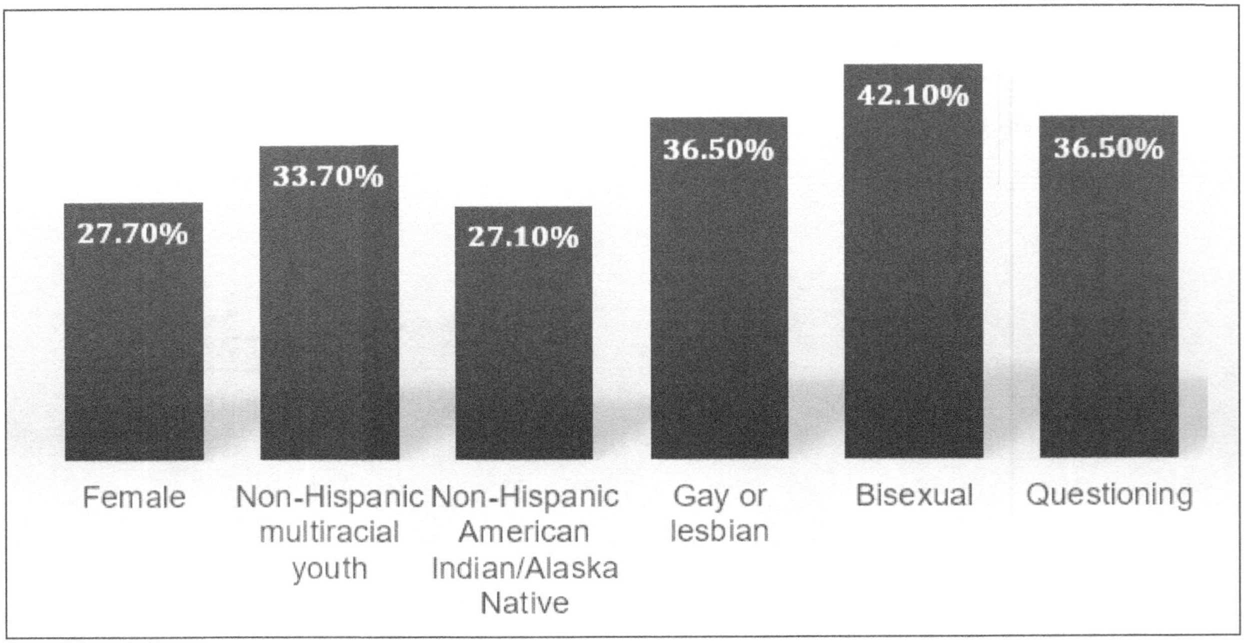

Adapted from Swedo et al., 2024

Adults

The content in this subsection represents one reality: Much of the research for adults exposed to trauma has been compiled through population-based studies. Also note that actual incidence of trauma is likely greater than what is reported. Trauma is often viewed as a subjective experience, which means it can be denied or buried within a person's subconscious. A patient's response to a well-intended, straightforward question such as, "Have you ever been exposed to trauma?" may not yield an accurate reply. This is one reason evidence-based screening tools to assess patients in a given moment have become so valuable to case managers.

Military members and veterans. Trauma-related diagnoses for adults have been studied most often in military and veteran populations. Seven percent of veterans experience some form of PTSD annually, compared with 5 percent of the general adult population (National Center for PTSD, 2025b). Figure 10.7 shows the percentage of veterans diagnosed with PTSD according to service era. Readers should note that the numbers may be lower than expected due to the history of stigma associated with mental health issues and PTSD within the military.

Figure 10.7: *Veterans with PTSD by service era*

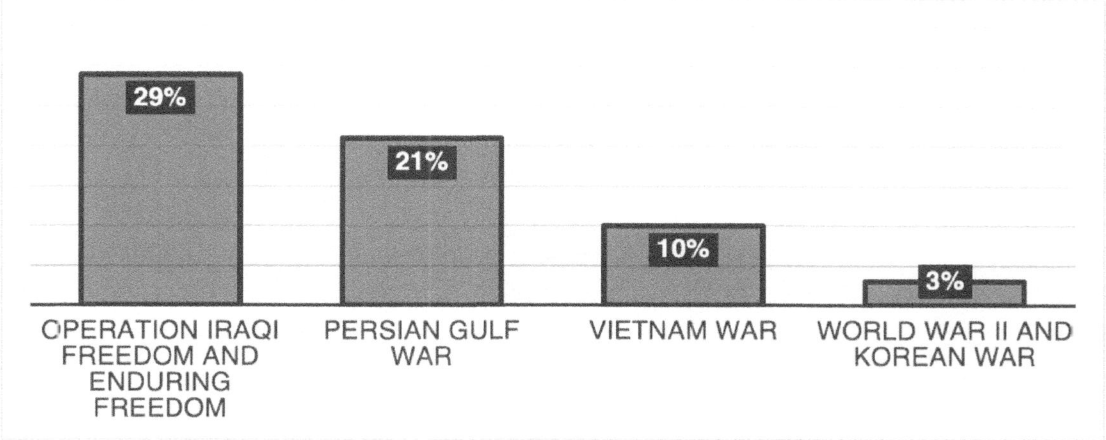

Data adapted from National Center for PTSD, 2025b

Gender, PTSD, and acute stress disorder. Persons who identify as female are twice as likely to develop PTSD and other trauma-related disorders, compared with male counterparts. Research often attributes this difference to females' increased exposure to sexual abuse, an issue that has historically impacted 40 percent of women (Farahi & McEachern, 2021).

Data on sexual abuse of males is limited, though there has been a recent shift to understand the stigma men experience when they identify as victims of domestic violence and sexual assault. Recent data shows relatively equal occurrence of intimate partner violence (IPV) between genders, close to 47 percent for women and 43 percent for men (Leemis et al., 2022). Research is also examining IPV in same-sex relationships. Table 10.6. shows some ways IPV presents across society.

Table 10.6: *Types of intimate partner violence*

Type	Example
Physical violence	Hitting, pushing, grabbing, biting, choking/strangulating, shaking, slapping, kicking, hair-pulling, restraining
Sexual violence	Attempted or actual sexual contact when a partner does not want to or is unable to consent (e.g., when affected by alcohol or illness)
Threats of physical/sexual abuse	Causing fear through words, looks, actions, or weapons
Physical or emotional abuse	Name-calling, humiliating, devaluing, isolating from friends and family, bullying, controlling where a person goes or what they wear

Type	Example
Stalking	Following, harassing, or unwanted contact that makes the victim feel afraid
Psychological aggression	Expressive aggression (insulting, humiliating, or making fun of a partner in front of others) and coercive control and entrapment, which includes behaviors intended to monitor, control, or threaten an intimate partner

Adapted from Leemis et al., 2022; National Center for PTSD, 2025c

The National Intimate Partner and Sexual Violence Survey (NISVS) is a continuing survey that collects comprehensive national- and state-level data on intimate partner violence, sexual violence, and stalking victimization in the U.S. (Centers for Disease Control and Prevention, 2025). Access to survey data and reports is available through the primary survey website, found in the chapter resources.

Prevalence of adjustment disorder. Upwards of 20 percent of patients who experience a Type I traumatic event are diagnosed with an adjustment disorder (O'Donnell et al., 2016). Take a moment to consider every patient you know who endured a traumatic or life-threatening diagnosis or prognosis. Next, think of the family and friends involved in the patient's care and treatment. The ripple effect of trauma means countless persons have potential to develop an adjustment disorder. Case managers should keep this fact in mind during each patient interaction.

Older adults

Studies reveal upwards of 90 percent of all older adults have experienced at least one trauma in their lives, though only 3 percent of the population acknowledge this fact (Kluwert et al., 2013; National Center for PTSD, 2025d). This discrepancy can be explained by the identification and acceptance of psychological trauma as a recent phenomenon, only within the past several decades.

Another reason posed to explain this discrepancy is resilience by the aging population (Lima et al., 2023). Many are unwilling to seek or accept a diagnosis or a mental health treatment. Some older adults may view trauma as unworthy of mentioning, or they may reframe the event as a cultural norm. For example, countless older adults experienced historical traumatic events, like war, the Holocaust, or civil rights protests. They can detail the oppression and horrors they experienced. Yet these individuals often view their involvement as a collective generational experience everyone endured, rather than a traumatic event (National Center for PTSD, 2025d).

A third consideration involves how trauma experiences that occurred early in life may be buried in an older adult's subconscious. As we have also noted, may people simply do not identify an incident as a trauma but rather an unfortunate occurrence that a person has moved past. My gut says you know people who view emphasis on trauma as wasted time and energy.

While case managers may not encounter many older adults who consider themselves as having PTSD or even PGD, it does not mean traumatic experiences don't impact their quality of life. A trauma can be retriggered at any point and increase isolation, impede seeking medical treatment, or prompt self-medicating through substance use. This point transitions us to the novel approaches to assure sensitivity to traumatic experiences, past or present.

BRIEF INTERVENTIONS FOR TRAUMA

Trauma-informed interventions are among the most sought-after strategies to improve patient trust and enhance engagement and treatment adherence. Improvement in workforce retention outcomes have also been identified in organizations where focus is placed on trauma-directed leadership and psychological safety (Fink-Samnick, 2022; Oral et al., 2020).

Think about the people you interact with at work. How many might have been exposed to trauma during their lives? Consider the types of traumas and the examples provided in this chapter. My gut says trauma directly intersects with your patient population, and quite possibly, your colleagues' experiences. Maybe you or a colleague have dealt with bullying or gaslighting behaviors from a superior. Furthermore, many healthcare professionals are still reconciling workplace trauma experienced during the COVID-19 pandemic. Know that a universal truth exists for anyone who has experienced a traumatic event: The brain and body remember the trauma, whether the person knows it or admits it (Van Der Kolk, 2014).

TRAUMA-INFORMED CARE

The workplace moves quicker than ever these days, regardless of the practice setting. This leaves case managers finite time to engage with and address the vast incidence of trauma experiences that patients present with. If not handled carefully, however, *retraumatization* can occur, when a person relives a previous trauma and feels as if it is happening again. Furthermore, power and oppression are fraught elements of many trauma experiences, affecting patients' ability to form trusting and reciprocal interactions with providers. For the provider, however, a patient's inability to engage can be misunderstood as treatment reluctance or non-adherence.

Thus, how one responds to another person's trauma can make all the difference in building rapport and trust in the treatment relationship, independent of how or when the trauma was initially experienced. Harris and Fallot (2001) developed *trauma-informed care* (TIC) as a phased approach to intervention that accounts for trauma and the potential for retraumatization during a treatment experience. Each phase involves actions to advance patient and family rapport, trust, and psychological safety within the intervention space. Through TIC, they build the trust that is vital to patient motivation and satisfaction with care, one of several reasons trauma-informed approaches are increasingly popular.

By being cognizant of every patient's potential for a trauma history, case managers can bring empathy to every patient encounter. Consider first approaching a patient with grace, rather than antagonism or assumption. Imagine you offer patients the choice of:

- What name they want to be known by
- The pronouns the person will use, or if they wish to use a pronoun
- Who they want in the treatment space with them
- Who they want notified about their treatment experience
- The race, gender, and/or ethnicity of the person assigned to render care

Implementation of TIC by healthcare organizations yields higher levels of patient and family engagement and satisfaction and more successful outcomes (Brown, 2018; Oral et al., 2020). The tenets of TIC appear in Figure 10.8.

Figure 10.8: *The tenets of trauma-informed care*

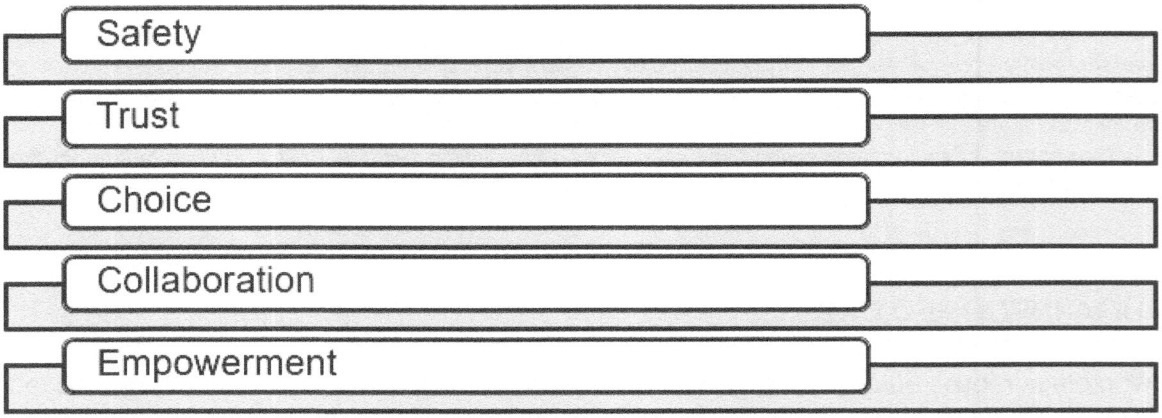

Adapted from Harris & Fallot, 2001

CUES MODEL OF TRAUMA-INFORMED CARE FOR SEXUAL ASSAULT

Imagine a person who enters the treatment space. He presents as guarded and hypersensitive to noises. His injuries do not appear consistent with his story. Maybe another person hovers around the patient and answers for him, even when your clinical questions are directed to the alert and oriented patient. Your clinical gut alerts when the patient says he tripped down the steps, particularly since the marks you see indicate something else. Case managers who are clinically astute may be concerned the patient is a victim of intimate partner violence, other domestic assault, or human trafficking.

The CUES model for sexual assault is a trauma-informed approach grounded in psychoeducation. It provides case managers a template to engage, built rapport, assess, intervene with, and refer patients who may have experienced sexual abuse or assault. Prevention is at the core of the model. The stigma of abuse is addressed with sensitivity and respect. Patients are afforded access to support as needed. Each letter of the acronym represents a phase of the model, as shown in Table 10.8.

Table 10.8: *The CUES model for sexual assault*

Confidentiality	Ensure a private space for patients to discuss sensitive issues Clearly communicate the limits of confidentiality
Universal education	Provide information on healthy relationships, the effects of violence, and available resources to all patients, and not just to those who have disclosed experiencing abuse
Empowerment	Empower individuals by providing them with psychoeducation (knowledge and resources) to make informed decisions about their safety and well-being
Support	Connect patients with appropriate resources, such as counseling, advocacy services, or legal aid Offer ongoing support through the process

Adapted from American Academy of Pediatrics, 2016

SCREENING AND ASSESSMENT TOOLS FOR TRAUMA

Many screening tools now do better at gauging the presence and severity of trauma in youth and adults. These valuable offerings are expanding on a regular basis. Tables 10.9 and 10.10 provide a sampling of these tools to advance your assessment mastery.

Table 10.9: *Screening tools for trauma (adults)*

Instrument	Focus	Source
Acute Stress Disorder Scale (ASDS)	A 19-item self-report checklist to evaluate acute stress reactions in adults or older teens. Measures 4 symptom clusters: 1. Dissociation 2. Re-experiencing 3. Avoidance 4. Arousal Respondents rate symptoms experienced within the past 2 weeks post-traumatic event using a 5-point Likert scale	Bryant, R.A., Moulds, M.L., & Guthrie, R.M. (2000). Acute stress disorder scale: A self-report measure of acute stress disorder. *Psychological Assessment, 12*(1), 61-68. https://doi.org/10.1037/1040-3590.12.1.61

Instrument	Focus	Source
Posttraumatic Adjustment Scale (PAS)	A 10-item screening tool frequently used in EDs and urgent care to identify individuals at risk for developing PTSD and depression after a traumatic injury It assesses: • Pretrauma factors (e.g., psychiatric and trauma history, social support) • Peritrauma factors (e.g., severity of the event) • Posttrauma factors (e.g., acute pain, cognitive responses, and coping self-efficacy)	O'Donnell, M.L., Creamer, M.C., Parslow, R., Elliott, P., Holmes, A.C.N., Ellen, S., Judson, R., McFarlane, A.C., Silove, D., & Bryant, R.A. (2008). *Post-traumatic Adjustment Scale (PAS)* [Database record]. APA PsycTestsPsycTESTS. https://doi.org/10.1037/t08802-000
Primary Care PTSD Screen for DSM-5 (PC-PTSD-5)	A 5-item screening tool to identify adults at risk for PTSD in primary care and general medical settings	Prins, A., Bovin, M.J., Kimerling, R., Kaloupek, D.G., Marx, B.P., Pless Kaiser, A., & Schnurr, P.P. (2016). The Primary Care PTSD screen for DSM-5 (PC-PTSD-5): Development and evaluation within a veteran primary care sample. *Journal of General Internal Medicine, 31*(10), 1206-11. doi: 10.1007/s11606-016-3703-5. PMID: 27170304; PMCID: PMC5023594.
PTSD Checklist for DSM-5 (PCL-5)	A 20-item self-report measure to assess the presence and severity of PTSD per DSM criteria, and grouped into 4 clusters of: 1. Intrusion 2. Avoidance 3. Negative alterations in cognition and mood 4. Alterations in arousal and reactivity Symptoms rated on a 5-point Likert scale	Blevins, C.A., Weathers, F.W., Davis, M.T., Witte, T.K., & Domino, J.L. (2015). The post-traumatic stress disorder checklist for *DSM-5* (PCL-5): Development and initial psychometric evaluation. *Journal of Traumatic Stress, 28*(6), 489-498. https://doi.org/10.1002/jts.22059
Short Post-Traumatic Stress Disorder Rating Interview (SPRINT)	An 8-item self-report measure that assesses the core symptoms of PTSD: • Intrusion • Avoidance • Numbing • Arousal • Somatic malaise • Stress vulnerability • Role and social functional impairment Symptoms rated on 5-point Likert scales	Connor, K., & Davidson, J. (2001). SPRINT: A brief global assessment of post-traumatic stress disorder. International Clinical Psychopharmacology, 16(5), 279-284.

Instrument	Focus	Source
SPAN Self-Report Screen	A 4-item self-report PTSD screening tool developed to rapidly identify individuals who may have PTSD SPAN encompasses the first letters of the 4 assessed symptoms: 1. Startle 2. Physiological arousal 3. Anger 4. Numbness Items are rated on a 5-point Likert scale	Davidson, J. (2002). SPAN Addendum to DTS Manual. Multi-Health Systems Inc. New York.
Traumatic Grief Inventory-Adults	18- or 22-item tools developed as self-report measures to assess for symptoms of traumatic grief associated with PGD and previously-diagnosed Persistent Complex Bereavement Disorder	Lenferink, L.I.M., Eisma, M.C., Smid, G.E., de Keijser, J., & Boelen, P.A. (2022). *Traumatic Grief Inventory--Self Report Plus (TGI-SR+)* [Database record]. APA PsycTests.
Trauma Screening Questionnaire (TSQ)	A 10-item symptom screen designed for use with survivors of all types of traumatic stress Based on the PTSD Symptom Scale - Self Report (PSS-SR) with 5 items to address re-experiencing items and 5 items on arousal	Brewin, C.R., Rose, S., Andrews, B., Green, J., Tata, P., McEvedy, C., Turner, S., & Foa, E.B. (2002). Brief screening instrument for post-traumatic stress disorder. The British Journal of Psychiatry, 181, 158-162.

Table 10.10: *Screening tools for trauma (youth)*

Instrument	Focus	Source
Acute Stress Checklist for Children (ASC-Kids)	A 29-item self-report checklist, or a 3- or 6-item brief screening version, to evaluate acute stress reactions or potential to develop PTSD in youth 8-17 years old Based on the DSM criteria for acute stress disorder to assess one-month post-trauma for: • Dissociation • Re-experiencing • Avoidance • Arousal • Functional impairment	Kassam-Adams, N., Gold, J.I., Montaño, Z., Kohser, K.L., Cuadra, A., Muñoz, C., & Armstrong, F.D. (2013). Development and psychometric evaluation of child acute stress measures in Spanish and English. *Journal of Traumatic Stress, 26*(1), 19-27. doi: 10.1002/jts.21782. PMID: 23371337; PMCID: PMC4646425.

Instrument	Focus	Source
Child and Adolescent Trauma Screen (CATS)	A standardized tool done by self-report or caregivers, to assess exposure to traumatic events and the presence of post-traumatic stress symptoms in youth 7-17 years old Two sections: 1. Trauma exposure checklist: Screens for a range of traumatic experiences (e.g., abuse, accidents, disasters) 2. PTSD symptom scale: Measures symptoms based on DSM-5 PTSD criteria (intrusion, avoidance, negative mood/cognitions, and hyperarousal)	Sachser, C., Berliner, L., Holt, T., Jensen, T.K., Jungbluth, N., Risch, E., Rosner, R., & Goldbeck, L. (2017). International development and psychometric properties of the Child and Adolescent Trauma Screen (CATS). *Journal of Affective Disorders, 210,* 189-195. https://doi.org/10.1016/j.jad.2016.12.040
Child PTSD Symptom Scale (CPSS)	A 24-item self-report or interviewer-administered checklist that assesses PTSD or monitoring of symptoms and impairment in youth 8-18 years old who have experienced a traumatic event Two main components: 1. PTSD symptom items: 17 items that align with DSM PTSD criteria (re-experiencing, avoidance, and hyperarousal) 2. Functional impairment items: 7 items assessing how symptoms affect areas of life, such as school, relationships, and daily activities Provides a total symptom severity score and a functional impairment score	Foa, E.B., Asnaani, A., Zang, Y., Capaldi, S., & Yeh, R. (2018). Psychometrics of the Child PTSD Symptom Scale for DSM-5 for trauma-exposed children and adolescents. *Journal of Clinical Child and Adolescent Psychology, 47*(1), 38-46. https://doi.org/10.1080/15374416.2017.1350962
Child Stress Disorders Checklist (CSDC) (CSDC-Short Form)	A 35-item checklist completed by a parent (or provider) to assess for acute stress or PTSD symptoms in youth The short version contains 4 items to assess children 5-12 years old and is based on caregiver observations	Bosquet Enlow, M., Kassam-Adams, N., & Saxe, G. (2010). The Child Stress Disorders Checklist-Short Form: A four-item scale of traumatic stress symptoms in children. *General Hospital Psychiatry, 32*(3), 321-7. https://doi.org/10.1016/j.genhosppsych.2010.01.009. PMID: 20430237; PMCID: PMC2862234.
Child Trauma Screening Questionnaire (CTSQ)	A 10-item screening tool for early identification of trauma in youth 7-16 years old who have been injured and may be at higher risk for developing PTSD Typically administered within the first month following the traumatic event	Kenardy, J., Spence, S.H., & Macleod, A.C. (2006). *Child Trauma Screening Questionnaire. (CTSQ)* [Database record]. APA PsycTests. https://doi.org/10.1037/t04843-000

Instrument	Focus	Source
Hospital Mental Health Risk Screen (HMHRS)	A 10-item self-report screen that predicts mental health risk in youth 10-17 years of age, after a recent trauma Particularly beneficial in ED and other ambulatory or outpatient settings	Carlson, E.B., Palmieri, P.A., Barlow, M.R., Macia, K., Bruns, B.R., Shieh, L., & Spain, D.A. (2023). Development and initial performance of the Hospital Mental Health Risk Screen. Journal of the American College of Surgeons, 238(2), 147-156. https://doi.org/10.1097/XCS.0000000000000009044
Traumatic Grief Inventory-Kids (TGI-K)	A clinician-administered instrument of 16 items that aligns with the DSM-5-TR criteria for PGD	Van Dijk, I., Boelen, P.A., de Keijser, J., & Lenferink, L.I.M. (2023). Assessing DSM-5-TR and ICD-11 prolonged grief disorder in children and adolescents: Development of the Traumatic Grief Inventory - Kids - Clinician-Administered. *European Journal of Psychotraumatology*, *14*(2), 2197697. https://doi.org/10.1080/20008066.2023.2197697

CONCLUSION

This chapter wraps up Section 2 and its comprehensive view of the conditions and diagnoses commonly faced by case managers. Exposure to trauma has countless implications for patients and their families, as well as the practitioners who render and intervene in their care.

Section 3 will provide three chapters to continue your learning journey. Get ready for general knowledge on assessment and treatment planning. You also won't want to miss Chapter 13, with ten complex case scenarios.

CONTEMPLATION QUESTIONS

1. Trauma can trigger many emotions for case managers and other healthcare professionals. Review the types of traumas listed in Tables 10.2, 10.3, and 10.4.
    a) Which types of trauma are you most familiar with?
    b) Which drivers of trauma are you most familiar with?
    c) Reflect on how your familiarity with these types of traumas impacts your work with patients and their families.

2. Review the content and Figures 10.1 and 10.2 on ACEs.
    a) What surprises you about the original study?
    b) Reflect on the ACE Pyramid and your professional and personal experiences.
3. Use the following case scenario for the questions below.

A patient presents to urgent care appearing nervous and on high alert. While being screened by the nurse, the patient comments, "This all started after I witnessed my sister being used as a punching bag by some guy she was dating." Later, when the patient is forced to wait, she lashes out at team members, then apologizes profusely 10 minutes later. "I am so sorry. My sister left that guy, but still. I just haven't been able to right myself since. It's been a few months."

    a) Considering the diagnoses in Table 10.5, which do you think would be most applicable and why?
    b) Review Figure 10.8 on trauma-informed care. Imagine you are interacting with this patient. What actions would you take to implement each of the five tenets of the model with this patient?

1. Access any two screening tools for trauma from Tables 10.8 and 10.9. If possible, choose ones that are unfamiliar to you.
    a) Review the screening tool.
    b) Complete the screening tool for a patient you are working with.
    c) Reflect on how use of a standardized tool for trauma will inform your future efforts.
2. As the case manager for a rural, federally-qualified health center, you are assigned to meet Marco. Marco is a 55-year-old patient who presents for treatment for injuries sustained in a fight with their partner. Marco is new to the area and requests to meet with a provider who can be "discreet" in this small town.
    a) Considering use of trauma-informed care, how would you set a safe treatment environment to engage Marco in treatment?
    b) Use Case Management's Behavioral Health Conversation Map in Table 1.4 to script your interactions with Marco.

RESOURCES

- **ACES Aware: Screening Tools**
  https://www.acesaware.org/learn-about-screening/screening-tools/
- **Administration for Children & Families: Trauma-informed resources for persons with disabilities**
  https://acf.gov/trauma-toolkit/people-disabilities
- **American Academy of Pediatrics: The CUES Model**
  https://www.aap.org/en/patient-care/intimate-partner-violence/cues-confidentiality-universal-education--empowerment-support/

- **American Psychiatric Association: Stress and Trauma Toolkit for Treating LGBTQIA in a Changing Political and Social Environment**
  https://www.psychiatry.org/psychiatrists/diversity/education/stress-and-trauma/lgbtq
- **Centers for Disease Control and Prevention: CDC-Kaiser ACE Study**
  https://www.cdc.gov/violenceprevention/aces/about.html
- **Center for Healthcare Strategies: Trauma-Informed Care Implementation Resource Center**
  https://www.traumainformedcare.chcs.org
- **EMDR International Association**
  https://www.emdria.org/
- **IPV Health**
  https://ipvhealth.org/
- **Military One Source: Combat Stress and PTSD**
  https://www.militaryonesource.mil/military-basics/wounded-ill-injured-and-caregivers/understanding-and-dealing-with-combat-stress-and-ptsd/
- **National Center on Domestic Violence, Trauma, and Mental Health**
  https://ncdvtmh.org/
- **National Domestic Violence Hotline**
  https://www.thehotline.org
- **National Human Trafficking Hotline**
  https://humantraffickinghotline.org/en
- **National Intimate Partner and Sexual Violence Survey (NISVS)**
  https://www.cdc.gove/nisvs/about/index.html
- **National Network for Youth**
  https://nn4youth.org/
- **National Sexual Violence Resource Center**
  https://www.nsvrc.org/blogs/resources-and-support-transgender-survivors
- **SHE Recovers Foundation**
  https://sherecovers.org/

U.S. Department of Veterans Affairs

- **National Center for PTSD**
  https://www.ptsd.va.gov/index.asp
- **Partners of Veterans with PTSD**
  https://www.ptsd.va.gov/family/effect_partners_vets.asp

- **Traumatic Stress in Women**
  https://www.ptsd.va.gov/professional/treat/type/trauma_female_veterans.asp
- **Wounded Warrior Project**
  https://www.woundedwarriorproject.org/

REFERENCES

- American Academy of Pediatrics. (2016). CUES: Confidentiality, Universal Education + Empowerment, Support. Retrieved August 10, 2025, from https://www.aap.org/en/patient-care/intimate-partner-violence/cues-confidentiality-universal-education--empowerment-support/
- American Psychiatric Association. (2013). *Diagnostic and Statistical Manual of Mental Disorders* (5th ed.).
- American Psychiatric Association. (2022). *Diagnostic and Statistical Manual of Mental Disorders* (5th ed., text rev.).
- Borda Bohigas, J.P., Carrillo, J.O., Garzón, D.F., Ramírez, M.P., & Rodríguez, N. (2015). Trauma histórico. Revisión sistemática de un abordaje diferente al conflicto armado [Historical trauma. Systematic review of a different approach to armed conflict]. *Revista Colombiana de Psiquiatria*, *44*(1), 41-49. https://doi.org/10.1016/j.rcp.2014.09.005
- Bowe, C., Thomas, C., & Mackey, P. (2025). Perspective to practice: Theoretical frameworks explaining intergenerational trauma, violence, and maltreatment and implications for the therapeutic response. *International Journal of Environmental Research and Public Health*, *22*(3), 321. https://doi.org/10.3390/ijerph22030321
- Brown, V.B. (2018). *Through a Trauma Lens: Transforming Health and Behavioral Health Systems*. Routledge.
- Brzozowska, A., & Grabowski, J. (2025). Hyperarousal, dissociation, emotion dysregulation and re-experiencing—Towards understanding molecular aspects of PTSD symptoms. *International Journal of Molecular Sciences*, *26*(11), 5216. https://doi.org/10.3390/ijms26115216
- Centers for Disease Control and Prevention. (2021). About the CDC-Kaiser ACE study. Retrieved August 5, 2025, from https://www.cdc.gov/violenceprevention/aces/about.html
- Cruz, D., Lichten, M., Berg, K., & George, P. (2022). Developmental trauma: Conceptual framework, associated risks and comorbidities, and evaluation and treatment. *Frontiers in Psychiatry*, *13*, 800687. https://doi.org/10.3389/fpsyt.2022.800687
- Davis, L.L., Schein, J., Cloutier, M., Gagnon-Sanschagrin, P., Maitland, J., Urganus, A. Guerin, A., Lefebvre, P., & Houle, C.R. (2022). The economic burden of posttraumatic stress disorder in the United States from a societal perspective. *Journal of Clinical Psychiatry*, *83*(3), 21m14116. doi: 10.4088/JCP.21m14116. PMID: 35485933.
- Dhabhar F.S. (2009). A hassle a day may keep the pathogens away: The fight-or-flight stress response and the augmentation of immune function. *Integrative and Comparative Biology*, *49*(3), 215-236. https://doi.org/10.1093/icb/icp045

- Edmondson, A.C., & Bransby, D.P. (2023). Psychological safety comes of age: Observed themes in an established literature. *Annual Review of Organizational Psychology and Organizational Behavior, 10*(1), 55-78. https://doi.org/10.1146/annurev-orgpsych-120920-055217
- Farahi, N., & McEachern, M. (2021). Sexual assault of women. *American Family Physician, 103*(3), 168-176.
- Felitti, V.J., Anda, R.F., Nordenberg, D., Williamson, D.F., Spitz, A.M., Edwards, V., Koss, M.P., & Marks, J.S. (1998). Relationship of childhood abuse and household dysfunction to many of the leading causes of death in adults. The Adverse Childhood Experiences (ACE) Study. *American Journal of Preventive Medicine, 14*(4), 245-58. doi: 10.1016/s0749-3797(98)00017-8. PMID: 9635069.
- Ferriante J., & Sharma N.P. (2023). Acute and Chronic Mental Health Trauma. [Updated 2023 Aug 2]. StatPearls Publishing: Treasure Island, FL.: Available from https://www.ncbi.nlm.nih.gov/books/NBK594231/
- Fink-Samnick, E. (2022). Collective occupational trauma, health care quality, and trauma-informed leadership: Intersections and implications. *Professional Case Management, 27*(3):107-123. doi: 10.1097/NCM.0000000000000559. PMID: 35363656.
- Frawley, C., Babb, K., & Lambie, G.W. (2023). Predictors of trauma symptoms among children referred for behavioral school-based mental health counseling. *Journal of Child & Adolescent Trauma, 16*(3), 597-605. https://doi.org/10.1007/s40653-023-00522-4
- Geronimus, A.T., Hicken, M., Keene, D., & Bound, J. (2006). "Weathering" and age patterns of allostatic load scores among blacks and whites in the United States. *American Journal of Public Health, 96*(5), 826-833. https://doi.org/10.2105/AJPH.2004.060749
- Glickman, K. (2021). Prolonged grief disorder in a diverse college student sample. *Frontiers in Psychology, 11*, 604573. https://doi.org/10.3389/fpsyg.2020.604573
- Goldstein, E., Chokshi, B., Melendez-Torres, G.J., Rios, A., Jelley, M., Lewis-O'Connor, A. (2024). Effectiveness of trauma-informed care implementation in health care settings: Systematic review of reviews and realist synthesis. *The Permanente Journal, 28*(1):135-150. doi: 10.7812/TPP/23.127. Epub 2024 Mar 6. PMID: 38444328; PMCID: PMC10940237.
- Hagenaars, M.A., Stins, J.F., & Roelofs, K. (2012). Aversive life events enhance human freezing responses. *Journal of Experimental Psychology: General, 141*(1), 98-105. https://doi.org/10.1037/a0024211
- Harris, M., & Fallot, R.D. (2001). Envisioning a trauma-informed service system: A vital paradigm shift. In M. Harris & R.D. Fallot (Eds.), *Using Trauma Theory to Design Service Systems* (pp. 3-22). Jossey-Bass/Wiley.
- Hirschberger G. (2018). Collective trauma and the social construction of meaning. *Frontiers in Psychology, 9*, 1441. https://doi.org/10.3389/fpsyg.2018.01441
- Ito, A., Sato, K., Yumoto, Y., Sasaki, M., & Ogata, Y. (2022). A concept analysis of psychological safety: Further understanding for application to health care. *Nursing Open, 9*(1), 467-489. https://doi.org/10.1002/nop2.1086

- Jaramillo, S., Suffoletto, B., Callaway, C., & Pacella-LaBarbara, M. (2019). Early screening for posttraumatic stress disorder and depression among injured emergency department patients: A feasibility study. *Academic Emergency Medicine*, *26*(11), 1232-1244. https://doi.org/10.1111/acem.13816
- Kar, S.K., & Singh, S. (2023). Anomic suicides on rise during recently emerging crises: Revisiting Durkheim's model. *CNS Spectrums*, *28*(6), 655-656. https://doi.org/10.1017/S1092852923002341
- Korovynskyi, I., Volnova, L., Yuryk, O., Borysova, O., & Manchuk, V. Cognitive-behavioral therapy methods in the treatment of post-traumatic stress disorder and their role in mental health recovery. *Georgian Medical News*, (362), 51-60. PMID: 40737648.
- Kuwert, P., Pietrzak, R.H., & Glaesmer, H. (2013). Trauma and posttraumatic stress disorder in older adults. *Canadian Medical Association Journal, 185*(8), 685. https://doi.org/10.1503/cmaj.120866
- Kwon, H.J., Leem, J., Kim, D.W., Kwon, C.Y., & Kim, S.H. (2023) Effect of acupuncture on patients with major psychiatric disorder and related symptoms caused by earthquake exposure: Protocol for a scoping review of clinical studies. *PLoS One 18*(1), e0281207. https://doi.org/10.1371/journal.pone.0281207
- Lannert, B.K., Garcia, A.M., Smagur, K.E., Yalch, M.M., Levendosky, A.A., Bogat, G.A., & Lonstein, J.S. (2014). Relational trauma in the context of intimate partner violence. *Child Abuse & Neglect*, *38*(12), 1966-1975. https://doi.org/10.1016/j.chiabu.2014.10.002
- Lawrence-Sidebottom, D., Huffman, L.G., Beam, A.B., Guerra, R., Parikh, A., Roots, M., & Huberty, J. (2024). Rates of trauma exposure and posttraumatic stress in a pediatric digital mental health intervention: Retrospective analysis of associations with anxiety and depressive symptom improvement over time. *JMIR Pediatrics and Parenting*, *7*, e55560. https://doi.org/10.2196/55560
- Leemis R.W., Friar N., Khatiwada S., Chen M.S., Kresnow M., Smith S.G., Caslin, S., & Basile, K.C. (2022). *The National Intimate Partner and Sexual Violence Survey: 2016/2017 Report on Intimate Partner Violence.* National Center for Injury Prevention and Control, Centers for Disease Control and Prevention.
- Lima, G.S., Figueroa, A.L.G., Caravalho, E.C., Kusumota, L., & Caldera, S. (2023). Resilience in older people: A concept analysis. *Healthcare, 11*(18), 2491. https://doi.org/10.3390/healthcare11182491
- Maercker, A., Cloitre, M., Bachem, R., Schlumpf, Y.R., Khoury, B., Hitchcock, C., & Bohus, M. (2022). Complex post-traumatic stress disorder. *The Lancet*, *400*(10345), 60-72. https://doi.org/10.1016/S0140-6736(22)00821-2
- Maercker, A., & Eberle, D.J. (2022). Disorders specifically associated with stress in ICD-11. *Clinical Psychology in Europe, 4*(Spec Issue), 1-16.
- Meiser-Stedman, R., McKinnon, A., Dixon, C., Boyle, A., Smith, P., & Dalgleish, T. (2017). Acute stress disorder and the transition to posttraumatic stress disorder in children and adolescents:

Prevalence, course, prognosis, diagnostic suitability, and risk markers. *Depression and Anxiety*, *34*(4), 348-355. https://doi.org/10.1002/da.22602

- Merriam-Webster. (2025). Compassion Fatigue. Retrieved August 10, 2025, from https://www.merriam-webster.com/dictionary/compassion%20fatigue.
- Mohr, D.C., Elnahal, S., Marks, M.L., Derickson, R., & Osatuke, K. (2025). Burnout trends among U.S. health care workers. *JAMA Network Open*, *8*(4), e255954. https://doi.org/10.1001/jamanetworkopen.2025.5954
- National Center for PTSD. (2025a). PTSD: How Common Is PTSD in Children and Teens? Retrieved August 10, 2025, from https://www.ptsd.va.gov/understand/common/common_children_teens.asp
- National Center for PTSD. (2025b). How Common Is PTSD in Veterans? Retrieved August 10, 2025, from https://www.ptsd.va.gov/understand/common/common_veterans.asp
- National Center for PTSD. (2025c). Intimate Partner Violence. Retrieved August 10, 2025, from https://www.ptsd.va.gov/understand/types/violence_ipv.asp
- National Center for PTSD. (2025d). Older Adults and PTSD. Retrieved August 10, 2025, from https://www.ptsd.va.gov/understand/what/aging_veterans.asp
- O'Donnell, M.L., Alkemade, N., Creamer, M., McFarlane, A.C., Silove, D., Bryant, R.A., Felmingham, K., Steel, Z., & Forbes, D. (2016). A longitudinal study of adjustment disorder after trauma exposure. *The American Journal of Psychiatry, 173*(12), 1231-1238. https://doi.org/10.1176/appi.ajp.2016.16010071
- Oral, R., Coohey, C., Zarei, K., Conrad, A., Nielsen, A., Wibbenmeyer, L., Segal, R., Wojciak, A. S., Jennissen, C., & Peek-Asa, C. (2020). Nationwide efforts for trauma-informed care implementation and workforce development in healthcare and related fields: A systematic review. *The Turkish Journal of Pediatrics*, *62*(6), 906-920. https://doi.org/10.24953/turkjped.2020.06.002
- Pfaltz, M.C., & Schnyder, U. (2023). Allostatic load and allostatic overload: Preventive and clinical implications. *Psychotherapy and Psychosomatics*, *92*(5), 279-282.
- Schlote S. (2023). History of the term 'appeasement': A response to Bailey et al. *European Journal of Psychotraumatology*, *14*(2), 2183005. https://doi.org/10.1080/20008066.2023.2183005
- Strauss, J.L., Lang, A.J., & Schnurr, P.P. (n.d.). Complimentary and Integrative Health (CIH) for PTSD. PTSD: National Center for PTSD. VA Department of Veterans Affairs. Retrieved August 7, 2025, from https://www.ptsd.va.gov/professional/treat/txessentials/complementary_alternative_for_ptsd.asp
- Swedo, E.A., Holditch Niolon, P., Anderson, K N., Li, J., Brener, N., Mpofu, J., Aslam, M.V., & Underwood, J.M. (2024). Prevalence of adverse childhood experiences among adolescents. *Pediatrics*, *154*(5), e2024066633. https://doi.org/10.1542/peds.2024-066633
- Van Der Kolk, B. (2014). *The Body Keeps the Score: Brain, Mind and Body in the Healing of Trauma.* Penguin Books.
- Van Dijk, I., Boelen, P.A., de Keijser, J., & Lenferink, L.I.M. (2023). Assessing DSM-5-TR and ICD-11 prolonged grief disorder in children and adolescents: Development of the Traumatic

Grief Inventory - Kids - Clinician-Administered. *European Journal of Psychotraumatology*, *14*(2), 2197697. https://doi.org/10.1080/20008066.2023.2197697

- Wang, S.K., Feng, M., Fang, Y., Lv, L., Sun, G.L., Yang, S.L., Guo, P., Cheng, S.F., Qian, M. C., & Chen, H.X. (2023). Psychological trauma, posttraumatic stress disorder and trauma-related depression: A mini-review. *World Journal of Psychiatry*, *13*(6), 331-339. https://doi.org/10.5498/wjp.v13.i6.331
- World Health Organization. (2022). *ICD-11: International Classification of Diseases* (11th revision). https://icd.who.int/
- World Health Organization. (2024). Post-traumatic Stress Disorder: Key Facts. Retrieved August 9, 2025, from https://www.who.int/news-room/fact-sheets/detail/post-traumatic-stress-disorder

SECTION 3

THE TREATMENT PROCESS

CHAPTER 11

IN THE TRENCHES ASSESSMENT

CHAPTER 12

INTERVENTIONS AND SHORT-TERM TREATMENT

CHAPTER 13

CASE SCENARIOS

INTRODUCTION TO SECTION 3

By this point in the book, you may be wondering what else you can learn about behavioral health. I reviewed the questions I've received from case management colleagues on this topic over the years and have tried to hit every critical query.

Chapter 11 provides an overview of many disruptive conditions case managers commonly face. These include management of personality disorders, psychiatric emergencies and de-escalation strategies, and a novel approach to the management of trauma, both for patients and the workforce. Chapter 12 contains information on short-term interventions and developing treatment plans. Chapter 13 is your opportunity to apply all you have learned by answering ten complex, critical-thinking questions. The questions will advance your proficiency in assessing, managing, and intervening with behavioral health conditions. Cues to answer locations may be found in the book are also provided.

CHAPTER 11

IN THE TRENCHES ASSESSMENT

INTRODUCTION

It is an understatement to say that case managers are often forced to face unpredictable, "in the trenches" moments on the job, including moments they may feel unprepared for. We can't predict the patients we'll encounter or the situations that will unfold during a treatment experience.

This chapter provides an overview of the most stressful situations case managers may face. Patients with personality disorders may present a host of challenging and disruptive behaviors. Some clinicians across the industry don't view them as formal mental illnesses, despite the impediment to a person's academic, social, occupational, and other functioning. But the behaviors associated with the most common personality disorders (including anti-social, borderline, histrionic, and narcissistic) are well-known to case managers and other industry professionals. They tax the most seasoned practitioner and obstruct outcomes, so I provide suggestions for strategic management of these traits, along with dedicated screening tools. The chapter also covers psychiatric emergency de-escalation, a skill now needed in practice settings.

BEHAVIORAL LEARNING OBJECTIVES

1. Identify the 5 Cs of Care Considerations for Case Management
2. Understand the 11 elements of mental status exams
3. Distinguish among types of mental status exams used across the industry
4. Examine personality disorders and how they are organized in the DSM
5. Articulate the 10 trauma-directed tactics to address disruptive behaviors
6. Integrate guidance to manage psychiatric de-escalation
7. Identify screening tools for personality disorders

ESSENTIAL TERMS

- 5 Cs of Care Considerations for Case Management
- Mental Status Exam (MSE)
- Mini-Cog
- Mini-Mental Status Exam (MMSE)
- Montreal Cognitive Assessment (MoCA)
- Personality disorder
- Personality disorder clusters
- Psychiatric de-escalation
- Psychiatric emergencies
- Social desirability bias
- Splitting
- Trauma-directed tactics

GENERAL ASSESSMENT

Case managers are frequently consulted to render interpretation of a patient's mental status—quite the slippery slope. Chapter 2 addressed the first step of assessing a patient's understanding of treatment: clinical capacity or informed consent. Once determined, attention should be paid to legal capacity, also known as competency. Legal capacity can be determined only by a judge or a court but requires taxing and time-consuming discussions and interactions for case managers, treatment teams, and their organizations.

In *The Ethical Case Manager: Tools and Tactics* (Fink-Samnick, 2023), I provided case managers a roadmap to sequence these decisions, called the 5 Cs of Care Considerations for Case Management. The process starts with defining clinical capacity, then legal capacity. The model appears in Figure 11.1. Each step is rooted in case management industry regulations, professional codes of ethics, and standards of practice, as well as other industry requirements, such as the patient bill of rights and Medicare Conditions of Participation. Case management's ethical principles of autonomy, beneficence, fidelity, integrity, justice, and nonmaleficence are also prioritized, with primary respect for patient self-determination and decision-making, and that of any involved family. Although the individuality of patient circumstance must always be considered, the 5 Cs provide a natural starting point for case management assessment. Quality, safe, and ethically-sound care coordination can only be implemented after case managers understand if their patients can participate in the decision-making process.

Figure 11.1: *The 5 Cs of Care Considerations for Case Management*

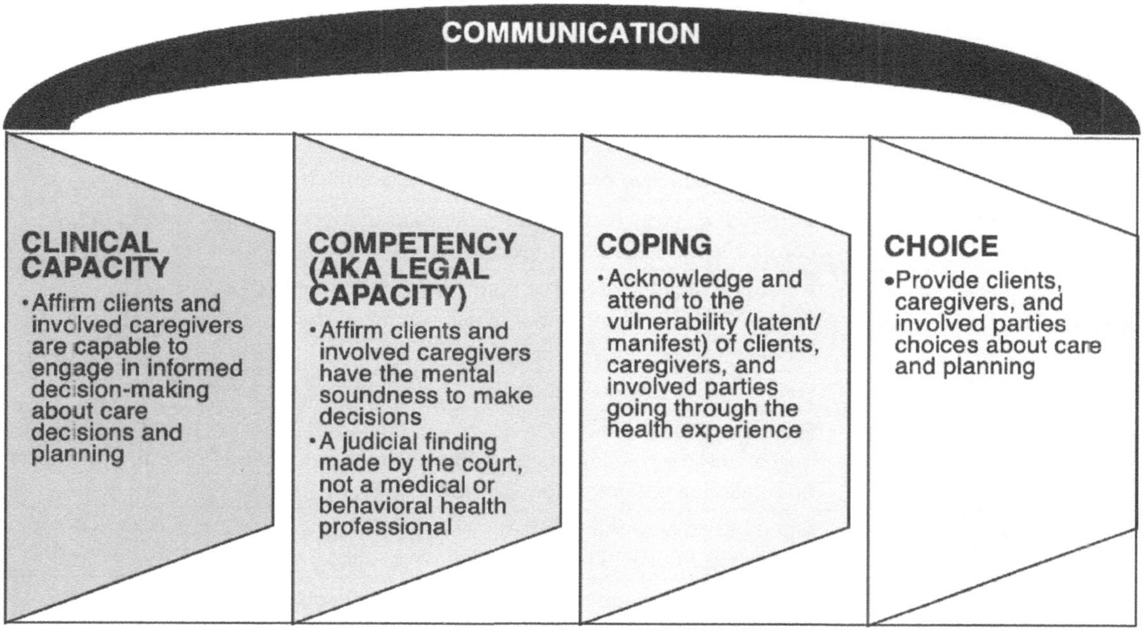

Adapted from Fink-Samnick, 2023

MENTAL STATUS EXAMINATIONS

A *mental status examination* (MSE) is a standardized evaluation of a patient's psychological, cognitive, and emotional functioning. MSEs focus on specific domains of functioning and whether they fall within normal limits. For example, is the patient alert and oriented to person and place but not consistently time? Does she claim to be happy but appear to be seething with frustration and anger? Does she think messages are coming through a bedside lamp and controlling others' actions? What about suicidal ideation? An MSE assesses these domains.

An MSE is presented as a comprehensive but concise paragraph or bullet-point list and paints a clear picture of a patient's functioning. Customary elements of an MSE appear in Table 11.1.

Table 11.1: *Elements of a mental status exam*

Element	Description
1. General appearance, attitude, and behavior	State of clothing and grooming as appropriate to season, disheveled or neat manner, whether engaging, cooperative, combative, or guarded
2. Characteristics of speech	Quantity, quality, and amount of language: rate, volume, ease and flow of communication; tone or emotional quality of speech
3. Affect	Observable facial or emotional state: blunted, flat, elated, or incongruent
4. Mood	An actual affective or emotional state: cheerful, happy, labile, sad
5. Thought content	Intrusive, disruptive, disorganized, obsessive or psychotic-thinking (e.g., compulsions, delusions, hallucinations, paranoia)
6. Imminent or foreseeable harm to self or public	Presence of suicidal and/or homicidal ideation; note if person engages in nonsuicidal self-injurious behaviors with type, frequency, and severity (e.g., burning, cutting)
7. Memory	Defined by presence and quality, short-term and long-term recall
8. Orientation	Based on four spheres: person, place, time, and situation; noted as alert and oriented x 4 (abbreviated 'AOx4'). When accounting for fewer spheres of orientation, it becomes, for example, 'AOx3, not place.'
9. Intellectual level	Often based on general observation of intelligence or IQ: noted by average, borderline, intellectual disability, above average, gifted
10. Insight	Ability to understand the issues at hand, as in diagnosis or reason for an interview or meeting; assessed as poor, fair, good, or improving
11. Judgment	Ability to understand and anticipate the benefits and/or consequences of one's actions; assessed as poor, fair, good, or improving

Mini-Mental Status Exam

The Mini-Mental Status Exam (MMSE) has been widely used for over 50 years. Soon after it was introduced, it became an industry favorite for its quick, simple, and standardized assessment of a patient's cognitive capacity. As discussed in Chapter 2, at the time many patients were being admitted for care, particularly to EDs, acute care hospitals, and nursing homes, due to deinstitutionalization. Some were aging, and many were military veterans; a majority had a history of SMI or acute onset of symptoms that warranted emergent stabilization. The MMSE helped clinicians triage the influx of patients.

MMSEs are traditionally divided into two sections, as shown in Table 11.2; part 1 evaluates orientation, memory, and attention, and part 2 assesses verbal and written ability (Folstein et al., 1975).

Table 11.2: *Mini-Mental Status Exam*

ELEMENT	DESCRIPTION
PART 1	
Orientation to time	Assesses awareness of the current date, day, month, year, and season
Orientation to place	Evaluates recognition of present location, such as country, state, city, building, or floor
Registration	Assesses ability to immediately recall information, usually words spoken by the examiner
Attention and calculation	Measures focus and basic arithmetic skills, use of tasks such as serial 7s or spelling words backwards
Recall	Checks short-term memory by asking a person to remember previously mentioned words
Naming	Determines ability to correctly name common objects presented by the examiner
Repetition	Assesses ability to repeat a phrase as stated by the examiner
PART 2	
Comprehension	Evaluates understanding and following of verbal or written instructions
Reading	Assesses ability to read and carry out a written command
Writing	Examines ability to write a complete sentence spontaneously
Drawing	Assesses visuospatial skills such as replicating a simple figure or design

Adapted from Folstein et al., 1975

Mini-Cog

If you have ever asked a patient to perform the four activities shown in Box 11.1, you are familiar with the *Mini-Cog* (Borsen et al., 2000). Increased industry attention to utilization and resource management in the early 21st century called for comprehensive but quick screening tools for acute and primary care settings. Practitioners, patients, and their caregivers were also eager for early identification of cognitive dysfunction, particularly for Alzheimer's and other types of dementia. A timelier diagnosis meant earlier access to the new generation of prescription medications that promised to delay cognitive deterioration.

Enter the Mini-Cog, which could be completed in 3 minutes or less, with 84 percent accuracy across populations (Abayomi et al., 2024). It was quickly adopted across the industry and set the standard for screening instruments to follow. The four simple steps thwarted influence from language, literacy, or educational levels, compared with other cognitive tests. It could be administered as easily in annual health and wellness screenings as by family members or homecare providers. The four steps appear in Box 11.1.

Box 11.1: Elements of the Mini-Cog

1. Obtain the person's attention
2. Give the person any 3 words to repeat and ensure understanding
    a. Cue the person that the words may be asked again later in the session
3. Ask the person to draw a clock
4. Ask the person to recall the initial 3 words

Adapted from Mini-Cog, 2025

Montreal Cognitive Assessment

The Montreal Cognitive Assessment (MoCA) is another popular and brief MSE standardized screening tool. It assesses and identifies patients with mild to moderate cognitive impairment and early dementia. The MoCA takes approximately 10-15 minutes to administer and is scored out of 30 points; a score of 26 or above is generally considered normal. The instrument is widely used in primary care and other clinical settings. The domains assessed appear in Box 11.2.

Other screening tools are also used to assess mental status and cognition across health conditions and populations. Many have been developed for digital devices and administration across virtual portals. A list of MSE tools appears in Table 11.3.

Box 11.2: Montreal Cognitive Assessment (MoCA) domains

- Attention and concentration
- Calculations
- Conceptual thinking
- Executive functions
- Language
- Memory
- Orientation
- Visuoconstructional skills

Nasreddine et al., 2005

Table 11.3: *Screening tools for general assessment of mental status and cognition*

Instrument	Focus	Source
Ascertain Dementia (AD) 8: The Washington University Dementia Screening Test	An 8-item informant-based tool of yes/no questions used to detect early signs of dementia • A family member, close friend, or caregiver is asked if the person has had changes in memory, problem-solving, judgment, or daily functioning. • Examples include difficulty remembering appointments, handling finances, or learning to use new tools, gadgets, or devices.	Galvin, J.E., Roe, C.M., Powlishta, K.K., Coats, M.A., Muich, S.J., Grant, E., Miller, J.P., Storandt, M., & Morris, J.C. (2005). The AD8: A brief informant interview to detect dementia. Neurology, 65(4), 559-564. https://doi.org/10.1212/01.wnl.0000172958.95282.2a
Addenbrooke's Cognitive Examination-III (ACE-III), and Mini-ACE	A brief bedside cognitive screening test that takes 15-20 minutes to administer; assesses cognitive function in individuals with suspected dementia or other cognitive impairments • Evaluates key cognitive domains: o attention o memory o language o visuospatial abilities o verbal fluency	Beishon, L.C., Batterham, A.P., Quinn, T.J., Nelson, C.P., Panerai, R.B., Robinson, T., & Haunton, V.J. (2019). Addenbrooke's Cognitive Examination III (ACE-III) and mini-ACE for the detection of dementia and mild cognitive impairment. The Cochrane Database of Systematic Reviews, 12(12), CD013282. https://doi.org/10.1002/14651858.CD013282.pub2
Computerized Cognitive Screen (CoCoSc) (digital)	A 15-min computerized cognitive screen administered on a touchscreen device covering: • memory • executive functions • orientation • attention and working memory • prospective memory	Wong, A., Fong, C.H., Mok, V.C., Leung, K.T., & Tong, R.K. (2017). Computerized Cognitive Screen (CoCoSc): A self-administered computerized test for screening for cognitive impairment in community social centers. Journal of Alzheimer's Disease, 59(4), 1299-1306. https://doi.org/10.3233/JAD-170196

Instrument	Focus	Source
General Practitioner Assessment of Cognition (PCoG)	A 2-part screening tool to help PCPs identify patients with cognitive impairments, potentially dementia • Combines a brief cognitive test administered to the patient with a short interview by a caregiver or informant.	Brodaty, H., Pond, D., Kemp, N.M., Luscombe, G., Harding, L., Berman, K., & Huppert, F.A. (2002). The GPCOG: A new screening test for dementia designed for general practice. Journal of the American Geriatrics Society, 50(3), 530-534. https://doi.org/10.1046/j.1532-5415.2002.50122.x
Geras Solutions Cognitive Test (digital)	A 16-item screening instrument assessing multiple domains: • cognition • attention • executive functioning • memory • language • visuospatial skills • social cognition The tool quickly identifies cognitive decline in clinical populations, particularly motor neuron disease and mild neurocognitive disorders.	Bloniecki, V., Ulfvarson, J., Javanshiri, K., Hagman, G., Freund-Levi, Y., & Nordström, A. (2023). The Geras Solutions Cognitive Test for assessing cognitive impairment: Normative data from a population-based cohort. The Journal of Prevention of Alzheimer's Disease, 10(2), 207-211. https://doi.org/10.14283/jpad.2023.9
Informant Questionnaire on Cognitive Decline in the Elderly (IQCODE)	A 16- to 26-item screening tool that assesses changes in an older adult's cognitive functioning over time, based on information provided by someone who knows the person well (e.g., family member, close friend, caregiver) • The informant rates how the person's memory and thinking skills have changed over the past 10 years (or a shorter time frame, based on the version used). Focuses on: o Everyday cognitive abilities (e.g., remembering recent events, learning new things, handling finances) o Managing daily activities	Jorm, A.F., & Korten, A.E. (1988). Informant Questionnaire on Cognitive Decline in the Elderly (IQCODE) [Database record]. APA PsycTests. https://doi.org/10.1037/t03166-000

Instrument	Focus	Source
Memory Impairment Scale (MIS)	A 4-item cued-recall test designed to screen for memory problems, such as early Alzheimer's and other dementias • Uses controlled encoding with category cues to ensure poor recall is due to memory impairment rather than lack of attention or comprehension.	Buschke, H., Kuslansky, G., Katz, M., Stewart, W. F., Sliwinski, M.J., Eckholdt, H.M., & Lipton, R.B. (1999). Screening for dementia with the Memory Impairment Screen. Neurology, 52(2), 231-238. https://doi.org/10.1212/WNL.52.2.231
Rowland Universal Dementia Assessment Scale (RUDAS)	A 6-item tool to assess cognitive domains: • memory • praxis • language • judgement • drawing • body orientation	Storey, J.E., Rowland, J.T.J., Conforti, D.A., & Dickson, H.G. (2004). The Rowland Universal Dementia Assessment Scale (RUDAS): A multicultural cognitive assessment scale. International Psychogeriatrics, 16(1), 13-31. https://doi.org/10.1017/S1041610204000043

IN THE TRENCHES CONSIDERATIONS FOR CASE MANAGERS

Case managers strive to engage patients and their support systems in care and to build positive therapeutic relationships. But challenging and disruptive behaviors can obstruct their efforts, and personality disorders are marked by these types of behaviors, which can directly influence how patients form relationships, participate in the care process, and respond to interventions. Another difficult situation for case managers is emergent escalation of a patient's mental health condition. Case managers are being called into emergency situations with greater frequency and should learn to navigate them proficiently.

PERSONALITY DISORDERS AND CHARACTER TRAITS

Over 10 percent of the world's population has at least one *personality disorder* (Winspear et al., 2020), though it can feel like more when you're in the thick of it. The intense behavioral presentation of personality disorders and the tense dynamics that result can contribute to burnout, leading to healthcare workforce attrition and turnover.

When teaching social work master's students about personality disorders, I often frame them like this: I explain that every person is born with traits of each disorder. For example, as youth, we can all be a bit anxious, avoidant, dependent, or guarded. Teens can be a bit dramatic about life decisions or a bit obsessive over details. Let's face it, most of us like to do things in a certain way, at a certain time, and in a certain order.

The developmental life cycle teaches that individuals outgrow the extreme presentation of these personality attributes over time, as they move through each life stage. Children typically learn how to play and socialize with others and leave behind the 'my way or the highway' mindset. As adolescents progress to young adulthood, their egos develop to a more mature state.

Yet the maturation process doesn't always go as planned. Life stressors, adverse childhood experiences, and traumas can impede ego maturation, and behavioral traits of youth become ingrained parts of one's personality. This is when a personality trait becomes a personality disorder. Some individuals become so rigid in their likes and dislikes that any shift can cause them profound discomfort. Others have trouble reconciling information received from multiple sources; they assume one perspective is on-target and another is completely missing the mark. They can see no gray area.

Personality disorders are organized across three clusters: A, B, and C, according to shared characteristics and symptoms. The organization also supports healthcare workers to align the complex patterns of behavior and thinking. Table 11.4 shows the varied personality disorders and their categorization by cluster.

Table 11.4: *DSM-5-TR diagnoses for personality disorders, by cluster*

DSM-5-TR Diagnosis	Code
Cluster A: Odd, eccentric behaviors and thinking patterns	
Paranoid personality disorder	F60.0
Schizoid personality disorder	F60.1
Schizotypal personality disorder	F21
Cluster B: Dramatic, emotional, or erratic behaviors and thinking patterns	
Antisocial personality disorder	F60.2
Borderline personality disorder	F60.3
Histrionic personality disorder	F60.4
Narcissistic personality disorder	F60.81
Cluster C: Anxious or fearful behaviors and thinking patterns	
Avoidant personality disorder	F60.6
Dependent personality disorder	F60.7
Obsessive-compulsive personality disorders	F60.5
Other personality disorders	
Personality change due to another medical condition	F07.0
Other specified personality disorder	F60.89
Unspecified personality disorder	F60.9

American Psychiatric Association, 2022

DISRUPTIVE BEHAVIORS AND THEIR IMPACT ON TREATMENT

Patients with personality disorders commonly respond reactively to the care team, particularly when their ego feels threatened or they perceive their voice isn't valued. Even well-intended case managers can be unaware they present as dictating care to the patient, rather than collaborating as a treatment partner. It is critical case managers approach these patients with grace instead of confrontation. The literature validates the importance of mutual understanding, shared goals and priorities, and respectful communication (Moreno-Leal et al., 2024; Rothstein, 2011).

Patients with personality disorders may compensate for feeling out of control of their care or for not feeling heard. In doing so, the traits of their personality disorder come to the forefront. For example, persons with anti-social and borderline personality disorder (BPD) may have intense emotional reactions to receiving information from multiple members of the care team. They may engage in *splitting,* viewing one provider as all right and another as all wrong. Or they may push the boundaries of a practitioner-patient relationship by sharing intimate personal details, trying to schedule social outings, or trying to connect on social media. Patients with histrionic personality disorder behave melodramatically, making out-of-the-ordinary requests, such as demanding extra prescriptions without evaluation or pleading through repeated, long messages via the patient portal. Patients with dependent personality disorder may push providers to make treatment decisions for them by feigning overwhelm or powerlessness. Others may try to manipulate providers by giving compliments, positive reviews on social media, or gifts.

TRAUMA-DIRECTED TACTICS

Case managers often tell me that their priority in the trenches is managing the disruptive behaviors that obstruct the care process, rather than rendering a mental health diagnosis. Motivational interviewing and other short-term interventions enhance management of disruptive behaviors. Chapter 12 will review these valued counseling techniques.

Another innovative approach to managing difficult behaviors is *trauma-directed tactics.* The ten tactics in Box 11.3 embed the tenets of trauma-informed care from Table 10.8. The steps also align with the Behavioral Health Conversation Map in Table 1.4.

Box 11.3: Ten trauma-directed tactics to manage disruptive behaviors

1. Set safety and inform patients why you are meeting
2. Engage patients with empathy and authenticity to build trust
3. Respect patient autonomy to advance choice
4. Talk to and with patients rather than down to or at them
5. Forge collaboration to avoid power struggles with patients
6. Establish clear boundaries in the provider-patient relationship
7. Respect the patient perspective to promote self-efficacy and empowerment
8. Assess for suicidality and immediate self-harm
9. Evaluate for psychopharmacological interventions
10. Recognize and address co-occurring conditions which can complicate treatment (e.g., anxiety, depression, substance use)

SCREENING AND ASSESSMENT TOOLS FOR PERSONALITY DISORDERS

The strong drive to name and categorize behaviors and diagnoses has led to numerous screening tools for personality disorders, many of them self-report tools and accessed online through social media and consumer platforms. Self-report measures for personality disorder are imperfect, however, due to *social desirability bias*, when people respond in ways they perceive as favorable. This bias can lead to faulty assessments. Evidence-based recommendations appear in Table 11.5.

Table 11.5: *Screening tools for personality disorders (youth and adults)*

Instrument	Focus	Source
Diagnostic Interview for Personality Disorders (DIPD)	A structured clinician-administered interview of > 200 questions to assess the presence of personality disorders based on DSM criteria, with their duration and impact on: • Current functioning: recent behaviors and experiences • Lifetime history: patterns and onset of traits • Rule-out criteria: Symptoms due to other mental or medical conditions	Zanarini, M.C., Frankenburg, F.R., Sickel, A.E., & Yong, L. (1996). The Diagnostic Interview for DSM-IV Personality Disorders (DIPD-IV). Belmont, MA: McLean Hospital.
International Personality Disorder Examination (IPDE)	A semi-structured clinical interview to assess personality disorders per DSM and ICD-criteria with 2 components: • a self-administered screening questionnaire • a clinician-administered interview The tool emphasizes cultural adaptability and standardized administration to ensure reliability across varied settings.	Loranger, A.W., Sartorius, N., Andreoli, A., Berger, P., Buchheim, P., Channabasavanna, S.M., Coid, B., Dahl, A., Diekstra, R.F.W., Ferguson, B., Jacobsberg et al. (1994). The International Personality Disorder Examination: The World Health Organization/ Alcohol, Drug Abuse, and Mental Health Administration international pilot study of personality disorders. *Archives of General Psychiatry, 51*(3), 215-224. https://doi.org/10.1001/archpsyc.1994.03950030051005
McLean Screening Instrument for Borderline Personality Disorder (MSI-BPD)	A brief, 10-item self-report questionnaire of yes/no questions to quickly screen for the likelihood of borderline personality disorder (BPD): A score of 7 or higher notes probable BPD	Semaan, F., & Croarkin, P.E. (2025). The McLean Screening Instrument for borderline personality disorder: A review. *Journal of Psychiatric Practice, 31*(1), 20-23. https://doi.org/10.1097/PRA.0000000000000827
Narcissistic Personality Inventory (NPI)	A 40-question self-report questionnaire to assess the presence of narcissistic personality traits	Raskin, R.N., & Hall, C.S. (1979). *Narcissistic Personality Inventory (NPI)* [Database record]. APA PsycTests. https://doi.org/10.1037/t00001-000

Instrument	Focus	Source
Pathological Narcissism Inventory (PNI)	A 52-item, self-report, Likert scale questionnaire to assess the traits of pathological narcissism. 7 subscales: 1. Contingent self-esteem: dependence on external validation 2. Exploitativeness: manipulation or taking advantage of others 3. Self-sacrificing self-enhancement: boosting self-image via perceived altruism 4. Hiding the self: avoidance of showing perceived flaws or weaknesses 5. Grandiose fantasy: preoccupation with fantasies of power, success, or idealized relationships 6. Devaluing: dismissing or belittling others to protect self-image 7. Entitlement rage: intense anger when expectations are unmet	Pincus, A.L., Ansell, E.B., Pimentel, C.A., Cain, N.M., Wright, A.G.C., & Levy, K.N. (2009). *Pathological Narcissism Inventory (PNI)* [Database record]. APA PsycTests. https://doi.org/10.1037/t00490-000
Structured Clinical Interview for *DSM-5* Personality Disorders	A semi-structured, clinician-administered interview to assess the 10 personality disorders in DSM-5, and presence and severity of traits: • Organized by disorder, with specific questions linked directly to each diagnostic criterion for paranoid, schizoid, schizotypal, antisocial, borderline, histrionic, narcissistic, avoidant, dependent, and obsessive-compulsive personality disorders • Uses a 3-point scale to denote symptom presence: absent, subthreshold, or threshold	First, M.B., Williams, J.B.W., Benjamin, L.S., & Spitzer, R.L. (2016). *Structured Clinical Interview for DSM-5 Personality Disorders (SCID-5-PD).* American Psychiatric Association Publishing. https://doi.org/10.1176/appi.books.9780890426807

Instrument	Focus	Source
Structured Clinical Interview for DSM-5 Alternative Model of Personality Disorders	A semi-structured interview to assess the Alternative Model for Personality Disorders (AMPD) in Section III of DSM-5. • Module I: Level of Personality Functioning Scale (self and interpersonal functioning) • Module II: Pathological Personality Traits (negative affectivity, detachment, antagonism, disinhibition, and psychoticism) • Module III: Hybrid Categorical-Dimensional Diagnosis (applies AMPD criteria to antisocial, avoidant, borderline, narcissistic, obsessive-compulsive, and schizotypal personality disorders; functioning rated on a 4-point scale, traits on a 3-point scale • Captures dimensional (severity and traits) and categorical parts of diagnosis	First, M.B., Skodol, A.E., Bender, D.S., & Oldham, J.M. (2018). *Structured Clinical Interview for the DSM-5 Alternative Model for Personality Disorders (SCID-5-AMPD).* American Psychiatric Association Publishing. https://doi.org/10.1176/appi.books.9780890427590

DE-ESCALATION OF PSYCHIATRIC EMERGENCIES

An epidemic of violence in healthcare settings has undermined efforts for occupational safety. Staff have been increasingly assaulted by patients displaying aggressive and disruptive behavior, often during psychiatric emergencies. Emotions can flair at any touchpoint of healthcare, though, often related to a new diagnosis, expectations for treatment, or misunderstanding of discharge options. Patients in psychiatric crisis warrant de-escalation tactics to keep patients and staff safe.

STAGES OF A PSYCHIATRIC EMERGENCY

Psychiatric emergencies can be frightening events for the care team. They generally refer to acute disturbances of thought, behavior, or mood that require immediate intervention to prevent harm to the patient, caregivers, or other members of the healthcare team. These situations often call for rapid assessment and stabilization of the patient's condition, though often without a clear clinical history. Case managers may be asked to step in during one of five psychiatric emergency stages displayed in Figure 11.2.

Figure 11.2: *Stages of a psychiatric emergency*

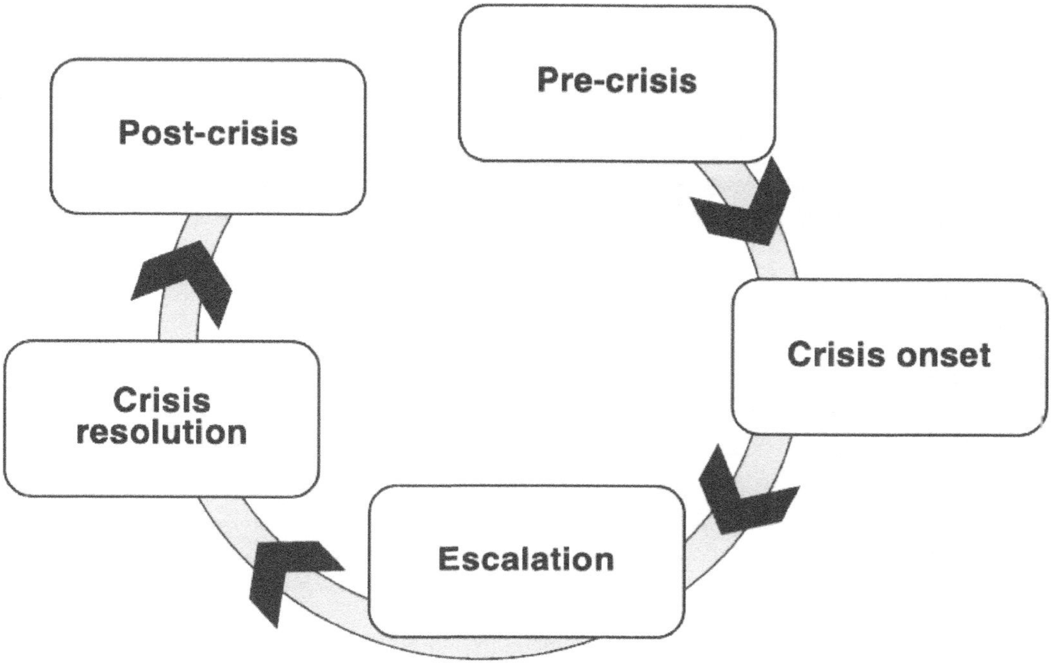

In the pre-crisis phase, a patient may present with subtle changes in behavior, mood, or thought patterns that can reflect potential escalation. There is no conventional way to identify these signs across all patients and conditions; a patient on the verge of psychiatric emergency may present in ways even healthcare workers don't expect, such as vocalizing increased sadness, withdrawal, or frequent worry about one's purpose in the world. But as discussed in Chapter 6, hypomania can be a clue for exacerbation of symptoms.

During onset of a crisis, the patient shows apparent deterioration in his or her behavior. Intense agitation and confusion can often be observed, and the individual appears disoriented to person, place, time, or sphere. Mania and self-destructive behaviors can manifest, possibly reflecting intentional self-harm or impulsivity with poor judgement, such as driving intoxicated or under the influence of substances. During crisis escalation, the patient's behaviors and actions pose an immediate risk to self or others. There may periods of self-harm, extreme aggression and violence, or attempted suicide.

As emergency intervention is rendered, the patient is stabilized though medication management or other therapeutic treatments. The final, post-crisis phase encompasses critical actions to minimize future crises and promote the patient's recovery through continued treatment, support, and monitoring.

PHASES OF PSYCHIATRIC DE-ESCALATION

Psychiatric de-escalation is a multifaceted approach and relies on dedicated steps. Assessment, communication, and respect for the patient's dignity and safety are critical elements, which align with case management regulations, accreditation, codes of ethics, and standards of practice. Box 11.4 displays seminal guidance for de-escalation over four phases, with a list of considerations included.

Box 11.4: Phases of psychiatric emergency de-escalation

1. **Recognize, assess, and triage**
   - Prioritize safety: Ensure your safety and that of others. This may involve having enough staff present or considering environmental factors.
   - Identify the stage of escalation for the patient: Early recognition of escalations in behavior allows for timely intervention.
   - Assess the patient's state: Consider potential triggers, underlying conditions, and history of aggression.
2. **Respond calmly and respectfully**
   - Maintain a calm manner: Avoid reacting with anger or frustration, which can escalate a situation.
   - Use a calm, soft voice: Avoid shouting or use of a condescending tone.
   - Use non-threatening body language: Maintain an open stance, avoid sudden movements, and make eye contact.
   - Respect personal space: Give the patient enough physical space to feel comfortable.
   - Validate feelings and concerns: Acknowledge the patient's emotions and perspective, even if you disagree.
3. **Ensure effective communication**
   - Listen actively: Pay attention to the patient's verbal and non-verbal interactions.
   - Use clear and concise communication: Use simple language and avoid jargon.
   - Avoid arguing: Seek common ground and solutions.
   - Offer choices and optimism: Empower the patient by offering choices and expressing hope for a positive outcome.
4. **Set limits**
   - Establish clear expectations: Communicate boundaries and expectations in a respectful yet firm manner.
   - Address inappropriate behavior: Clearly state what behavior is unacceptable and associated consequences.
5. **Other important considerations**
   - Environmental factors: Minimize noise, bright lights, and other triggers.
   - Staff training: Ensure staff are trained in de-escalation techniques and understand how their own attitudes and behaviors can aggravate a situation.
   - Debrief: Post-incident, debrief with the patient and staff to support all involved. Identify what worked well and what could be improved.

Adapted from Stubbe, 2023

CONCLUSION

Your mastery of working with behavioral health populations continues to grow. You now have the knowledge to manage mental status exams, personality disorders, and psychiatric de-escalation. We have one final practice area to address. On to Chapter 12 and brief interventions and treatment planning.

CONTEMPLATION QUESTIONS

1. Reflect on a patient from past or present.
   a) Review the elements of a Mental Status Exam in Table 11.1.
   b) Complete an MSE on your patient.
2. Reflect on your experience interacting with a patient diagnosed with a personality disorder shown in Table 11.4.
   a) What challenges did you face during the interaction?
   b) How did you reconcile those challenges?
   c) What was the outcome of the situation?
   d) Identify what information in this chapter would enhance your ability to manage that situation now.

Use the case scenario below for questions 3-5.

Let's revisit Jake, our animated and potentially manic young man from the Contemplation Questions in Chapter 7. He has been brought to a hospital ED for evaluation after his girlfriend, Carina, called the police. She reports that Jake became verbally and physically abusive toward her. Carina also shares the following information during intake:

- Jake's colleagues notice he is on a constant high. They have told Carina, "He has become verbally abusive to staff."
- Jake's mother shared with Carina, "I always told Jake he was the most important person in the world. His father was a real narcissist and used to tell Jake, 'You have to believe in your own value, or nobody will believe in you! You must enter every meeting showing your power and brains; YOU are in charge. You may not be the smartest person in that room but need to act like you are.' I always worried that messaging didn't teach Jake how to play well with others."
- At a recent party, Jake's boss told Carina, "Jake is getting arrogant, but he gets the job done. He has a promising future in the company if he keeps saving us this much money."
- Carina shares they have fought constantly since moving in together. "Jake's arrogance has turned to aggression, and he devalues others constantly. We fought last week about whether to go out for dinner or order in; such a small thing turned into such a big deal. He was furious, and at first I thought he was playing, but soon realized he wasn't. It was the first

time in all our years together that I was frightened. When he slapped me today, I called the police."

1. Review the stages of a psychiatric emergency in Figure 11.2. What stage do you think Jake is in, and why?
2. You have been asked to assess Jake with the clinical director of the ED. Craft a plan to approach Jake using the Phases of Psychiatric Emergency De-Escalation in Box 11.4. What would you do in each of the five phases?
3. Now walk through the Behavioral Health Conversation Map in Table 1.4.
    - Reflect on how you would move through phases 1-7.
    - Identify what you would you need to consider for each phase.

REFERENCES

- Abayomi, S.N., Sritharan, P., Yan, E., Saripella, A., Alhamdah, Y., Englesakis, M., Tartaglia, M.C., He, D., & Chung, F. (2024). The diagnostic accuracy of the Mini-Cog screening tool for the detection of cognitive impairment—A systematic review and meta-analysis. PloS One, 19(3), e0298686. https://doi.org/10.1371/journal.pone.0298686
- American Psychiatric Association. (2022). Diagnostic and Statistical Manual of Mental Disorders (5th ed., text rev.).
- Borson, S., Scanlan, J., Brush, M., Vitaliano, P., & Dokmak, A. (2000). The Mini-Cog: A cognitive 'vital signs' measure for dementia screening in multi-lingual elderly. *International Journal of Geriatric Psychiatry, 15*(11), 1021-1027. https://doi.org/10.1002/1099-1166(200011)15:11<1021::AID-GPS234>3.0.CO;2-6
- Folstein, M.F., Folstein, S.E., & McHugh, P.R. (1975). "Mini-mental state": A practical method for grading the cognitive state of patients for the clinician. Journal of Psychiatric Research, 12(3), 189-198. https://doi.org/10.1016/0022-3956(75)90026-6
- Fink-Samnick, E. (2023). The Ethical Case Manager: Tools and Tactics. Blue Bayou Press.
- Moreno-Leal, P., Leal-Costa, C., Díaz-Agea, J.L., Castaño-Molina, M.L.Á., Conesa-Ferrer, M.B., & De Souza-Oliveira, A.C. (2024). Disruptive behavior and factors associated with patient safety climate: A cross-sectional study of nurses' and physicians' perceptions. Journal of Nursing Management, 2024, 5568390. https://doi.org/10.1155/2024/5568390
- Mini-Cog. (2025). Step-by-Step Instructions: Mini-Cog. Retrieved August 11, 2025, from https://mini-cog.com
- Nasreddine, Z.S., Phillips, N.A., Bédirian, V., Charbonneau, S., Whitehead, V., Collin, I., Cummings, J.L., & Chertkow, H. (2005). The Montreal Cognitive Assessment, MoCA: A brief screening tool for mild cognitive impairment. Journal of the American Geriatrics Society, 53(4), 695-699. https://doi.org/10.1111/j.1532-5415.2005.53221.x

- Rosenstein, A.H. (2011). Managing disruptive behaviors in the health care setting: Focus on obstetrics services. American Journal of Obstetrics and Gynecology, 204(3), 187-192. https://doi.org/10.1016/j.ajog.2010.10.899
- Stubbe, D.E. (2023). Psychiatric emergencies: Empowering connections to de-escalate aggression. Focus (American Psychiatric Publishing), 21(1), 54-57. https://doi.org/10.1176/appi.focus.20220079
- Winsper, C., Bilgin, A., Thompson, A., Marwaha, S., Chanen, A.M., Singh, S.P., Wang, A., & Furtado, V. (2020). The prevalence of personality disorders in the community: A global systematic review and meta-analysis. The British Journal of Psychiatry, 216(2), 69-78. doi:10.1192/bjp.2019.166
- Widiger, T.A., Hines, A., & Crego, C. (2023). Evidence-based assessment of personality disorder. Assessment, 31(1), 191-198. https://doi.org/10.1177/10731911231176461

CHAPTER 12

INTERVENTIONS AND SHORT-TERM TREATMENT

INTRODUCTION

Imagine a patient sitting across from you who appears motivated to change his behaviors. He understands that increased activity will lower his weight and decrease strain on his joints and musculature. That, in turn, will lead to better management of the chronic pain and insomnia that has reduced his quality of life for decades.

Your employer's quality measures require you to focus on patient engagement. But neither the employer's measures nor accreditation requirements define what it means to engage a patient. Questions mount as you consider the critical next steps. What stage of engagement—or change—is the patient at? What short-term interventions can be implemented so the patient experiences sufficient improvement? What relaxation techniques could benefit the patient? With only two or three sessions to advance a treatment plan, what specific, measurable, achievable, relevant, and timely goals can you and patient develop?

Herein lies a case manager's consummate challenge: to effectively engage and partner with patients in a way that allows the execution of efficient short-term interventions and effective treatment plans. This shared process facilitates the creation of mutually determined goals that yield successful outcomes. These topics and other related themes are our focus in Chapter 12.

BEHAVIORAL LEARNING OBJECTIVES

1. Understand theories that support successful treatment planning
2. Distinguish between engagement of patients and patient engagement
3. Recognize the stages of change in the Transtheoretical Model
4. Identify the primary theme of each motivational interviewing phase

5. Utilize the 5 As framework of brief intervention with behavioral health
6. Understand various relaxation techniques used in short-term treatment
7. Explain the value of sleep hygiene to whole person health and wellness
8. Apply each letter of the SMART acronym for treatment planning
9. Apply Case Management's Behavioral Health Conversation Map to treatment planning

ESSENTIAL TERMS

- 5 As
- Decisional balance
- Engagement of patients
- Motivational interviewing
- Self-efficacy
- Sleep hygiene
- SMART goals
- Transtheoretical model (Stages of Change)

THEORETICAL FOUNDATION

Case managers must understand the theories that undergird the treatment relationship, treatment planning, and a brief intervention to achieve successful outcomes and meet employer expectations.

ENGAGEMENT OF THE PATIENT VERSUS 'PATIENT ENGAGEMENT' METRICS

The quality of rapport-building will dictate the success or failure of an entire treatment encounter (Fink-Samnick, 2021). This fact is independent of treatment setting or mode (e.g., in person, telephonic, or virtual). Yet many organizations treat patient engagement as an output of the care process, rather than the means to attain a successful treatment outcome.

This perspective on rapport does not alter the onus for behavioral change, which remains with the patient. It does, however, emphasize the case manager's duty to set a trusting, collaborative, and respectful atmosphere as the steadfast foundation of the practitioner-patient therapeutic alliance. Still, the scope of successful patient engagement isn't detailed in our industry's standards and reporting—while HEDIS includes measures on patient engagement in certain areas, the measure provides only a narrow view. True engagement with a patient or a population is a far broader concept. It starts with building a safe and trusting space to inform a person's healthcare decision-making and to promote self-management (Harris et al., 2011). Seminal research validates the profound impact of positive patient relationships and engagement with patients on quality of care (Marzaban et al., 2022).

Engaging with patients is among the primary competencies taught to members of the interprofessional care team. Social workers and other behavioral health professionals are weaned on this concept in academic coursework. But the concept is not taught equally or consistently across all healthcare disciplines. Onboarding processes for case managers may gloss over it, choosing to focus instead on regulations and requirements. As a result, many case managers inadvertently and unintentionally talk *at* patients rather than *with* them. The patient's or family's reluctance to accept treatment becomes misunderstood as refusal of care or non-adherence.

Case managers are constantly exposed to varied patient cultural perspectives, as well as continual need to reconcile mental health stigmas. This concept was explored in Chapter 1, though bears repeating at this point in the book. Case managers must prioritize learning about each patient's views and what matters most, especially in considering treatment planning.

ENGAGEMENT OF PATIENTS AS A PROFESSIONAL NORM

Professional standards of practice and ethical codes identify the importance of developing rapport with patients, their families, and support systems (American Nurses Association, 2025; Commission for Case Manager Certification, 2023; Case Management Society of America, 2022, 2024; National Association of Social Workers, 2021). Respect for patient autonomy is the core of patient-centric treatment. Reflect on the case scenario in Box 12.1.

Would you, or any case manager or healthcare practitioner you know, accept this quality of care? The limited communication and failure to respect Brent's unique situation does not meet the minimum standards of practice defined by any regulatory body, professional association, or credentialing entity. Yet Brent's experience is more the norm than the exception across every busy touchpoint of care. We can also expect that Brent will be judged by Elena and Dr. Jaqua as resistant to care. Respect for each patient's integrity and dignity should always be heeded to minimize the risk of a flawed treatment process.

Healthcare encounters are fraught with unexpected stress and emotion. Chapter 10 addressed the value of providing trauma-informed and directed treatment experiences. Respectful engagement of patients is an extension of this approach. Table 12.1 details guideposts to soundly implement this effort.

Box 12.1: How to not engage a patient

Elena is the behavioral health case manager for a community health clinic. She moves quickly through her day, helping one patient, then quickly moving on to help the next. Brent P. is a patient waiting in a treatment room and next on Elena's roster. She assumes Mr. P. will require only a quick visit, rather than a lengthy encounter.

When Elena enters the treatment room, she recalls meeting Brent earlier in the year. *Brent will remember meeting me, too,* she thinks, and skips her introduction. Elena scans her tablet for information and starts speaking, failing to make eye contact with Brent.

"Mr. P., Dr. Jaqua asked me to get you this list of mental health providers." Elena hands Brent a list of names, then leaves. The encounter lasts less than a minute.

Brent had no time to ask questions about the reason for the referral. He wanted to say that in his family, mental illness is a sin, only ever discussed privately with the family's spiritual leader. Brent wonders if Dr. Jacqua will see him again if he doesn't contact the mental health practitioner.

Table 12.1: *Engagement of the patient*

Open with empathy and respect
Use empathic communication and active listening
Speak *to*, not *at*, patients and their support systems
Be intentional, open, and honest
Use culturally-inclusive and sensitive practices
Engage patients and involved support system as partners
Ensure they understand diagnosis, prognosis, and treatment options
Create opportunities for them to ask questions
Educate according to health literacy
Assess for health literacy and digital health literacy
Explain treatment recommendations
Include other team members, specialists, and providers
Use patient education tools (e.g., infographics, apps)
Be dependable
Follow-up in a timely manner, as necessary
Communicate consistently
Define accountability
Designate responsibility for shared decisions
Describe follow-up actions (e.g., communications, meetings)
Work toward consensus
Prioritize patient autonomy
Agree to disagree as needed
Accept differing perspectives of treatment
Provide access to all health information
Demonstrate how to access patient portals and EHR, as needed
Access modes for accommodation, if needed (e.g., TTY systems)
Respond with patience first
Allow patients and support systems time to express emotions
Think: *How would I feel in this situation? What would I expect in this situation?*
Set limits, as appropriate
Don't take anything personally

THE TRANSTHEORETICAL MODEL AND STAGES OF CHANGE

The year 1983 was a monumental one in behavioral health. Aside from being the year I completed a master's degree in social work, it was when Prochaska and DiClemente introduced the industry to the *transtheoretical model* (TTM), or the *stages of change*. The model was originally developed to address smoking cessation though found broad application across other at-risk behaviors (e.g., substance use), behavioral health (e.g., management of anger, anxiety, depression, stress), and chronic health conditions (e.g., treatment adherence for chronic illness).

TTM remains part of the gold standard for understanding how and why individuals make intentional changes in their behavior, particularly when adopting healthier habits. It combines features of health promotion, mental healthcare, and case management. The original model included five stages, as shown in Figure 12.1. The sixth stage, relapse, was added later (Prochaska & DiClemente, 1992) to emphasize the cyclical nature of the model. The stages provide scaffolding for case managers to support patients as they work to modify their behavior. The effort for change is viewed as a non-linear series of forward and backward actions, rather than a steady forward-moving process. Any movement is viewed as an opportunity for growth and learning instead of a failure.

Decisional balance is an underlying tenet of TTM. It refers to the simple weighing of pros and cons for the person's actions and behaviors. The concept captures the natural **ambivalence** that individuals feel when they know that changing behavior may be their only option. Patients often say this ambivalence is the **biggest barrier to change** (Shtaynberger & Krebs, 2016). The decisional balance construct is also integral to patient *self-efficacy*. Patients who achieve decisional balance can assess their insight and strengths and advance their personal commitment to shifting behaviors they now see as detrimental.

Table 12.2: shows TTM in action. Reflect on the interaction between the case manager and a patient living with alcohol use. The patient's perspective and case manager role considerations should provide food for thought. Consider how you might work through this situation.

Figure 12.1: *The TTM and six stages of change*

Precontemplation
Not intending to take action within the next 6 months

↕

Contemplation
Intending to change with the next 6 months

↕

Preparation
Intending to take action in the immediate future (within the next month)

↕

Action
Making overt changes to their behavior in the moment

↕

Maintenance
Working to prevent relapse and consolidate gains

↕

Relapse
Acknowledging the cyclical nature of behavioral change

Adapted from Prochaska & DiClemente, 1983; Prochaska & DiClemente, 1992

Table 12.2: *TTM in action*

Precontemplation
• Patient mindset: "Drinking helps me relax; it's really not a big deal."
• Case manager's role: Build rapport, educate on health impacts, and explore values
Contemplation
• Patient mindset: "My drinking makes it tough to get up in the morning; those headaches are the worst. I just don't know if I can stop."
• Case manager's role: Use motivational interviewing to assess ambivalence, weigh pros and cons, and empower patient motivation.
Preparation
• Patient mindset: "I want to cut back. I'll try to drop from 8 drinks each night to 2 or 3."
• Case manager's role: Partner with the patient to set SMART goals, identify triggers, and connect with individual and group support (e.g., AA, counseling, medication-assisted treatment).

Action
• Patient actions: Actively reduces alcohol use; attends weekly counseling, builds sober support system, and avoids high-risk situations and going out only with friends who drink.
• Case manager's role: Provide ongoing support, encourage self-monitoring, celebrate successes, and troubleshoot barriers.
Maintenance
• Patient actions: Consistently reduces drinking for 6 months and has not been late to work since cutting back.
• Case manager's role: Reinforce coping strategies, help prevent relapse, and continue to support.
Relapse (as it occurs)
• Patient mindset: "This company merger is stressing me. When am I going to lose my job?" Over several weeks, increases alcohol consumption back up to 8 drinks each night.
• Case manager's role: Frames relapse as a learning opportunity, revisits triggers, and supports re-engagement in the process without judgment.

SHORT-TERM BEHAVIORAL TREATMENTS

MOTIVATIONAL INTERVIEWING

Motivational interviewing (MI) has become the industry standard to engage patients in short-term treatment, especially for management of behavioral health. Since MI is treated as a foundational intervention in academic coursework and continuing education programming, few healthcare workers are unfamiliar with it. Yet this chapter would be incomplete without a basic overview.

Although Miller and Rollnick (2023) initially developed MI to help individuals with substance use and misuse, the intervention has demonstrated success for populations managing chronic conditions, treatment non-adherence, and other issues. Over four phases, as shown in Figure 12.2, the practitioner uses open-ended questions to understand, in a non-judgmental way, how the patient views their condition, how it may or may not be impacting their life, and specific values and goals for treatment. By engaging in this way, the patient and practitioner build a trusting relationship and a constructive therapeutic alliance.

The success of MI lies in the patient-driven process, where the patient is acknowledged as the expert of their human condition. During MI, clinicians must acknowledge the ambivalence that accompanies change, accept a patient's resistance to it, and subdue their inclination to press for treatment expectations. Through these efforts, the clinician minimizes the risk of unintentionally superseding the patient's readiness for change.

Patients may present with a number of issues to address, which can be overwhelming to them and the change process overall. While the patient is viewed as the authority within their unique MI process, attention is still placed on the power of the therapeutic relationship. It serves as a means to activate the patient's intent and achieve goals. During an interview, a patient will hopefully be able to identify one or more areas or rationales for change. The original model of MI by Rollnick and Miller referred to this phase as "developing disparities." A clinician's unconditional regard supports and activates identified change within a trusting, patient-driven treatment relationship, and with a defined goal. As a result, patient *self-efficacy* toward behavioral modification is empowered, and the person becomes confident in the ability to change.

Figure 12.2: *Phases of motivational interviewing*

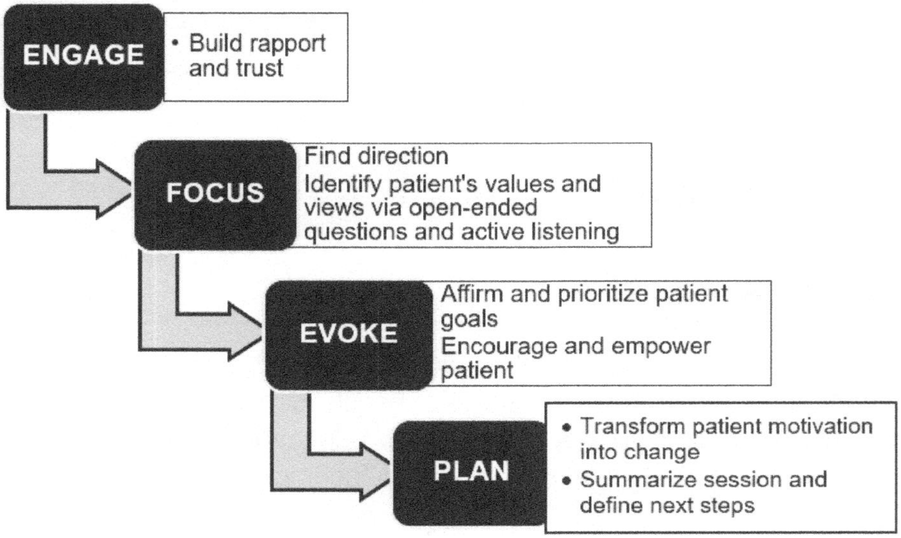

Adapted from Bischof et al., 2021; Miller & Rollnick, 2023

THE 5 AS

The *5 As model* is another established, evidence-based behavioral and cognitive-focused framework. Practitioners use the 5 As for managing at-risk behaviors and conditions, including depression, intense anxiety, panic disorder, insufficient physical activity, smoking, and weight management, and for promoting treatment adherence.

This framework, shown in Figure 12.3, encompasses five key steps: ask, advise, assess, assist, and arrange. Each step contributes to developing an individualized action plan. Iterations of the model weave in other short-term counseling interventions, such as MI, cognitive behavioral therapy, or solution focused brief therapy. A typical 5 As session lasts 30 minutes or less, which is one reason for the model's popularity across practice settings.

Figure 12.3: *The 5 As of short-term integrated care*

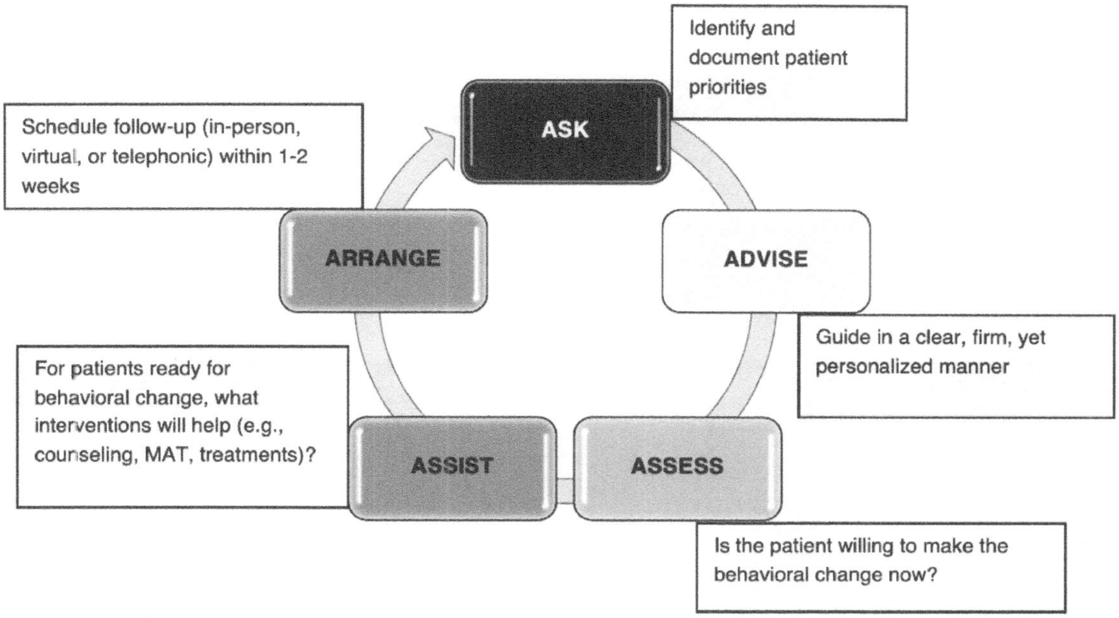

Information from Agency for Healthcare Research and Quality, n.d.

RELAXATION STRATEGIES

BREATHING TECHNIQUES

Breathing is among the body's most basic functions—perhaps why it's also among the easiest ways for individuals to control tension and anxiety from external stressors, even trauma. Several series of breathing exercises are favored by the workforce. They can be used to calm patients in the moment by reducing emotional angst and enhancing focus. Among these techniques are *box (or square) breathing and 4-7-8 breathing.*

Box breathing appears in Box 12.2. This technique promotes mindfulness while replenishing energy through defined actions. A person begins by inhaling, then pausing, during which fresh, oxygenated air is absorbed. On exhale, carbon dioxide is released, as are negative energy and tension, which activates the parasympathetic nervous system and the body's relaxation response. A final pause sets the breathing rhythm, then the person begins the four steps again.

Another favored relaxation practice is 4-7-8 breathing, which uses controlled breathing to calm the body and the mind, and is shown in Box 12.3. The person begins with a deep, calming breath, during which his intention is internally stated. Next, that breath is held for seven counts, which slows the heart rate and reduces tension. Finally, one last breath is discharged in an overt, loud exhale or *whoosh*, which releases energy and activates the parasympathetic nervous system. Focus and emotional regulation are enhanced by repeating the cycle two to four times.

Box 12.2: Box breathing

1. Inhale slowly through your nose and count to 4.
2. Hold your breath for another count of 4.
3. Exhale slowly through your mouth and count to 4.
4. Hold during a final count to 4, then repeat the process.

Box 12.3: 4-7-8 breathing

1. Find a comfortable and quiet place to sit.
2. Close your eyes as you feel able to do so.
3. Breathe in through your nose for 4 seconds.
4. Hold the breath for 7 seconds.
5. Exhale loudly through your mouth for 8 seconds.

SLEEP HYGIENE

Imagine you feel stress over managing a handful of challenging patients and families at work. You have difficulty shutting off your brain when your shift ends. At bedtime, you toss and turn for hours. At some point exhaustion takes over, and you drift off while watching a relaxing TV show, but you don't stay asleep. You wake up at 2 or 3 a.m., grab your phone and check emails, then lie in bed until your alarm goes off.

Most individuals strive to fall asleep easily, sleep soundly through the night, then wake up refreshed. Yet this pattern is disrupted by a host of factors discussed in this book: psychosocial stressors, trauma, or chronic illness, leading to insomnia and havoc on your physical and behavioral health. You experience headaches and brain fog from lack of sleep, so you compensate by increasing caffeine intake. You become increasingly anxious and feel crispy around the edges most days. Shifting this pattern requires a dedicated effort, and that's where sleep hygiene comes in.

Sleep hygiene refers to a collection of healthy habits, behaviors, and environmental practices that promote consistent, restful, and restorative sleep (Alanazi et al., 2023). The critical elements of this technique appear in Box 12.4. Considerable research shows that good sleep regulates circulation, enhances immune function, and improves mental health (Baranwal et al., 2023; De Pasquale et al., 2024; Irish et al., 2015). Well-rested people have higher workplace productivity, better self-esteem, and better cognitive functioning than fatigued persons, and they are better able to regulate emotions and cope with mood disturbances. Good sleep promotes superior memory, concentration, and decision-making capacity (Hyndych et al., 2025).

Box 12.4: Key elements of sleep hygiene

- **Develop a consistent schedule.**
  - Go to bed and wake up at the same time each day, including on weekends
- **Set a bedtime or 'wind-down' routine.**
  - Engage in relaxing activities before sleep (reading, meditation, gentle stretching, warm baths or showers).
  - Don't engage in tense or serious discussions in-person or via email, text, or messaging app during this time.
- **Keep a healthy sleep environment.**
  - Maintain a cool, dark, and quiet bedroom.
  - Use a comfortable mattress and pillow.
- **Limit stimulants.**
  - Avoid caffeine, nicotine, and alcohol close to bedtime.
  - Do not eat spicy foods in the evening.
- **Minimize screen use.**
  - Reduce blue-light exposure from phones, tablets, or TVs before bed.
    - Set devices on 'do not disturb' or 'silent,' or turn off, as able.
  - Store devices away from sleeping space, as possible, to avoid being awakened.
- **Sustain physical activity.**
  - Maintain a consistent schedule for exercise each day.
  - Do not exercise immediately before bedtime.
- **Use the bed only for sleep and intimacy.**
  - Avoid working, watching TV, or eating in bed.

Sourced from Baranwal et al., 2023; De Pasquale et al., 2024; Irish et al., 2015

DEVELOPING TREATMENT PLANS AND SMART GOALS

Many would argue that artificial intelligence (AI) can do everything these days, including develop appropriate treatment goals and plans for patients. However, technology was meant to enhance practice, rather than replace the keen acumen of clinical professionals. Unlike AI, humans question their output, considering, *Does the plan match the interventions this practice setting allows for? Are they within the context of this patient's needs?* These same reflection questions are how practitioners will discern if the latest AI tool has returned a treatment plan that is accurate, appropriate, realistic, and ethical for the setting and situation.

Students and newer professionals should learn how to develop sound treatment plans without AI assistance. A formal treatment plan transforms a patient's often vague intentions into realistic actions. Figure 12.4 provides the original framework for SMART Goals developed by Doran (1981).

Case managers should partner with patients to develop treatment plans, with patients contributing specific goals for themselves. Rein in patient goals when needed, so patients don't inadvertently sabotage their motivation and potential for success. Keep treatment goals within the patient's reach in the allotted time frame, reminding patients that sustainable change takes a marathon, not a sprint. Ensure also that goals match the patient's long-term priorities and are not driven by agency or organization mandates.

Treatment plans should leave nothing up for interpretation. Patients and other practitioners alike should be able to comprehend the action steps and explain the critical five Ws of implementation: who, what, when, where, and why. It can be difficult, however, to set measurable goals that match specific outcomes. The following prompts can help define clear benchmarks:

- How will a patient's progress be measured (e.g., patient log, sharing of vital signs through an app and/or patient portal, particular screening and assessment tool)?
- Over what time frame will the goals be met (e.g., weekly, monthly, between patient visits)?
- What metrics or patient reported outcomes measures will you and the patient use to define progress (e.g., DASS-21, PHQ-9 for depression screening, Patient Activation Measures, MoCA)?
- What data or indicators will show that change has occurred (e.g., amount of weight lost, decreased A1c values, increased time spent working out)?
- How close has the patient come to reaching their goal at specific points during treatment (e.g., able to complete 4 minutes of the 6-Minute Walking Test for Oxygen Saturation; improved score by one measure on their PHQ-9; reduced level of severity for depression, anxiety, or stress indicated by a DASS-21)?
- How much further does the patient have to go to achieve their goal (e.g., 5 lbs., 2 minutes, 1-2 points)?

Finally, remember that interprofessional care teams are deadline-driven. When a patient is scheduled for discharge, transportation and other arrangements occur within certain timeframes. Heeding goal deadlines promotes accountability for both case managers and patients. Consider the case scenario in Box 12.5, then reflect on the SMART Goals in Table 12.3.

Figure 12.4: *SMART goals framework*

SPECIFIC	• *What does the patient want to accomplish?*
MEASURABLE	• *How will the patient and I know when the goal is accomplished?*
ACHIEVABLE	• *How will the goal be accomplished?*
REALISTIC	• *Is the plan realistic for the patient?*
TIMELY	• *What timeframe will progress happen in?*

Box 12.5: Case scenario

Michael is a 62-year-old depressed widower. His wife, Jana, died 6 months ago from colon cancer. He has one adult son, Jared, who lives with his partner in another state. Jared is supportive, though his rigorous work schedule limits the time he's physically present with his dad.

Michael is employed full-time at a catering service. In the past he was a model employee, but he's been calling in sick more frequently. He blames insomnia and chronic fatigue for some of the issues. Michael also has a history of uncontrolled diabetes due to poor nutrition. "Jana used to take care of everything; she watched what I ate like a hawk. Oh, I always snuck cookies and other food at work, that stuff I shouldn't have but can't stop eating."

Table12.3: *SMART goals for Michael*

S: Specific
Attend one grief counseling or support group session weekly
• Practice sleep hygiene strategies 5 nights per week
• Track blood sugar levels daily and share with provider
• Prepare and eat one balanced meal per day, 4 days per week
• Engage in 15 minutes of light physical activity at least 3 times per week
• Meet with primary care provider/diabetes educator within 2 weeks
• Aim to reduce sick calls from work by 25 percent in 6 weeks
M – Measurable
• 25% reduction in sick calls in 6 weeks

S: Specific
• Daily blood sugar checks documented for 30 days
• Balanced meals 4 out of 7 days each week for 6 weeks
• 15 minutes of activity, 3 times weekly
• 30% reduction in depressive symptoms on PHQ-9 within 6 months
• Miss no more than 1 workday per month within 9 months
• Stable blood sugar 70% of the time within 6-9 months
• Two balanced meals per day, 5 days per week within 6 months
• 30 minutes of activity, 4 times weekly, within 12 months
A – Achievable
• Short, focused activities – 15-minute walks, one balanced meal daily
• Professional support – counseling, PCP/diabetes educator
• Gradual increases – from 15 minutes of activity to 30, from one balanced meal daily to two meals
• Realistic timeframes – 2 weeks for PCP visit, 6–12 months for long-term changes
R – Relevant
• Goals directly address depression, grief, insomnia, diabetes management, and nutrition
• Supports return to consistent work attendance and improved functioning
• Lifestyle changes to improve physical health (diabetes, sleep, nutrition) and mental health (grief, depression)
T – Timely
• 2 weeks: Meet with PCP/diabetes educator
• 30 days: Daily blood sugar tracking
• 6 weeks: Implement sleep hygiene; eat one balanced meal daily 4 days/week
• 8 weeks: Exercise 15 minutes, 3 times weekly
• 3 months: Attend grief counseling weekly
• 6 months: 30% reduction in depressive symptoms; two balanced meals daily
• 6-9 months: Stable blood sugar 70% of the time
• 9 months: Miss no more than 1 sick day per month
• 12 months: 30 minutes of activity, 4 times weekly

CONCLUSION

We have wrapped an enormous box of knowledge with an equally large bow. But don't wrap the bow too tightly. Although the short-term interventions and treatment information provided here will hold for some time, stay open to learning. This action will empower your effectiveness with patients, their families, and colleagues. Enjoy the contemplation questions that follow below. Then further engage your critical thinking by the case scenarios and questions in Chapter 13. Onward to behavioral health excellence!

CONTEMPLATION QUESTIONS

Use the following case scenario to complete questions 1-5.

As a health plan case manager, you are assigned to integrated-care population health management and are responsible for 30 patients who have chronic health conditions and behavioral health issue(s). One of your patients, Iris, is a 30-year-old Black female with new onset of weight gain, chronic pain, and agitation. She is a nurse newly employed at an urgent care center and recently transitioned from working days to overnight shifts. Over the past 3 months, Iris has experienced the following:

- Weight gain of 20 pounds, caused by eating fast food instead of her usual home-cooked meals
- Drinking a 30-oz. thermos of caffeinated coffee during each shift, with caramel creamer and 10 sugars
- Trouble falling asleep and staying asleep most days after her shift
- Feeling increasingly self-conscious about her looks and anxious about her work performance; she makes comments reflecting poor self-esteem during a virtual meeting with you
- Passive suicidal ideation

Iris's PCP is concerned about her elevated blood pressure, low endurance, and decreased activity level outside of work.

1. Use the 5 As model to craft a session and plan for Iris.
2. Identify a sleep hygiene plan for Iris to enhance her rest.
3. Use an AI tool of your choice to develop SMART treatment goals that promote Iris's whole health and wellness. Note: The following tools are named for example only and do not constitute endorsement: ChatGPT, Claude, or Google Gemini.
4. Review the SMART goals provided in the AI treatment plan, then consider the following:
    a) Do the goals reflect Iris's needs?
    b) Is there anything you would change to reflect Iris's priorities for treatment?
    c) Reflect on your feelings about using an AI tool for clinical assessment and treatment or intervention planning, including ethical, legal, or risk management concerns.
5. Use the Behavioral Health Conversation Map in Table 1.4 to craft a dialogue with Iris about the SMART goals and interventions required.

REFERENCES

- American Nurses Association. (2025). *The Code of Ethics for Nurses.* Retrieved August 18, 2025, from https://codeofethics.ana.org/home
- Agency for Healthcare Research and Quality. (n.d.). The 5 As: 5 Major Steps to Intervention. Retrieved August 16, 2025, from https://www.ahrq.gov/prevention/guidelines/tobacco/5steps.html
- Baranwal, N., Yu, P.K., & Siegel, N.S. (2023). Sleep physiology, pathophysiology, and sleep hygiene. *Progress in Cardiovascular Diseases*, *77*, 59-69. https://doi.org/10.1016/j.pcad.2023.02.005
- Bischof, G., Bischof, A., & Rumpf, H.J. (2021). Motivational Interviewing: An evidence-based approach for use in medical practice. *Deutsches Arzteblatt International*, *118*(7), 109-115. https://doi.org/10.3238/arztebl.m2021.0014
- Case Management Society of America. (2022, 2024). *Standards of Practice for Case Management* (revised to include Standard Q). Retrieved August 17, 2025, from https://cmsa.org/about/standards-of-case-management-practice/
- Commission for Case Manager Certification. (2023). The Code of Professional Conduct for Case Managers. Retrieved August 17, 2025, from https://ccmcertification.org/about-commissiontm/code-professional-conduct#
- De Pasquale, C., El Kazzi, M., Sutherland, K., Shriane, A.E., Vincent, G.E., Cistulli, P.A., & Bin, Y.S. (2024). Sleep hygiene - What do we mean? A bibliographic review. *Sleep Medicine Reviews*, *75*, 101930. https://doi.org/10.1016/j.smrv.2024.101930
- Doran, G.T. (1981). There's a S.M.A.R.T way to write management's goals and objectives. *Management Review, 70*(11), 35-36.
- Fink-Samnick, E. (2021). The social determinants of mental health: Assessment, intervention, and wholistic health equity: Part 2. *Professional Case Management*, *26*(5), 224-241. https://doi.org/10.1097/NCM.0000000000000518
- Harris, A.H., Reeder, R.N., Ellerbe, L.S., & Bowe, T.R. (2011). Validation of the treatment identification strategy of the HEDIS addiction quality measures: Concordance with medical record review. *BMC Health Services Research*, *11*, 73. https://doi.org/10.1186/1472-6963-11-73
- Hyndych, A., El-Abassi, R., & Mader, E.C., Jr. (2025). The role of sleep and the effects of sleep loss on cognitive, affective, and behavioral processes. *Cureus*, *17*(5), e84232. https://doi.org/10.7759/cureus.84232
- Irish, L.A., Kline, C.E., Gunn, H.E., Buysse, D.J., & Hall, M.H. (2015). The role of sleep hygiene in promoting public health: A review of empirical evidence. *Sleep Medicine Review, 22,* 23-36. https://doi.org/10.1016/j.smrv.2014.10.001
- Marzban, S., Najafi, M., Agolli, A., & Ashrafi, E. (2022). Impact of patient engagement on healthcare quality: A scoping review. *Journal of Patient Experience*, *9*. https://doi.org/10.1177/23743735221125439

- Miller W.R. (2023). The evolution of motivational interviewing. *Behavioural and Cognitive Psychotherapy*, *51*(6), 616-632. https://doi.org/10.1017/S1352465822000431
- Miller, W.R., & Rollnick, S. (2023). *Motivational interviewing: Helping people change and grow.* Fourth edition. The Guilford Press: New York, NY.
- National Association of Social Workers. (2021). *Code of Ethics*. Retrieved October 24, 2025, from https://www.socialworkers.org/About/EThics/Code-of-Ethics/Code-of-Ethics-Engl sh
- Prochaska, J.O., & DiClemente, C.C. (1983). Stages and processes of self-change of smoking: Toward an integrative model of change. *Journal of Consulting and Clinical Psychology*, *51*(3), 390-395. https://doi.org/10.1037//0022-006x.51.3.390
- Prochaska, J.O., & DiClemente, C.C. (1992). Stages of change in the modification of problem behaviors. *Progress in Behavior Modification*, *28*, 183-218.
- Shtaynberger, J., & Krebs, P. (2016). Associations between decisional balance and health behaviors among adult cancer survivors. *Journal of Cancer Education, 31*(4), 749-754. https://doi.org/10.1007/s13187-016-1097-z
- Stewart, V., McMillan, S.S., Hu, J., Collins, J.C., El-Den, S., O'Reilly, C.L., & Wheeler, A.J. (2024). Are SMART goals fit-for-purpose? Goal planning with mental health service-users in Australian community pharmacies. *International Journal for Quality in Health Care*, *36*(1). https://doi.org/10.1093/intqhc/mzae009

CHAPTER 13

CASE SCENARIOS

INTRODUCTION

Your behavioral health knowledge is now bolstered with a strong foundation of relevant theories, diagnoses, screening tools, and treatment considerations. The book's chapters have provided opportunities to apply this vast content. However, we could all use further case scenarios to broaden our exposure to realities we might face.

This chapter includes ten scenarios for you to consider the book's information. Each scenario is followed by five questions to guide thoughts or discussions. Choose to work solo, with colleagues, or in a virtual or in-person classroom. There are also cues to the chapters that will support your deliberations.

CASE SCENARIO 1

Marcus is a new case manager for the ED of a large health system. He has a novel assignment, which is to follow all patients with an SMI who are discharged from the ED with referrals to the health system's new outpatient behavioral health clinic. Given the lengthy waiting lists carried by most local mental healthcare providers, the clinic is trying to decrease fragmentation and delays in care. Before being discharge from the ED, all patients are scheduled to meet with a case manager for behavioral health intake assessment and care coordination, a psychiatrist for medication evaluation and management, and a psychotherapist for counseling. Most, but not all, of the patients were previously seen by ED case managers, whether Marcus or someone else.

1. Which phase of Case Management's Behavioral Health Conversation Map should Marcus start at, and why?
2. What diagnostic considerations might Marcus need to consider?
3. What regulations and requirements should Marcus consider for patients who refuse treatments?
4. Which quality measures should Marcus be monitoring for the population?

5. If patients or their families request referrals to alternate community treatment sites, what resources could Marcus refer them to?

Guidance can be found in Chapters 2, 3, 4, and 7.

****

CASE SCENARIO 2

A college student, Gerri, recently broke up with her intimate partner. Friends notice Gerri is sleeping more than usual, missing meals, and has stopped attending classes. Gerri has a history of cutting and NSSI (nonsuicidal self-injury), and friends are concerned about her potential for self-harm. Friends also found social media posts Gerri recently made that express desires to harm the ex-partner, who ended their relationship. As the behavioral health case manager for Gerri's health plan, consider the following questions:

a) Would you consider this a mandatory duty to report situation? If so, why? If not, why not?
b) Which law(s) in Chapter 2 might apply to this situation and a case manager's mandatory duty to report?
c) On a scale of 1-10, with 1 being the least comfortable and 10 being the most, define your comfort level in reporting this situation to local authorities.
d) As you learn more about Gerri's clinical presentation, what DSM diagnosis might you consider, and why?
e) What screening tool(s) would you use to assess Gerri's mental health?

Guidance can be found in Chapters 2, 6, and 9.

****

CASE SCENARIO 3

Adina is 27-year-old trans woman who has been unhoused for the past year, alternating between local shelters and squatting. She has been a polysubstance user for the past decade and is not interested in treatment. Adina was previously referred to MAT (medication-assisted treatment) on multiple occasions, but despite short-term success, relapsed within months after discharge. However, after witnessing several friends die in a short period, Adina is again considering treatment.

1. Based on what you know about Adina, what DSM diagnoses would you consider?
2. What treatment considerations might best align with Alina's needs?

3. What would be your biggest concern in approving a treatment plan for Alina?
4. What screening tool(s) would be most appropriate to assess Alina's current clinical status?
5. What principles of the Harm Reduction Model best address Alina's clinical presentation?

Guidance can be found in Chapter 8.

****

CASE SCENARIO 4

Jeritah is a married 34-year-old teacher who was in motor vehicle accident 10 years ago. During the accident, Jeritah had right of way in an intersection but was hit by a driver who drove through a red light. Both vehicles ended up in a ditch on the side of the road, and Jeritah climbed out of her car through the sunroof. She initially experienced nightmares about the crash and totally avoided driving. She also stayed at home and stopped socializing with friends. She was able to manage symptoms with a combination of medication management and weekly psychotherapy and successfully completed treatment.

Jeritah recently shared with her spouse that she's having those "familiar feelings" from after the accident. She is irritable at work, has increasing bouts of insomnia, and has begun declining dinner invitations from friends. Jeritah has increased her alcohol use from 1-2 glasses of wine on the weekends to nightly. "I can't imagine what's happening. Everything has been fine...I've even been able to scroll right past social media posts about car accidents without getting lost in the details."

1. Based on what you know of Jeritah's history, what DSM diagnoses would you consider?
2. What screening tool(s) would be appropriate to use in assessment of Jeritah's status and condition?
3. What short-term treatment strategies could Jeritah implement to enhance her functioning?
4. What SMART goals could you develop to guide Jeritah's treatment plan?
5. Use Case Management's Behavior Health Conversation Map to consider your interactions with Jeritah and her spouse.

Guidance can be found in Chapters 4, 8, 10, and 12.

****

CASE SCENARIO 5

Alfonso's partner, Jaden, is an active duty service member in the U.S. Army. The couple have been together for most of Jaden's 20 years of military service. Over the past decade, Jaden has been deployed repeatedly, with the couple moving on three separate occasions. Alfonso has managed every move with grace, even amid having to secure a new job with each transition and helping the couple's two children adjust to new schools and friends.

After the last deployment, Jaden noticed a major change in Alfonso. He was more distant and needed to increase the dose of his anti-depressant. Jaden also found a large supply of sedatives hidden in an empty garment bag in the bedroom closet.

1. Based on what you know of Alfonso and Jaden's history, what DSM diagnoses would you consider?
2. What protective factors can you identify for Alfonso and Jaden?
3. What screening tools would you use to assess Alfonso?
4. Would you consider this a mandatory duty to report situation? If so, why? If not, why not?
5. Use Case Management's Behavior Health Conversation Map to consider your interactions with Alfonso and Jaden.

Guidance can be found in Chapters 4, 8, 9, 10, and 12.

****

CASE SCENARIO 6

Brody has been actively followed by a pediatric pain management group for juvenile rheumatoid arthritis since his early onset of the condition at 13 years of age. He is now 16 years old. The embedded case manager at the pain management group meets with Brody regularly.

Brody has been increasing his opioid use to manage his symptoms, and the case manager is concerned. During a recent virtual visit with the case manager, Brody shared that he is engaged in NSSI daily. "Yeah, using this paper clip for a cut here and there, just lets me breathe." Brody expresses frustration about his "parents treating me like a child; they are so protective and give me no freedom." He went on to share, "Most kids my age are driving and able to go to concerts. They won't let me do anything! Then they get worried about my pain tolerance, even with all the meds I'm forced to use. I understand that they're worried, but they gotta let me grow up at some point. I'm just over it."

1. Based on what you know of Brody's history, what DSM diagnoses would you consider?
2. What risk factors and protective factors do you identify with respect to Brody?

3. What screening tool(s) would you use to assess Brody?
4. How would you distinguish if Brody's behavior reflected malingering or manipulation?
5. Use Case Management's Behavior Health Conversation Map to consider your interaction with Brody.

Guidance can be found in Chapters 4, 5, 8, 9, and 11.

****

CASE SCENARIO 7

Maddy is a 40-year-old female admitted to acute rehabilitation from a local hospital following a bout of paralysis in her lower extremities. One morning she wasn't feeling herself and called out sick from work. When she woke up from a nap, she could not physically get off the bed. Maddy texted her partner, Daniel, and he dropped everything to take her to the ED.

That was 3 months ago, and the final determination was that Maddy had a mysterious virus. Maddy had a series of diagnostic tests and labs, which all came back negative. While her inflammatory markers were slightly elevated, she was ruled out for autoimmune disorders, including lupus and multiple sclerosis, and neurocognitive disorders, including Huntington's, Parkinson's, and Lewy Body Syndrome. The interdisciplinary team was optimistic about Maddy's rehab potential, and a short stay in acute rehabilitation was approved by her health plan.

Daniel was an active part of the intake and treatment process, especially sessions with the neuropsychologist. During the rehabilitation intake session, the couple was asked if Maddy had any history of trauma, as a victim of a crime, intimate partner violence, or other violence. The couple hesitated, looked at each other, and quickly replied, "No."

The next day, Daniel asked to meet with the neuropsychologist separately. He stated, "So, Maddy doesn't like to discuss it, but she was raped in college by her roommate's boyfriend. But that was over a decade ago. Why would you ask that question? Could this event have anything to do with Maddy's condition? Come to think of it, her college roommate called about 3 months ago, out of nowhere. She and Maddy hadn't spoken for years, and the call happened a few days before this all started."

1. Based on what you know of Maddy's presentation and history, what DSM diagnoses would you consider?
2. What risk factors and protective factors do you identify with respect to Brody?
3. What screening tools would you use to assess Maddy?
4. What interventions could you use to support Maddy's treatment process?

5. Use Case Management's Behavior Health Conversation Map to consider your interactions with Maddy and Daniel.

Guidance can be found in Chapters 4, 10, and 12.

****

CASE SCENARIO 8

Dante is a 16-year-old who identifies as trans and has appeared at a local clinic requesting therapy. He admits to being deeply depressed about the current news and is constantly at odds with his family over differing political perspectives. He admits to suicidal ideation that occurs several times a week, though has no clear plan in place to act on his thoughts.

Dante shared with the intake case manager that he had hoped to start receiving gender-affirming care in the coming years and was ready to move in with relatives in another state. "I was exploring my rights to become an emancipated minor when the crazy all went down. I knew that my parents would never agree to this surgery, though my aunt and uncle have been uber-supportive. But it's all a pipedream now with these crazy laws being put in place. At least I can get counseling, right? My folks have told me no, but I have to be able to get some support, right?"

1. Based on what you know of Dante's recent history, what DSM diagnoses would you consider?
2. What risk factors and protective factors do you identify with respect to Dante?
3. What screening tools would you use to assess Dante?
4. What are Dante's options should he wish to proceed with accessing psychotherapy and counseling?
5. Use Case Management's Behavior Health Conversation Map to consider your interactions with Dante.

Guidance can be found in Chapters 2, 4, 6, and 9.

****

CASE SCENARIO 9

Jolie receives her primary care at James Center, a federally-qualified health center in a rural community. Usually a quiet and polite woman, Jolie presented one day looking very different from what the team at the center was used to. She was irritable, even agitated. When Jolie was asked to enter the treatment space, she became guarded and wouldn't share information with the male medical assistant. The medical assistant alerted the PCP, but also the center's case manager.

The case manager, Marge, entered the treatment room and the patient became a bit more at ease. Jolie had met Marge on several occasions over the past year, mostly to coordinate care for her perinatal depression. Jolie began to cry and said, "Marge, he did it again…I can't believe it…My husband dragged me up the stairs, locked me in the bedroom, and raped me. I can't have another baby…I'll kill myself…"

1. Based on Jolie's presentation, what DSM diagnoses would you consider?
2. What screening tools would you use to assess Jolie?
3. What short-term interventions could be helpful in this situation?
4. How would you implement a trauma-informed treatment approach with Jolie?
5. Describe specific actions you would you take across each of the model's five steps?
6. Use Case Management's Behavior Health Conversation Map to consider your interactions with Jolie.

Guidance can be found in Chapters 4, 9, 10, and 12.

****

CASE SCENARIO 10

You are case managing Martin, a 75-year-old man admitted to the hospital following a fall in the parking lot of his local grocery store. Martin suffered a left hip fracture and torn ligaments and tendons in his right ankle. He is now status-post a left hip replacement and a tendon repair in his ankle, but he can't safely return home.

Martin lived alone in an apartment prior to the hospitalization and was independent with most activities of daily living. His sister, Danielle, reports he has a long history of severe bipolar II with rapid cycling. She also reports Martin's disorder has been successfully managed with prescription medications, though 'he has his moments.' The physical therapist is optimistic about Martin's recovery and recommends rehabilitation. The care team feels strongly that the rehab should take place in a skilled nursing facility, as Martin is non-weight bearing on his right ankle for 6 weeks, and weight-bearing as tolerated on his left leg.

1. Based on what you know of Martin's mental health history, does this information need to be shared with the skilled nursing facility?
2. If so, what documentation requirements would you need to comply with to assure understanding of Martin's current and potential mental health treatment needs?
3. Would Martin require a Psychiatric Advanced Directive? If so, why? If not, why not?
4. What screening tool(s) would you use to assess Martin's diagnosis?
5. Use Case Management's Behavior Health Conversation Map to consider your interaction with Martin and his sister, Danielle.

Guidance can be found in Chapters 2 and 7.

EPILOGUE

If there is one constant in behavioral health, it is the ever-shifting responses to the times. This book took me far longer to write than I ever imagined because of the universal state of flux we seem to constantly experience, perhaps more than has ever been experienced to date.

Each chapter of this book was a reminder of how upstream—sociopolitical, economic, and environmental—factors underscore the chronic systemic inequities that unleash a raging river of downstream, adverse individual and population-based behaviors. Their collective upstream force ravages the Quintuple Aim by placing excessive obstacles at every touchpoint of care. What results is a fragmented and burdensome system that fails to meet the needs of patients, their families, and the case managers who strive to care for them.

Yet let's remember that knowledge is power! My biggest hope is that this book provides you the fundamental knowledge you require to maneuver through these turbulent waters. As you embark on those critical mental health journeys with patients, let this text be the life raft that transports you both to safety. Let the content support your every effort and ensure you attain the most productive outcomes for every person you intervene with and any organization you represent.

Each individual case manager is part of a greater collective power: our case management profession. Stay committed to achieving the highest level of practice excellence possible by demonstrating your commitment to lifelong learning. No specialty area will provide as much opportunity to advance your practice proficiency as behavioral health. Utilize the expertise of every professional on the interdisciplinary teams you are part of. These actions will foster your learning to effect true whole-person care for your populations.

Behavioral Health for Case Management is my sixth authoritative text for our workforce, and I can't wait to hear your feedback. As you read, jot down thoughts, then send them to me at efssupervision@me.com. I am already hard at work on my seventh book, editing a text with colleagues on the exciting topic of integrated care. It's due for publication in 2026.

Where should I dedicate my energies next? My successful text, *The Ethical Case Manager: Tools and Tactics* will be due for a second edition by late 2026. But I know how case managers have keen perspectives on their learning needs, so I'd love to hear from you. Email me those thoughts at efssupervision@me.com! Your messages will provide a running list of themes for me to choose from.

INDEX

SYMBOLS

A

B

C

D

E

F

G

H

I

J

K

L

M

N

O

P

Q

R

S

T

U

V

W

Y

Made in United States
Cleveland, OH
09 November 2026

47973503R00224